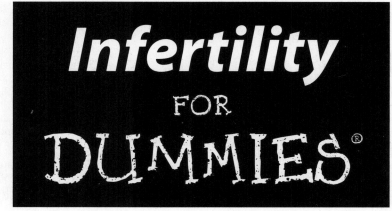

Infertility FOR DUMMIES®

by Sharon Perkins, RN and
Jackie Meyers-Thompson

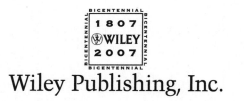

BICENTENNIAL
1807
WILEY
2007
BICENTENNIAL

Wiley Publishing, Inc.

Infertility For Dummies®

Published by
Wiley Publishing, Inc.
111 River St.
Hoboken, NJ 07030-5774
www.wiley.com

WILEY

About the Authors

Sharon Perkins has spent the last twenty years working as an RN, raising five children and spoiling two grandchildren. Following her Air Force pilot husband from state to state, she's lived from Arizona to South Carolina, and still enjoys traveling from Arizona to Texas to Michigan to Virginia to visit kids, grandkids, and mom.

Sharon's ambition to be a writer dates back to grade school, if not earlier, and her desire to be a nurse (okay, she originally thought it would be nice to be a doctor but changed her mind) goes back at least that far. Amazingly enough, she found a way to combine nursing and writing in a way she would never have dreamed possible, thanks to a patient (Jackie) with the persistence and drive to make it happen.

Jackie Meyers-Thompson is managing partner of Coppock-Meyers Public Relations/JD Thompson Communications Inc. and a "professional" fertility patient (seeking "early retirement" however!) It's been said that we make plans . . . and the gods laugh. Jackie has heard that laughter often. It took her longer than she expected, and yielded more than a few laughs, and tears, before she met her husband-to-be, Darren Thompson. But by 35, she was newly married and deliriously happy and felt that the rest of the story would soon fall into place . . . Jackie can be a slow learner.

Nonetheless, she can also be an industrious worker. She loved writing and, as a result, carved her path in marketing and public relations. She had a loving husband and a successful business, so the only things left to add were a few cherubic children and her own Great American Novel. Three years and a slew of physicians later, Jackie had more than a few doubts whether her future would ever include children. But her persistence and focus paid off. *Infertility For Dummies* is, in part, Jackie's story of the journey that landed her a book and her beautiful baby daughter Ava Rose, who at $3\frac{1}{2}$, doesn't want to be called a baby anymore. When not writing, working, or watching her daughter grow, Jackie spends her time making plans. Some things never change.

Dedication

From Sharon: To my father, who always thought I could do anything, and my mother, who kept all our dreams alive.

From Jackie: This book is dedicated to my *still* wonderful and Darling Husband (DH!), Darren Thompson, who has now added DF (Darling Father) to his 'resume' as well! And to Ava Rose Thompson, our long awaited child, who reminds me daily of the miracles in life that so often come when you least expect them.

Authors' Acknowledgments

From Sharon: It's hard to say thank you to everyone in the world, and yet I feel I would have to thank everyone from third grade teachers to babies I cared for in the NICU, because every one has taught me something useful and helped me become who I am today—both a nurse and a writer!

So I'll settle for thanking my family, including children, husband, in-laws, sisters, brothers, nieces, nephews and of course my grandchildren. I can't leave out my friends, work buddies, and every patient I've ever cared for, as well as my church family and various writing groups who have been supportive and encouraging over the years. And, last but not least, Jackie — for having the vision and optimism to see that we really could accomplish this, even when we hardly knew each other outside of the nurse-patient relationship. Without her, I never would have tried this, and we've long since left the nurse-patient thing behind for genuine friendship. To quote St. Paul, "I thank God for all of you."

From Jackie: I don't believe I would have gotten to this point had it not been for the wonderful care and treatment that I received through Dr. Jerome Check and the Cooper Center for In Vitro Fertilization in Marlton, New Jersey. It was also at the Cooper Clinic that I met Sharon Perkins. Her humor, caring, and expertise make her as great a nurse as they do a writer and most importantly a friend.

I have so much to be grateful for in the support of family and friends. Cousin Sandy searched and researched and learned as much about fertility as his own field of medicine in helping us through the maze of doctors and protocols. My mother Larissa Meyers who helped us through the highs and lows in every way she knew how along with the rest of our families, the Thompsons, the Jaffes, the Cicecklis, and the Perlsteins. To my friends Melissa, Camille,

Courtenay, Susan, Leslie, Irene, Erin, Liz, Judy, Donna, Patty, Angie, Cheron, Leora, Margaret and Maureen, who were there for me during some of the most difficult and glorious times, unfailing in their encouragement and always providing a shoulder to cry on or a voice to laugh with.

In the writing of this book, a number of professionals became friends as well. Jennifer R. Bloome, founder and president of Anji, Inc. and The Anji Connection, provided me with great insight into the power of mind and body when trying to conceive. To Rachel Glasser who listened and helped me learn. To Lisa, Evan, Dan and all the great folks at Follas Laboratories who celebrated every good result with me.

And a special thanks to Dr. Garry Cutting and his staff at Johns Hopkins University who gave their time and expertise when we hit another brick in the wall during our efforts to conceive. Thanks as well to Dr. Martin Schwarz, who became a friend and great source of information on the 'other side of the pond' and Steven Keiles and Dr. Luke Padwick, who helped provide us with some crucial pieces to our puzzle.

From both of us: Wiley took a chance on us six years ago, and we thank you all for your faith in us and your support. Our acquisitions editor Lindsay Lefever's enthusiasm for this book was infectious; our project editor, Jen Connolly, has been a pleasure to work with.

Immense thanks to Dr. Richard Paulson, who has been a marvelous source of information and guidance for this book; he kept our hyperbole under control and made sure we had our facts straight!

Publisher's Acknowledgments

We're proud of this book; please send us your comments through our Dummies online registration form located at www.dummies.com/register/.

Some of the people who helped bring this book to market include the following:

Acquisitions, Editorial, and Media Development

Project Editor: Jennifer Connolly

Acquisitions Editor: Lindsay Lefevere

Copy Editor: Jennifer Connolly

Technical Editor: Richard Paulson, MD

Editorial Manager: Michelle Hacker

Editorial Supervisor: Carmen Krikorian

Media Development Manager: Laura VanWinkle

Editorial Assistants: Erin Calligan Mooney, Joe Niesen, Leeann Harney

Cover Photos: © Matthias Kulka/Corbis

Cartoons: Rich Tennant (www.the5thwave.com)

Composition Services

Project Coordinator: Heather Kolter

Layout and Graphics: Claudia Bell, Carl Byers, Laura Pence, Alicia B. South

Anniversary Logo Design: Richard Pacifico

Proofreaders: Jessica Kramer, Susan Sims

Indexer: Techbooks

Publishing and Editorial for Consumer Dummies

Diane Graves Steele, Vice President and Publisher, Consumer Dummies

Joyce Pepple, Acquisitions Director, Consumer Dummies

Kristin A. Cocks, Product Development Director, Consumer Dummies

Michael Spring, Vice President and Publisher, Travel

Kelly Regan, Editorial Director, Travel

Publishing for Technology Dummies

Andy Cummings, Vice President and Publisher, Dummies Technology/General User

Composition Services

Gerry Fahey, Vice President of Production Services

Debbie Stailey, Director of Composition Services

Contents at a Glance

Table of Contents

Introduction

*I*nfertility is a medical problem for more than 7.2 million Americans, yet insurance companies often deny that it's a disease, many people (the "just relax and you'll get pregnant" crowd) don't understand its biological origins, and a few (the "take this magic pill and you'll get pregnant, guaranteed!" group) even exploit those suffering from it. If you're dealing with infertility, you may feel alone, confused and depressed over the potential loss of the dream you cherished since childhood: the dream of having a baby of your own.

There is good news on the infertility front, however; not only are medical treatments for infertility making great gains, but there's also more awareness of the emotional effects of infertility.

Infertility For Dummies was conceived by combining Jackie's knowledge of infertility from a patient's viewpoint, Sharon's wealth of information as an infertility nurse, and both of their personal experiences. We wrote this book so that patients dealing with infertility will know that they're not alone. We hope it finds its way to the bookshelves and nightstands of all the patients who need it to help find their road to their baby. And, as Sharon and Jackie found out along the way, anything can happen!

About This Book

This book is our attempt to help those of you who want to walk into the doctor's office and not walk out feeling foolish and out of control of your fertility. Our vision is to provide fertility patients — both those at the starting line and those close to the finish — and the people who love them, with as much information as we can on the options available to them. We discuss topics ranging from the scientific to the spiritual.

You can read through this book from front to back and feel confident that you can find the answer to just about any fertility issue, from natural family planning to cloning. But if you're like most people, you'll probably look through the Table of Contents, zero in on the chapters that affect you, and jump directly to them. This book is meant as a resource, which means that you can go back to it whenever a new issue or question arises and find the answer you need without reading through everything that comes before. This book is meant for people with every degree of fertility expertise, from the novice to the jaded, been-there-done-that patient. The no-tech and low-tech fertility chapters come first, so you can skip them if you're already a veteran and move right into high-tech and *really* high-tech stuff found in the second half of the book.

We intersperse personal stories throughout the book; these (we hope!) make interesting reading from the viewpoint of either Sharon (an infertility nurse) or Jackie (an infertility patient). If you skip them, you won't miss any essential information, although you may miss a few humorous sidelines or "I did it, so you can too" stories.

Conventions Used in This Book

To help you pick out information from a page, we use the following conventions throughout the text to make elements consistent and easy to understand; the last thing we want to do is confuse you!

- ✔ Any Web addresses appear in `monofont`.
- ✔ New terms appear in *italics* and are closely preceded or followed by an easy-to-understand definition.
- ✔ **Bold** highlights the keywords in bulleted lists.
- ✔ Sidebars, which look like text enclosed in a shaded gray box, consist of information that's interesting to know but not necessarily critical to your understanding of the topic.

What You're Not to Read

We think every word in this book is interesting and educational, but we understand that sometimes you just need a quick answer to a burning question. Other times you want to discover everything possible about infertility, even the technical stuff. We've designated some information as *interesting-but-not-essential-to-read*. Feel free to read it, but if you skip it, you're not missing anything vital. Optional sections are:

- ✔ **Text in sidebars:** Shaded boxes that appear throughout the book. The information they contain may be anything from personal stories to technical information. The common denominator is that the information isn't essential to understanding or dealing with endometriosis.
- ✔ **Anything with a Technical Stuff icon attached**: This information is interesting, but not essential — unless you're planning on doing your doctorate thesis on endometriosis. (For more information on icons, check out "Icons Used in This Book" later in this Introduction.)
- ✔ **The stuff on the copyright page:** The attorneys require that we have this information. Unless you're an aspiring lawyer, feel free to skip it.

Foolish Assumptions

We assume that you're reading this book because you want to know more about infertility and because, despite your hopes to the contrary, you and/or a loved one, are dealing with infertility on one level or another, be it your first child or your fifth. We also assume that you want to:

- Understand the biologic causes of infertility
- Discover what you can do to overcome infertility, from proper timing to changing underwear!
- Be up-to-date on the latest medical and surgical treatments for infertility
- Learn about high tech options for conception
- Pursue options for parenthood if the traditional roads fail you, from donor egg to use of a surrogate

Infertility is not the end of the road, or the end of your dream of parenthood. There is help available, and we're here to help you find the resources you need, whether your infertility issues are simple to solve or complex.

How This Book is Organized

Infertility For Dummies is divided into six parts. As with every *For Dummies* book, this one is designed to help you find the information you need quickly and easily, without having to read the book cover to cover. The following explanations can help you find the information you need with a minimum of effort.

Part 1: Are We There Yet? Wondering Why You're Not Pregnant

If you're a newcomer to the wonderful world of baby making, we suggest that you start reading here. In this part, we explain male and female anatomy (including everything you ever wanted to know about reproductive organs), look at the logistics of getting pregnant, and review behaviors you should change — or not — before trying to get pregnant.

Part II: Stepping Up Your Efforts

This part helps you fine-tune your conception efforts by using methods to predict ovulation and helps you understand how complicated getting pregnant, whether infertility is involved . . . or not, really is. We also guide you through your initial gynecology visits for simple infertility treatment. Next we take a look at some alternative approaches to pregnancy, from herbs to acupuncture, discuss the special issue of secondary infertility, and last but not least, help you avoid the emotional pitfalls that can be the most painful part of infertility.

Part III: Asking for Directions: Finding the Problem

This part explains the tests you may be doing to find out why you haven't gotten pregnant yet; we explain what the tests are and what the results may mean. We also give male factor issues a chapter of their own. We give you information about miscarriage; why it occurs and what you can do emotionally and physically to overcome recurrent miscarriage.

Part IV: Moving Up to High-Tech Conception

This part explains what high-tech infertility treatments are, from injections to in vitro fertilization. We guide you through the complicated maze of finding the right clinic and take you through the stimulation process and the egg retrieval itself. We visit the embryology lab after your egg retrieval and give advice on how to get through the "two week wait" for your pregnancy test without losing your mind. We also discuss the dollars and cents of infertility, what different processes may cost, and how to maximize your funds, your insurance, and your resources.

Part V: The Road Less Traveled . . . So Far!

In this part, we look at nontraditional families and methods of conception, including donor egg and surrogacy. We also help you decide when "enough is enough" and discuss the possible alternatives to biological parenthood. Finally, we peer into the future for a look at what's on the horizon for infertility treatment.

Part VI: The Part of Tens

Want to know the ten most annoying things people say when you're trying to get pregnant? Want to know where to find fertility medications for reasonable prices and find out exactly what a gonadotropin is? Need to navigate your way through an infertility chat board? Then this is the part for you.

Icons Used in This Book

Icons are the strange-looking symbols that appear occasionally in the margins next to the text. We include them to let you know that a topic or information is special in some way. *Infertility For Dummies* includes the following icons:

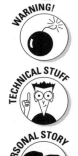

This icon identifies information that's helpful and can save you time or trouble.

This icon highlights key points in the section you're reading.

This icon stresses information that describes potentially serious issues, such as side effects to medication or other dangerous problems. Pay attention to warnings — they can keep you out of trouble!

This icon signals information that's interesting but not essential to understanding endometriosis, unless you're a scientist or medical student.

If either of us has a personal story that is funny, informative, inspirational, or otherwise interesting, we identify it with the Personal Story icon. These anecdotes are never essential reading, but they're usually entertaining!

Where to Go from Here

If we'd written the great American novel, we'd want you to start at Chapter 1 and read straight through. But it's not a novel, and it's not a textbook, where each chapter builds on the one before. You can open this book at any point and be able to understand the information there.

The early chapters of this book deal with infertility issues that can be solved fairly easily, like timing. If you don't have a basic understanding of human biology, Chapter 2 can help you understand the complexity of the human reproductive system. On the other hand, if the emotional aspects of infertility are impacting your relationships, Chapter 9 may be more what you need to read.

The point is, you don't have to read everything (although you certainly can, and you may discover something you never knew before)! Just flip to the Table of Contents or index, find a subject that interests you, and turn to that chapter. It's not essential to read everything — just what interests you and helps you.

Infertility For Dummies is a resource, a guide that presents the practical information in a fun, easy-to-read-and-understand format. Read a chapter a day or a chapter a year, or keep it in the bathroom for frequent browsing. But however you choose to use this book, we hope it's helpful.

Part I
Are We There Yet? Wondering Why You're Not Pregnant

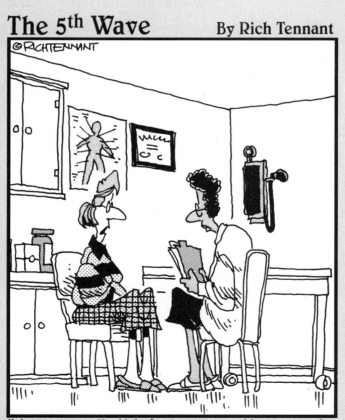

The 5th Wave   By Rich Tennant

"Actually, I didn't become dizzy and nauseous until I started inhaling the scent strips in the waiting room magazines."

In this part . . .

*I*f you're a newcomer to the wonderful world of baby making, we suggest that you start reading here. In this part, we explain male and female anatomy (including everything you ever wanted to know about reproductive organs), look at the logistics of getting pregnant, and review behaviors you should change — or not — before trying to get pregnant.

Chapter 1

Where, Oh Where, Can My Baby Be?

*I*f you're reading this book, the odds are good that you want to have a baby. You may actually have been trying to have a baby for a while without success, and maybe you're becoming frustrated, annoyed, and a little scared — are you *ever* going to have the family you've dreamed of?

We want to help make this process easier for you — less stressful and more successful. In this chapter, we tell you the official definition of infertility (it may surprise you!), show you statistics on infertility today, show you how to shake your family tree for genetic problems and talk about the cost of infertility — the emotional cost as well as the monetary cost.

Defining Infertility

Infertility as defined by the experts may surprise you. According to guidelines established by infertility specialists, you're not considered to be infertile until you've been trying to get pregnant for one year, if you're under age 35. That means that trying to get pregnant last week and not having signs of pregnancy this week does *not* mean that you're infertile.

However, since the modern world is one of immediate gratification, it can be hard — if not downright impossible — to try to get pregnant for a full year without getting impatient, discouraged, or just plain panicked. There's nothing wrong with going to see your gynecologist to talk about why you're not getting pregnant after just a few months; in fact, your co-authors, being fairly impatient people themselves, would consider you to be a candidate for sainthood if you could wait a year without talking to your doctor. One year is, however, the official definition.

Infertility in America — Looking at the Statistics

Most women know that the older you get, the harder it is to get pregnant. But what about race, socioeconomic status, geography and heredity as fertility factors? In the next sections we look at how infertility affects different groups.

Making babies: An inefficient process at best

You may think of Mother Nature as a pretty efficient woman, but the truth is, the path to pregnancy is an inefficient one even under the best of circumstances. For example, out of 100 couples under the age of 35 trying to conceive, only 20 will get pregnant in any given month, and of those 20, 3 will miscarry. In other words, if you're under 35, every month you have a 17 percent chance of walking out of the maternity ward with a baby nine months later. Obviously, nature is not as efficient as people think.

Looking at 100 women under age 35 trying to get pregnant, the breakdown will look like this:

- 80 will be pregnant within one year
- 10 more will be pregnant after two years of trying without medical intervention.
- 10 won't get pregnant without some help from the medicine man.

High-tech infertility treatments, such as in vitro fertilization, claim a success rate of about 50 percent for those under age 35, which means 5 out of 100 women will not become pregnant, even with medical intervention.

Age and infertility

If you're over 35, you're in good company; 20 percent of all first-time moms in the United States are over 35! Despite this, Mother Nature doesn't make it easy to get pregnant past age 35. (We look more at age and infertility in Chapter 6.)

For example:

- By your late thirties, 10 percent will get pregnant in any given month and 17 percent of those will miscarry.

- If you're over 40, the pregnancy rate, per month, slips to 5 percent, with 34 percent of those miscarrying.

- By age 45, your chance per month of conceiving is less than 1 percent, and 53 percent of those will miscarry.

Race and infertility

Does your racial background affect your chance for pregnancy? There is a slight difference in infertility rates, with Hispanic women under 35 experiencing a 7 percent infertility rate, Caucasians a 6.4 percent infertility rate, and African American women recording a 10.5 percent rate of infertility. These differences could be due to socioeconomic factors, such as poverty, poor nutrition, or lack of physician care, rather than strictly racial issues.

High-tech treatments and infertility

If you're already frantically reading your insurance booklet and shaking the piggy bank in hopes of finding a few spare thousand dollars to pay for high tech infertility treatments, you might take comfort in the following statistic: only around 3 percent of infertile couples end up doing high tech treatment like in vitro fertilization IVF) to get pregnant. (You can find everything you need to know about IVF in Chapters 15 to 18.)

Shaking Down the Family Tree

It may seem silly to look to your family tree for signs of infertility that could be inherited; after all, *you're* here, so how could your parents have had fertility issues?

Putting together a family birth history

Most of us don't ask our parents about their road to parenthood until we're trying to become parents ourselves. But you might be surprised to learn that it took your parents a number of years to have you or your siblings. It's also possible that people in your family tree may be adopted or the product of artificial insemination, issues that often weren't discussed a few decades ago.

While family lines who are completely infertile tend to die out in a generation (for obvious reasons), some families may be sub-fertile, with less than average sperm counts or ovulation issues, and still manage to have a child or two.

Ask the most talkative member of your family for a family "birth history." You may be surprised what you learn. And remember, sometimes a vehement denial, such as "there's never been any problem in _our_ family," may be a clue to dig a little deeper and find out why everyone is so defensive.

Finding out important information

Researching your family history can provide valuable information. For example, you may learn of family genetic tendencies that could cause problems on your own reproductive road. Or you may find out that everyone in your family took six months to get pregnant, a fact that may put your mind at ease, particularly around month number five of trying without success.

Before trying to get pregnant, you'll want to know whether any diseases occur more than once on your family tree. This disease may be caused by a dominant gene that you could pass on, if you carry it, even if your partner doesn't carry it. Depending on how open your family is, finding out this information can be difficult. Many families don't discuss anything related to pregnancy, especially not problems getting pregnant, pregnancy losses, or genetic defects. Just a few generations ago, parents of children with genetic abnormalities were encouraged to put them in a home and tell the relatives the baby had been stillborn.

If your family tree does hold a genetic problem or a birth defect that shows up more than once, you'll probably want to have genetic testing done. A gene map, which can be done from a blood test, will show whether you carry abnormal genes that could cause problems for your child.

Sometimes the only thing you learn from family records is nonspecific, such as "all the Smith boys died young." Try and pin down why they all died young: Did they have hemophilia or muscular dystrophy, or did they all fall out of the same apple tree?

You may also want to ask your mother whether she took any pills during her pregnancy, or whether her doctor gave her anything to prevent miscarriage. Women whose mothers took DES, a synthetic estrogen hormone, to help prevent miscarriage may have a T-shaped uterus, which may make it difficult to carry a pregnancy. Almost 5 million women were given DES by their doctors between 1938 and 1971, and as many as 50 percent of their daughters may have infertility issues related to DES exposure. Studies are now beginning to be done on problems that affect DES sons and their fertility. The following male problems may be linked to DES:

- ✔ **Varicocele:** An enlarged vein in the testicles that can affect sperm production
- ✔ **Undescended testicles:** Testicles that fail to descend into the scrotum
- ✔ **Hypospadias:** A misplacement of the opening on the end of the penis

REMEMBER

Don't be too hard on Mom for not telling you everything. Many women aren't even aware that they took DES until their children enter their reproductive years and begin experiencing problems. Asking the doctor what was in the pills he gave you wasn't something many women did in the 1950s and 1960s.

WARNING!

If you and your partner are blood relatives, it is especially important to see a genetic counselor before getting pregnant. You may carry more of the same abnormal genes than unrelated partners would, which may make you more likely to have a child with a genetic problem. The risk for serious birth defects is 1 in 20 for second cousins and 1 in 11 for first cousins.

Checking the stats of your race

Even if you're not aware of genetic illnesses in your family, certain populations tend towards specific issues. For example, while sickle cell anemia occurs in 1 of 8 African Americans, cystic fibrosis can be found in 1 out of 26 Caucasians and at an even higher percentage among Ashkenazi Jews. Other diseases such as Tay-Sachs and Gaucher are also prevalent among the Jewish population.

Many OB/GYNs suggest screening for the most likely diseases based on your heritage. It doesn't hurt to get this done *before* you become pregnant. While many genetic diseases are recessive, meaning that both parents must carry the gene in order for the baby to develop the disease itself, should you turn up to be a carrier, your partner can be tested right away. If both you and your partner are carriers, each child from your union holds a 25 percent chance of inheriting both genes and thus the disease. Fifty percent of your children will be carriers of the disease and twenty-five percent will not have *or* carry the disease.

Remember, these are all statistical numbers. Some families where both parents carry a recessive gene disorder have multiple children in a row who have the disease, despite the 25 percent odds per child. Other families don't. Statistics are based on large numbers of people and the likelihood of any one event occurring. You and your family may fall into the statistical pattern or not.

The good news about inherited diseases

When it comes to inherited diseases, you have options your grandmother and mother never did. You can receive pre-pregnancy genetic counseling or have early pregnancy testing of the fetus for abnormalities. Your grandmother, who may have had children well into her 40s, was more likely to have a baby born with chromosomal abnormalities. Such problems are more common in women over 35, and there was no way to test for them during pregnancy in earlier generations. Your mother may have been afraid to have more than one child if she knew there was a family history of cystic fibrosis or muscular dystrophy. The problem that your aunt had during pregnancy from an inherited bleeding disorder is now a condition that can be diagnosed and treated during pregnancy, increasing your chances of having a healthy full-term baby. Rh factors may have caused fetal death just two generations ago, but they can now be easily prevented by an injection of RhoGAM, which prevents the growing fetus from having its blood cells attacked in utero.

In the case of diseases such as cystic fibrosis, just because you don't see evidence in your family tree doesn't mean it isn't there. Eighty percent of families who give birth to a child affected with cystic fibrosis have never had an incidence of the disease in their family. That's because recessive disorders require two carriers in order to produce the disease in their offspring. Even if two carriers do reproduce, there is still only a 25 percent chance per child that any given baby will have the disease itself. Thus, carrier status can be passed along for generations without ever showing up as the disease itself. Testing is the only way to know for sure.

If you do uncover a "bad" or questionable gene through testing, don't panic. This is the reason for testing in the first place. Before you make out a will or go hunting down your mother, father, or great-great-aunt to give them a piece of your mind, remember this:

- ✔ Not all gene mutations are disease causing. Some are merely benign changes. These differences are what make us all unique individuals.
- ✔ If you're a carrier of a recessive genetic disorder, you're carrying only one gene and will not get the disease. You're simply a potential conduit.

What Causes Infertility?

Infertility has many causes, and figuring out which applies to you may be very simple — or very difficult. Although women used to bear the brunt of blame for infertility, the truth is that male and female factors share equally in infertility. Consider the following statistics:

- One third of infertility is caused by female factors
- One third of infertility is caused by male factors
- Around 20 percent of infertility is unexplained
- Around 10 to 15 percent of infertility is caused by a combination of male and female factors

Among women, the main causes of infertility are:

- Ovulatory disorders — no ovulation or irregular ovulation
- Tubal disorders — blocked or infected tubes
- Uterine issues — fibroids, polyps or adhesions

For men the most common causes of infertility are:

- Low sperm count
- Decreased sperm motility
- Abnormally shaped sperm
- No sperm at all in the ejaculate

Each of theses categories of infertility can be caused by a number of things; for example, a decreased sperm count can be caused by a disease such as diabetes, by a birth defect, or by trauma. A woman can have blocked tubes from endometriosis, pelvic inflammatory disease, or from a congenital malformation. Anovulation can be caused by polycystic ovarian syndrome, premature ovarian failure, or by over-exercising. While it may be fairly obvious what the problem is, finding the reason for the problem may be more difficult.

Diagnosing Infertility

You may think this is a no-brainer: If you're not getting pregnant, it seems like you've already diagnosed yourself with infertility! However, diagnosing a lack of pregnancy is the easy part; figuring out why you're not getting pregnant is the hard part.

After reading through Chapter 5, which discusses simple techniques for increasing your pregnancy odds, or Chapter 10, which explains some of the tests used to diagnose infertility, of this book, you may be able to diagnose the reason for your difficulty in getting pregnant without any help from your doctor. For example, you might be having sex at the wrong time of the month — your "infertility issue" may be solved with a calendar, a thermometer and an ovulation predictor kit! Or you may not have realized how irregular your periods were — 35 days apart one month, 40 the next, 60 the next — maybe you're not ovulating on a regular basis.

Your gynecologist can run a few simple blood tests to help determine whether or not you're ovulating. Ovulation is, after all, the first step in getting pregnant, and usually blood tests or observation of your own cervical mucus and temperature (see Chapter 4 for ways to figure this out) can help you figure out when you're ovulating so you can time sex accordingly.

If you're still not pregnant after six months of "hitting the mark," it's time for more testing; your doctor may suggest a test to see if your tubes are open and testing on your partner to see if "his boys can swim."

This process of looking for the problem and then seeing if it's fixed can take a few months. Only 20 percent of infertile couples never have a definite answer to why they can't get pregnant, so the odds are your favor.

Getting Pregnant: More Difficult Today than Yesterday?

Sometimes things seemed easier in Grandma's day. Large families were common, and it appeared that everyone had children. In fact, getting pregnant may be harder today, for several reasons:

- **People are having children later in life.** Over age 25, there is a slight but definite decrease in fertility in women, a decrease that increases dramatically over age 35. Men are also less fertile at older ages.

- **Due to better medical management, people are living longer and getting pregnant (or trying to) despite the presence of serious chronic disease, such as diabetes or lupus.** In the past, just the *presence* of these conditions would have precluded the possibility of pregnancy.

- **Male infertility, related to decreased sperm counts, has increased.** Many theories circulate as to why this is occurring, with environmental factors being carefully studied.

- **The incidence of sexually transmitted diseases has increased.** Some of these diseases, such as chlamydia, cause serious damage to the reproductive organs.

✔ **More men and women have had either a vasectomy or a tubal ligation at a young age and then decided to have another child.** Needless to say, they immediately face fertility issues due to their previous choices.

✔ **It may seem as if everyone had children years ago, but start asking questions and you'll get a different story.** You may find out that Uncle Charlie wasn't really Aunt Jo's son; he was her sister's child, whom she raised after his mother died young, and on and on. Everyone may have been raising children, but many of those children may have been extended family members.

✔ **People today talk more.** Just because you never heard about your grandmother's stillborns or your mother's miscarriages doesn't mean they didn't happen. Pregnancy talk today is big business, and everyone in the world seems to be in the news talking about their babies, lack of babies, adopted babies, and how they got pregnant. This focus puts a constant in-your-face emphasis on pregnancy. It also makes you feel, when you're trying to get pregnant, like everyone else is doing it — and doing it better than you are!

Relax, this is only the beginning for you, and we do our best to help you start baby making with the best of them.

Calculating the Cost of Infertility

Infertility costs a lot. We're not just talking money here; the emotional toll is usually much higher and longer lasting than any hit to your pocketbook. In the next sections, we look at the costs of infertility on your self esteem, your marriage, and last of all (because it's really the least important) on your wallet.

The emotional costs of infertility

Infertility is not for the faint of heart. Will it test your mental, physical and spiritual strength? Um, possibly. Will you come out a better person than before? No guarantee, but as with all of life's challenges, the better prepared you are going in, the more likely your psyche is to survive and thrive.

In this book, we discuss a lot about support, be it your partner, friends, family, professionals, or online networks. It doesn't matter in what shape it comes, everyone needs a little help from their friends, no matter who those friends may be.

You might decide to let just a few close confidantes know of your situation with trying to conceive. You might tell anyone who will listen. Regardless, know that at some point, someone will say something wrong. Set the ground rules now. If you don't want to be asked how *things* are going (secret speak for "Are you pregnant yet?"), tell your network up front that you will let them know when there is something to know. Their over-enthusiasm may annoy you time and again, but they are probably almost as excited as you are to hear about your success.

While you don't want to anticipate a long, arduous battle with your fertility, or lack thereof, don't set yourself up to expect that within a month you'll be shopping online for maternity clothes. Decorating the baby's room at this point is probably not a great idea either. If all goes well and success finds you early, that's great . . . and we promise you that you'll have plenty of time to find the perfect maternity wardrobe and baby collection. If not, you will only set yourself up for disappointment, and the goal is to keep that to a minimum as best you can, in the areas over which you do have control. Your thinking is one of them.

And it's not just you!

Whether the infertility issues are yours, your partner's, or something you share, be certain that you most likely will share the ups and downs of baby making. Infertility is tough on the most resilient of individuals and couples. It will find the weak spots in you and your relationship. Steady yourself and your union for what could be turbulent waters ahead (this includes success *and* a new baby!).

When it comes to baby making, sooner is often better than later, but keep in mind that this is from a biological perspective. And although you may hear the biological clock ticking away, ready-or-not is not the best way to make your decision about when to conceive. The state of your union is an issue we revisit throughout this book, as it is one of the most important aspects in dealing with fertility, infertility, and baby makes three (or more). And although biology is a key issue in deciding when and if you're ready to conceive, maturity, financial security, and stability are equally important, whether your challenge is trying to get pregnant or trying to raise said baby in a difficult and expensive world.

The quality of your partnership is the foundation for your family. Take the time to make sure that it's solid before moving on to the next level. Re-visit it often to make sure it's staying secure through the ups and downs of trying to conceive.

Just keep talking! As with all other areas, communication is key in the decision to add on to your family, whether you're successful right away or not. If you find yourselves at an impasse, enlist the help of an outside party: a member of the clergy, a therapist, or a physician to help you sort out feelings and facts.

The costs of treatment

Talk about rubbing salt on a wound. Infertility treatments can be difficult enough. Now throw in the "opportunity" to spend anywhere from a few hundred to tens of thousands of dollars, and you have the makings for a truly bitter pill.

Like everything, infertility costs vary and can depend on where you live, which physician/practice you see and most importantly, whether your treatment is small, medium, or large.

When you're starting out, expect to pay $10 to $15 for an ovulation predictor kit and about the same for home pregnancy kits. A basal body thermometer will run you about $10 to $20. This is the easy stuff. We haven't brought in the professionals yet.

What about insurance you ask? "What about it?" we answer. Only 15 states have mandated coverage for infertility, meaning that for those who aren't fortunate enough to live in one of these areas, infertility treatments are paid for out of pocket . . . yours that is. Even if you have insurance coverage, you may be amazed to see how little of your bill is covered. Some insurance plans cover only monitoring, meaning the frequent blood draws and ultrasounds. Because these can run well over $2,000 per cycle, this coverage is a help. Other plans cover only the medications, which is a help, but not by any means relief from the total cost.

Many insurance plans, however, will cover the tests and procedures related to diagnosing your particular infertility problem. This can be very helpful as well because many cases of infertility require blood work, ultrasound, and even exploratory surgical procedure, to determine a cause for infertility . . . a mere starting point for treatment. This generally applies to both you and your partner, but double-check this with your insurance company prior to signing up for the "party platter" of tests.

Once diagnosed, and even if you escape diagnosis (20 percent of infertility is unexplained), that's when the real costs can kick in. Should your problem be resolved quickly and easily, you may get by with the cost of a few months' worth of Clomid (a pill that causes super ovulation in order to push your ovaries into producing one or more follicles that can be fertilized), a few ultra-sounds (which generally cost anywhere from $200 to $500 depending on where you live and which physician practice you frequent) and approximately $200 per blood draw for the basic tests needed to monitor your cycle. If you need IUI (Intrauterine Insemination), the cost is generally $500 per insemination.

If you are to be monitored via blood work and ultrasound throughout the month, some clinics offer "package" prices which can range from $900 to $1500 for blood work and ultrasounds for one month.

If your cycle require injectable gonadotropins (Repronex, Follistim, Gonal F to name a few), you are looking at a cost of $50 per vial. Most of these drugs are sold in five-vial boxes, although some are available in larger multidose containers. You could use as few as one vial per day for 5 to 10 days of your cycle or as many as six vials per day for 12 days. It all depends on your issues, protocol, physician, and response.

If you are also adding in luteal support (which occurs after the egg has supposedly been fertilized), progesterone and estrogen may run you a few hundred dollars per cycle (a bargain compared to other costs!).

Keep in mind that these are all approximate costs. Later on in the book, we discuss places to purchase medications that may offer better deals and other methods that you can use to cut your costs.

If you move up to the big time, keep in mind that the average IVF cycle costs between $8,000 and $15,000. Of that, about $4,000 to $5,000 is spent on medication, and another $4,000 to $10,000 goes to your clinic.

But, for now, let's take it one step at a time. You've bought this book and if you get pregnant from the information you find here, consider it a great bargain!

Chapter 2

Understanding Your Anatomy

*Y*ou may think that you know how to get pregnant. Doesn't everybody? Not necessarily! In this chapter, we review basic male and female biology, educate you on the inner workings of your menstrual cycle, and teach you about sex and conception. Then we peer into your genes — what they are, how they affect you and your future child, and what scientists currently know about them.

Biology 101: Reviewing Male and Female Anatomy

Were you paying attention in Biology 101? You may have taken a quick peek at the film on the miracle of birth and announced loudly to all your friends, "Eww, gross, I'm never having kids!" And yet here you are, some undisclosed number of years later, wishing you had paid more attention back then. Don't worry; we're here to fill in the gaps in your reproductive education.

The human body has the basics and the accessories — just like at Macy's! When you buy an outfit, you can be dressed with just the basics, but the accessories really pull your outfit together. When you're trying to have a baby, the parts that you don't see — the "accessories" —determine whether you can get pregnant.

Looking at the female accessories (besides shoes)

A naked woman is pretty unrevealing, from a reproductive viewpoint. You can't see the organs that count in childbearing, so you can't tell at a glance whether yours are present and functioning. Take a look at what should be inside every woman, starting from the outside and working your way up. (See Figure 2-1.)

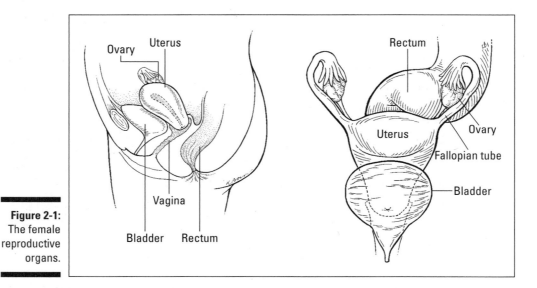

Figure 2-1: The female reproductive organs.

The vagina

The vagina mostly serves as a passageway, first for the penis to deliver sperm up near the opening of the uterus, and later for the delivery of the baby. If you have a very small vaginal opening, intercourse may be uncomfortable. If your vaginal opening is large, as it may be after having a baby, sex may be less pleasurable. Neither condition, however, will have any effect on your ability to get pregnant.

The vagina secretes fluid during sexual arousal, making it easier — and a lot more enjoyable! — for a penis to enter the vagina. Sometimes, (especially when you have to have sex at a particular time), the lubrication function may not work as well as it should. In these cases, you may need a personal lubricant. This is much better for your vagina than trying to have a "dry experience," which causes abrasion of the vagina, and will make intercourse that much more uncomfortable the next time.

Some women are born without a vagina; usually the uterus is also missing in these women. The formal name of this syndrome is Rokitansky-Kuster-Hauser-Mayer, and it's the second most common cause of *amenorrhea,* or lack of periods starting by age 16. This condition is usually diagnosed when you don't start your periods by age 16.

Found at the entrance to the vagina, the *hymen* is a nonfunctional piece of circular tissue; the bleeding many women have the first time they have sex comes from the tearing of the hymen. The hymen is not a solid piece of tissue; 99 percent of baby girls already have openings, or perforations, in the hymen. An *imperforate hymen,* one that has no holes, can cause blood to back up behind the small opening; this blood can be forced back up into the fallopian tubes. Women with an imperforate hymen have a higher incidence of endometriosis, a disease that can affect your ability to get pregnant in several ways. (See Chapter 6 for more on endometriosis in this book, and check out *Endometriosis For Dummies*, by Joseph Krotec. MD and Sharon Perkins, RN [Wiley 2006], for all you ever wanted to know about endometriosis.)

The cervix

The *cervix* is the lower part of the uterus. It keeps the baby from falling out of the uterus when you're pregnant because it's a tight, muscle-like tissue. The cervix also guards against infection because it's filled with mucus that forms a barrier between your vagina and the inside of the uterus. If you have an *incompetent cervix,* it means that the cervix doesn't stay tight and closed when you're pregnant but starts to open up from the weight of the growing baby. An incompetent cervix is usually stitched with a suture called a *cerclage* in early pregnancy to keep the baby where it belongs.

The uterus

The *uterus,* or womb, is a pear-shaped organ designed to hold and nourish a baby for nine months. Every month the lining of the uterus, called the *endometrium,* thickens to make a nourishing bed for an embryo. If you don't get pregnant that month, the lining breaks down and is shed as your *menstrual flow,* or *period.*

Many women have a uterus that doesn't conform to the standard upside-down pear shape you've all seen in pictures marked "this is your uterus." If you're one of these women, your uterus is flopped forward, toward your pubic bone. Twenty percent of women have a tipped or retroverted uterus, which, contrary to what many women believe, does not cause problems getting pregnant.

Around 2 to 3 percent of women have an abnormally shaped uterus. The most common variation is a *septate uterus,* which means that a band of tissue *(septum)* partially or completely divides the inside of the uterus. This tissue can be surgically removed. A T-shaped uterus is often a side effect of your mom's taking DES, a drug given from the 1940s to the 1960s to prevent miscarriage.

Bicornuate (two-horn) and *unicornuate* (one-horn) uteri have either one (uni) or two (bi) narrower-than-normal cavities. Women with T-shaped, bicornuate, and unicornuate uteri have higher-than-normal miscarriage rates.

It's also possible to have two separate uterine cavities, called a *didelphys uterus;* such women usually also have a second cervix. You may need to have a cesarean section (a surgical delivery) if you have a double cervix, meaning that more isn't always better.

Even if the shape of your uterus is normal, it may contain some unwanted "accessories" — growths such as polyps and fibroids — which may decrease the chance that a fetus can implant and grow in your uterus. Polyps are easily removed and don't cause any complications after they're gone. Removing fibroids is more complex. Small ones may be removed through the vagina by entering the uterus through the cervix in an outpatient surgicenter, but large ones may require an abdominal incision and a hospital stay of a couple of days. Removing fibroids can leave scar tissue in the cavity that can make it harder to get pregnant because the fetus won't be able to implant in the scarred area. You may also need a cesarean section after fibroid removal.

Scar tissue can also form in your uterus after a dilation and curettage (D&C for short). If there's a lot of scar tissue, nearly filling the uterus, it's called Asherman's syndrome. This scar tissue can also be removed surgically to make it easier for you to get pregnant.

The ovaries

Most women have two ovaries, which contain the most important accessory of all — eggs! How many eggs? Less every year, since every day of your life, eggs are lost through *atresia,* which means that they die off because they're not being stimulated to mature. For example:

- Before birth, a girl fetus's ovaries contain around 3.5 million eggs
- A newborn baby girl's ovaries contain about 1 million eggs
- By puberty, only 300,000 to 400,000 eggs remain
- Every month, 500 to 1,000 eggs are lost, along with the one or possibly two eggs that mature and are released each month.
- By age 50, only 1,000 or so eggs remain, and many are abnormal because the "good" eggs get used up first.

The eggs

You may wonder what eggs contain to make them into your potential scream-ing newborn. The answer is chromosomes — 23 chromosomes, to be exact. Each chromosome contains the genes that determine whether your baby is tall or short, blond or brunet, and, to some extent, fat or thin. (See the section "Recognizing genetic diseases that can impact fertility" for more information on chromosomes and genes.)

Of course, there's more to an egg than chromosomes. Three protective layers surround the egg, starting with the *cumulus layer.* That's the nourishing and protecting fluffy layers of cells that completely surround the egg. Moving inward, you'll see the *corona radiate,* the protective single layer of cells covering the *zona pellucida,* the "shell" of the egg. A mature, ready-for-fertilization oocyte, or egg, has a small attachment called a *polar body,* which is the remnant left after the egg divides (a process called *meiosis*) so that it contains only 23 chromosomes. The polar body also contains 23 chromosomes.

All cells in the human body besides eggs and sperm have 46 chromosomes. Eggs and sperm each have 23, so the baby they create has 46.

Each month, one egg is released from one of your ovaries. The decision about which one ovulates (right or left) is random; they do not necessarily alternate. If you have only one ovary, either because you were born that way or because one was surgically removed, your one ovary takes over egg making each month, so that you still ovulate each month.

The fallopian tubes

You should have two fallopian tubes, one near each ovary. Tubes are kind of like a pickup bar — a place where sperm and egg should meet and, it is hoped, go on to create something bigger and better: a baby! When an egg is released from the ovary, little projections called *fimbriae* on the end of the tube move back and forth to "entice" the egg into the tube. Once in the fallopian tube, the egg needs a few days to shimmy down to the uterus. One hopes along the way it meets Mr. Sperm and fertilizes, thereby transforming into an embryo by the time it reaches the uterus. Damaged tubes, usually damaged from infection but sometimes from endometriosis or surgery, are a very common cause of infertility. We talk about this in depth in Chapter 11.

The egg does not have to be picked up by the fallopian tube nearest the ovary. As much as one-third of the time, the opposite tube can do the job. So if you only have one open tube, and you ovulate from the opposite ovary, pregnancy can still occur.

The breasts

Breasts aren't necessary for getting pregnant; women who have had breasts removed can get pregnant. The normal number of breasts, of course, is two. Nipples are a different matter. As many as 1 in 20 people have more than two nipples. The extras may be nothing more than reddish brown, rough pieces of skin, often found in line with the main nipples. Check yourself out!

Controlling your hormones

You can have all the reproductive organs you need, and all in perfect order, and still have no chance of getting pregnant. You can't get pregnant unless your organs are all synchronized to produce an egg and prepare a proper "landing spot" for it in the uterus at the proper time. What you need to orchestrate the process are *hormones,* which are chemical substances released from one part of the body that cause a reaction in another part of the body.

The three female hormone-control systems that work together to orchestrate your menstrual cycle are:

- ✔ The **hypothalamus** (the small structure in the middle of the brain that regulates the nervous and endocrine systems, as well as body weight and temperature)
- ✔ The **pituitary** (an endocrine gland at the base of the brain below the hypothalamus that secretes several hormones, including FSH and LH which are critical for reproduction; the pituitary gland used to be called the "master gland")
- ✔ The **ovary** (the female reproductive organ that produces estrogen, progesterone, and eggs)

These three hormone systems work together in a feedback system called the Hypothalamus-pituitary-ovarian axis, which simply means that they function together to produce a seamless masterpiece — your menstrual cycle.

The main female hormones are:

- ✔ Estrogen
- ✔ Luteinizing hormone (LH)
- ✔ Follicle-stimulating hormone (FSH)
- ✔ Progesterone

Putting All Your Reproductive Parts Together: Your Menstrual Cycle

All the components of your reproductive tract — the vagina, uterus, ovaries, fallopian tubes, and the glands that orchestrate your hormones — have to work together perfectly for you to be able to get pregnant. (Yes, you need sperm, too, but we get to that in a later section, "Hanging Out with the Guys.")

Although your menstrual cycle seems simple enough, a lot of things, unfortunately, can go wrong. We not only address how your cycle works but also how it may not work in the next few sections.

Checking out how your cycle runs

The hormone-secreting systems work to create your menstrual cycle like this:

1. **Follicular phase:** The old uterine lining breaks down and passes through the vagina as menstrual flow. This process takes one to five days. *Follicle-stimulating hormone (FSH)* is released from your pituitary gland.

   In the ovary, 10 to 15 follicles, called antral follicles, begin to grow. The cells surrounding each egg secrete a liquid, forming a follicle, a fluid-filled sac. Each follicle contains one egg. During this time period an egg matures.

   In response to FSH and *luteinizing hormone (LH),* the follicle is released from the pituitary gland, and begins to produce *estrogen.* In the ovary, one egg-containing follicle is growing and producing estrogen. In the uterus, the estrogen produced by the ovary is making the lining thicken. This is called the *proliferative phase* of the uterus.

   One follicle becomes dominant, growing faster than the others. As the dominant follicle grows, it produces more estrogen. The amount of FSH released decreases, and the smaller follicles stop growing.

   A large amount of LH, called an *LH surge,* is released from the pituitary gland as the estrogen rises. This makes the egg inside the dominant follicle mature.

2. **Ovulation:** The follicle bursts; the egg is released (*ovulation*) and is picked up by one of the fallopian tubes.

3. **Secretory phase:** After meeting up with the lucky sperm, the resulting embryo begins to travel down the fallopian tubes, a journey of several days. The uterine lining is now thick enough to support embryo implantation and its glands secrete proteins which help guide the embryo to the correct spot.

4. **Luteal phase:** The leftover part of the follicle, now called the *corpus luteum,* produces *progesterone* to help an embryo implant.

   The embryo floats in the uterus for several days and then implants in the thickened uterine lining and starts to grow. If you're not pregnant, the lining will break down two weeks after ovulation, and your cycle will begin again.

The importance of regular periods

Do your periods always come every 28 days like clockwork? If they do, you're a rarity; only one in ten women fall into what we've been conditioned to think of as a "normal" menstrual pattern. Most women have cycles 25 to 31 days apart.

When your doctor asks you how long your cycles are, he's asking how many days are between day one of one period and day one of the next period. When he asks how long your period is, he's asking how many days you bleed. Day one of your period is the first day of normal (for you) flow, not the day when you have light or irregular spotting before your period starts.

If you are on, or have been on, birth control pills, be sure to note that in charting your menstrual pattern. The pill chemically coordinates your cycle to come at the same time each month (provided you take the pill correctly!). Determining your *actual* menstrual pattern can only be done after you've been off the pill for at least three months.

What's regular for you may not be regular for someone else, but having some sort of pattern to your periods is important, because it indicates that you're producing and releasing eggs on a regular basis. This isn't, however, a hard-and-fast rule; some women with periods like clockwork aren't making eggs at all, but that's a rarity.

It normally takes between 10 to 14 days to mature a good egg and release it, so you normally ovulate sometime between day 10 and day 14 of your cycle. How do you know if you've ovulated? Some women experience a sharp pain when they ovulate, called *mittelschmertz* (see the section "Recognizing signs of ovulation" for tips on knowing when you're ovulating).

The most consistent part of your period should be the time between ovulation, or release of the egg, and the start of your next period. This time period should be between 13 to 14 days; if you're getting your period 12 days or less after ovulation, you may not be making enough progesterone to support a pregnancy.

If you're cycles are very long, or very irregular, you may not be producing eggs often, or at all! See "Malfunctioning menstrual cycles" for more on how irregular cycles affect your chance of getting pregnant.

Wanna know what's in that flow?

Just before your period starts, your uterine lining is approximately 10 millimeters thick. Your period starts when the lining, or endometrium, starts to break down. Menstrual flow consists of endometrial tissue mixed with blood from the torn blood vessels, cervical mucus, and cellular debris. This all adds up to a little more than 30 milliliters (an ounce) of discharge, although it certainly seems like a lot more! More than 80 milliliters (a little less than 3 ounces) of discharge is abnormal.

Menstrual blood normally doesn't clot, unless your flow is very heavy. Sometimes the lining is shed in large fragments (sometimes called *decidual casts*) that can look like an early miscarriage.

Don't assume that you're having a miscarriage if you pass some tissue and blood, even if it's not the right time to have a period. If you can, bring the tissue to your doctor (a zipper baggie or a plastic tub is fine), and even if you can't, you can still get a pregnancy test to see if you were or were not pregnant. This information may be very helpful to your doctor (and to you) in the future.

Timing and fertility

Timing is everything when it comes to getting pregnant. Many women miss the mark month after month because of mistaken ideas about the best time to get pregnant.

Sperm and eggs both have a short "shelf life"; eggs are capable of being fertilized for around 24 hours and sperm can live up to four days in the proper environment, such as the fluid that fills the fallopian tubes. That means that if you don't have sex within a few days before ovulation, you're not going to get pregnant.

Many women have been conditioned to believe that ovulation occurs on day 14; they have sex on days 12, 13, or 14 in hopes of hitting the right time. But the most consistent thing about your menstrual cycle should be that ovulation occurs 14 days before your period begins. So if your cycles are 28 days, you ovulate on day 14. But if your cycles are short, say 25 days, you're actually ovulating on day 11, and having sex starting on day 12 will be too late to achieve a pregnancy.

On the other hand, if your cycles are long, say 34 days, you don't ovulate until day 20. Having sex on day 14 will be way too early, since sperm don't live for a week.

So timing sex correctly when you want to get pregnant is dependent on a solid knowledge of when you're ovulating. We discuss the ways ovulation can be predicted in Chapter 4.

Sperm live longer in your body than the egg, so err on the early side when deciding when to start having sex. Every other day is enough, and there is no harm in having extra sperm around. When in doubt, just do it!

Malfunctioning menstrual cycles

Although it may seem like your menstrual cycle runs like clockwork, always appearing on the expected day, the likelihood is that at least part of the time, your cycle is out of synch, showing up too early, too late, or not at all, even though you're not pregnant. Irregular periods not only make it hard to determine when you ovulate; they can also indicate that your reproductive system is in need of fine tuning. In this section, we discuss all the ways cycles can get out of synch, what it can mean, and how your doctor might suggest fixing them.

Menstrual cycles that don't fall into the norm can indicate that you're not ovulating at all, or that you're only ovulating occasionally. An occasional irregular cycle can be brought about by stress, a change in routine, exercise, eating patterns, or illness, but periods that are "never the same length twice," consistently shorter than normal or longer than normal, should be evaluated by your doctor.

Bleeding too often — short cycles

If your cycles are very short — less than 25 days apart on a regular basis, you may be ovulating too soon. Since the period between ovulation and the start of your period should consistently be 14 days, if your periods are short, it usually (but not always — we discuss the alterative in this section) means that you have a short follicular phase, the time between you period and your ovulation.

A short follicular phase can mean that the egg doesn't have time to develop properly before it's being released; this is called *premature luteinization.* (See Chapter 11 for more about premature luteinization.) Short follicular phases can occur when your ovarian reserve, the number of eggs you still have in your ovaries, is starting to decrease.

Just realizing that you're ovulating before day 14 may result in pregnancy if your cycles are short. However, if your cycles are very short because you're ovulating very early, on day 6 or so, your uterine lining may not have time to build up enough for an embryo to implant by the time you ovulate. You need to see your doctor in this case, to help prolong your follicular phase with hormones. (See Chapter 14 for how this can be done.)

Your cycles can also be short if the secretory phase, the time between ovulation and your next period, is shorter than 14 days. This is called *luteal phase defect,* and usually indicates that the corpus luteum isn't making enough progesterone to sustain an embryo's growth into the uterine lining. You may need progesterone supplements if your progesterone is too low and your periods are coming too quickly after ovulation.

Bleeding too infrequently or skipping periods

Cycles that are very long, over 35 days apart, can indicate that you're not ovulating regularly. This can be a factor of stress, exercise, weight change, or other factors, but can also be caused by Polycystic Ovarian Syndrome, or PCOS. PCOS can cause changes in hormone ratios that can be diagnosed by your doctor, as well as physical changes such as excessive hair, weight gain, and acne. (See Chapter 5 for more on PCOS.)

Endometriosis, premature ovarian failure (see Chapter 5 for more on both of these), abnormal thyroid levels, or high prolactin levels (see Chapter 11 for the details on diagnosing infertility causes through blood tests) can also cause irregular or absent periods.

Bleeding between periods

Bleeding between periods can indicate that something is wrong inside your uterus, or that your hormones are out of balance. Some of the things that can go wrong with your uterus to cause irregular bleeding are:

- ✔ **Cervical irritations or infections:** Possible causes of cervical bleeding

- ✔ **Fibroids:** Benign growths found in the uterine wall

- ✔ **Polyps:** Small fleshy growths found on the endometrium, the lining of the uterus, or the cervix

Bleeding too heavily (menorrhagia)

Bleeding too heavily and passing clots can be "normal" for some women, especially in women who are overweight. Fibroids, PCOS, and irregular periods can be related to heavier than normal bleeding. Heavy bleeding can also be a sign of recurrent early miscarriage (see Chapter 13).

Women who bleed heavily every month are at risk for becoming *anemic* (having a decreased number of red blood cells). Anemia can lead to fatigue and weakness, so heavy periods should be checked out with your doctor. A simple blood test can diagnose anemia.

Having scant periods

If your period is very light, it could be a normal variant, (in which case, lucky you!) or it could be a sign that your uterine lining isn't getting as thick as it should. Scant periods are typical if you're usingbirth control pills or have just stopped using them, or if your periods have just started. If your lining isn't thickening properly, you may not be ovulating normally, so seeing your doctor is a good idea.

Experiencing painful periods (dysmenorrhea)

Up to 40 percent of women experience pain with their periods, called *dysmenorrhea*. Dysmenorrhea falls into two categories:

- ✔ **Primary dysmenorrhea** has no other underlying cause besides the release of *prostaglandins,* (chemicals made by cells that have specific functions such as controlling body temperature, stimulating smooth muscle, and influencing heat cycles) in the uterus, which cause uterine contractions.

- ✔ **Secondary dysmenorrhea** is caused by disease present in addition to the normal release of prostaglandins, such as endometriosis, fibroids, or infection.

Because painful periods can be caused by diseases that can interfere with getting pregnant, such as endometriosis, you should always see your doctor if you have painful periods. Dysmenorrhea is the most common symptom of endometriosis, which affects over 5 million women in North America and causes infertility in 30 to 40 percent of its sufferers.

The release of prostaglandins that cause cramping can also cause nausea, diarrhea, and exhaustion, just to make you feel really terrible during your periods. Taking anti-inflammatory medications such as ibuprofen can help with the symptoms.

Hanging Out with the Guys

Compared to women, guys let it all hang out, reproductively speaking. That's a good thing because "hanging out," at least as far as testicles are concerned, is necessary to keep the developing sperm from getting too warm. Take a look at what every guy should have. See Figure 2-2 for a graphic portrayal of your average man.

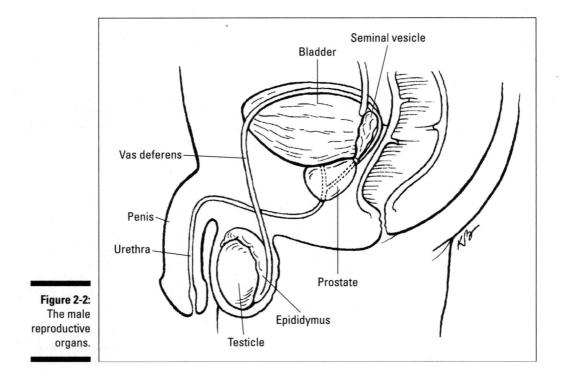

Figure 2-2:
The male reproductive organs.

The penis

The number-one guy concern is probably related to penis size: How do I compare to everyone else? For those obsessed, here are the standards: normal length when flaccid, or limp, 3.9 inches; stretched (still limp), 4.8 inches; erect, 5 to 7 inches. We hope that bit of info made most of you fellows feel better. A small penis, less than 1.9 inches limp, is usually able to impregnate as long as it can get the sperm into the vagina, up toward the cervix. Size is rarely an issue in infertility.

Size may not matter, but function does. If you watch Viagra commercials, you may be comforted to know that even athletes and famous men have problems with erectile dysfunction, also known as *impotence.* As nice as it is to know that you're not alone, this condition can be an embarrassing detriment to getting pregnant. Impotence, the inability to have or sustain an erection, is more common as men get older; as many as 50 percent of men between the ages of 40 and 70 have had problems with impotence. Impotence can be caused by diseases such as diabetes or by chronic conditions, such as alcohol abuse, or it can be a side effect of medications. (We discuss impotence in Chapter 12.)

The opening that lets both urine and sperm out of the penis should be at the tip of the penis, located dead center. Two types of variations can cause problems getting pregnant. One in around 300 men has *hypospadias,* which means that the opening is on the underside of the penis. In 20 percent of cases, this problem is hereditary. Epispadias occurs far less frequently; only 1 in approximately 100,000 men has epispadias. In *epispadias,* the opening is on the top of the penis. Both conditions are associated with an unusual curvature of the erect penis; it curves up in epispadias and down in hypospadias. Both conditions can prevent the sperm from getting exactly where they need to be. Surgical correction is possible, and inseminations can also help get the sperm to where they need to go.

The testicles

Testicles are the sperm production and warehouse site. Here, as in many other places on the human body, nature has been generous and given two of the same body part (testicles, in this instance), in case something happens to one. Testicles first develop inside the abdomen and gradually descend outside the body by the time a baby boy is born. At birth, about 4 in 100 boys have undescended testicles, properly called *cryptorchidism.* Testicles need to be kept a few degrees cooler than 98 degrees for sperm to develop properly, so to prevent future infertility, doctors usually recommend surgery to lower the testicles outside the body as soon as the baby is a year old.

The testicles are contained in a pouch of skin called the *scrotum.* In about 80 percent of men, the left testicle is bigger and hangs lower. Sometimes the testicles are abnormally large, which can be caused by a *hydrocele,* which is a collection of fluid inside the scrotum, or by a *varicocele,* which is the condition of dilated or varicose veins in the testicle. These conditions can be surgically corrected. If left alone, they can raise the temperature of the testes and cause infertility.

Sperm are produced every day, but it takes about 70 days for the new sperm to fully mature. Sperm production starts in the testes. FSH and LH, the same hormones that develop eggs, are needed to begin sperm production. LH stimulates production of testosterone, another male hormone. The sperm mature in the epididymis and travel through the vas deferens up to the seminal vesicle and the prostate, where they're bathed in the fluid known as semen. They're then ejaculated through the urethra during male orgasm.

Sperm — 200 million of them!

Here comes one egg — or maybe two eggs, if it's a good month — tooling down the fallopian tubes. The egg is about the size of a pencil point dot — in other words, barely visible. All of a sudden the egg meets up with about 200 sperm, the sole survivors of an ejaculate of over 100 million sperm a few hours before — talk about an embarrassment of riches. The sperm are much smaller than the egg, so small that all the sperm needed to repopulate the earth could sit on an aspirin tablet. There's enough room for all of them to attach their heads to the egg and try to beat down the door. Ideally, only one will succeed, and the others will be shut out immediately.

Why are there so many more sperm than eggs? Because it's a *long* way through the uterus and up the tubes, and because only 50 percent (of a *good* sperm sample) of the sperm know how to swim forward, *and* because some of them are barely moving, a tremendous number of sperm are needed to ensure that a few hundred will get through to the egg. Their journey is like one of you trying to swim across the Pacific Ocean. If there were 200 million of you, maybe a few hundred would make it. Imagine if you had to fertilize an egg when you finally got there! (We talk about sperm and male factor issues much more in Chapter 12.)

Putting Male and Female Parts Together: Having Sex (At the Right Time)

Now that you know how all your parts work, are you ready to have a baby? Yes? Then it's time to have sex. No, not right now. It's important to have sex when the timing is right. How do you know when the timing is right? This is more than just mood lighting and foreplay. To get pregnant, you need to be close to ovulation.

Recognizing signs of ovulation

You may be able to tell that you're ovulating in a few simple ways, just by watching the calendar and being observant about your bodily functions.

Usually the mucus from your cervix increases around the time of ovulation. It also becomes very thin, clear, and stretchy; you can easily stretch it out a couple of inches. Rising estrogen levels from a developing follicle create this mucus, which is easier for sperm to swim through than your usual thicker mucus and also has an alkaline pH, which helps the sperm live longer. At other times of the month, cervical mucus is acidic. Be sure that you're not confusing cervical mucus with semen from previous sex or increased secretions from sexual arousal.

Some doctors believe that taking antihistamines may decrease cervical mucus. To be on the safe side, avoid antihistamines around ovulation time.

If you have no objection to feeling around inside your vagina, you'll also notice that your cervix becomes softer, slightly open, and easier to locate with your fingers when you're about to ovulate. At other times of the month, the cervix is found farther back in the uterus, feels firmer to the touch, and is tightly closed.

If you know how long your cycles are, count back 14 days from the length of your cycle to figure out when you're probably ovulating. For example, if your cycles are 29 days, you ovulate on day 15. If your cycles are 26 days apart, you ovulate on day 12.

About 20 percent of women have pain called *mittelschmertz* (German for "middle pain") when they ovulate. The pain seems to be caused by blood and fluid irritating the tissues around the ovary after it releases from the follicle. Sometimes a small amount of vaginal bleeding occurs with ovulation too.

Some women have headaches around the time of ovulation, and others complain of bloating or breast pain. You're probably already aware of your personal ovulation indicators, but you may have just never paid much attention to them. Now you should. They're a big help in choosing when to have baby sex.

Conceiving a Baby: How Sex Should Work

The time is right, the moon is bright, and it's time to get pregnant. Here's what needs to happen:

1. It's near ovulation; an egg is about to release from its follicle.

2. You and your partner become aroused. Your vagina produces secretions that make it easier for the now erect penis to enter the vagina.

3. During the man's orgasm, several million sperm are forcefully ejaculated into the vagina. As they pass through the cervix into the uterus, the cervical mucus "filters" the sperm so that they're ready to penetrate an egg.

4. Your egg releases from the follicle and enters one of your fallopian tubes.

5. The sperm swim through the uterus up to the fallopian tubes; half choose the wrong tube to enter.

6. The next day your egg meets up with several hundred sperm in the fallopian tube, and the sperm all attach themselves to the egg, trying to beat down the door.

7. One sperm breaks through the outer layer of the egg, and the egg immediately becomes impenetrable to the rest of the sperm.

8. The genetic material of the egg and sperm combine, and the newly created embryo drifts down the fallopian tube to the uterus.

9. The embryo implants in the uterine wall and grows, and you miss your period.

10. You're pregnant! Congratulations.

After sex, just lie there for a while. Don't jump up and go to the bathroom right away. Let gravity help those little swimmers get to where they need to be. Some doctors advocate placing a pillow under the hips during sex to give gravity a little edge in directing the sperm where they need to be. Doing so probably isn't necessary. You can also choose whatever position is best for you and your partner. There is no "best" position for making babies.

Figuring Out How Often to Have Sex

When you're trying to get pregnant, you need to strike a balance between too much sex and not enough. Too much sex decreases sperm counts, but if you have too little sex, you may miss the right moment for conception. Not having sex for more than five days may raise the number of sperm but decrease their motility (the active movement). Sex less than two days apart may decrease the sperm count. So how do you figure out when the right time is?

When you're close to ovulating, have sex at least every other day; every day is okay, but more than once per day is probably too much. Most doctors recommend the two days before and the day you ovulate as the best time for conception.

Getting Into Your Genes

Everyone should inherit 23 chromosomes from each parent, for a total of 46 chromosomes, arranged in 23 pairs. Genes are found in standard locations on different chromosomes.

Genes are an important, although normally invisible, part of your anatomy. Genes are sections of DNA that occupy certain locations on chromosomes; they determine the characteristics that make you "you," like the color of your eyes, your height, and your predisposition to certain diseases. The sections that follow explore some of the diseases based on genetics as well as the basics about genetic testing.

Recognizing genetic diseases that can impact fertility

Certain inherited diseases can interfere with getting pregnant. You may already know you have an infertility-causing disease, , or may you just find out when you start trying to get pregnant.

Genetic diseases such as Turner Syndrome in women, Kleinfelter Syndrome in men and cystic fibrosis can cause infertility. Less easily recognized problems, such as deletion of part of the Y chromosome in males, may not be recognized until a fertility workup is done.

About 1 in 500 people has a chromosomal translocation. Translocation of chromosomes may cause an individual no problem and isn't usually obvious but may cause recurrent miscarriage if passed on by either parent. This is because the translocation in an individual is usually balanced — one piece of a chromosome has been exchanged for another. When the chromosome is passed on, however, it may be "unbalanced," causing miscarriage or abnormal pregnancy.

Factoring in your genes

Back in 1990, scientists began a project called the Human Genome Project, designed to map the location of every gene present on the 23 pairs of human chromosomes, and to sequence the over 3 billion DNA base pairs that make up the chromosomes. A daunting task — but the Human Genome Project announced the completion of this task in 2001, after the identification of 30,000 (give or take a few) genes. The Human Genome Project makes it possible to test for very specific changes on chromosomes that can cause diseases such as cystic fibrosis and Tay-Sachs diseases.

Understanding inherited genes

Genetic disease inheritance is complicated and falls into several different patterns; the four most common are:

- ✔ **Autosomal recessive:** A child must inherit the mutation from both parents to have the disease. A child whose parents both carry the gene has a 25 percent chance of having the disease, a 50 percent chance of being a carrier of the disease but not having it, and a 25 percent chance of not inheriting the gene at all. Cystic fibrosis and sickle cell anemia are examples of autosomal recessive diseases. Approximately 80 percent of children born with an autosomal recessive disorder have no evidence of the disease itself in their families. That's because family members can carry a gene for autosomal recessive disease for generations . . . or forever, without the disease showing up, if no one marries a partner with the same recessive gene. Without two copies of the mutation, one from each parent, a child will not be born with the actual disease.

- ✔ **Autosomal dominant:** The child will have the disease even if only one parent passes on the mutation. Huntington's chorea is an example of this disease. Huntington's chorea can be passed on because its carriers usually survive long enough to have children and pass on the gene.

- ✔ **X-linked dominant:** An X-linked disease is a mutation of the X chromosome. Females are more often affected because they have two X chromosomes. Men can only pass an X chromosome to a daughter (girls have XX sex chromosomes, boys have XY, and mom always passes on one of the Xs) so men can't pass X-linked disease to their sons. Fragile X Syndrome is an example of this disease.

- ✔ **X-linked recessive:** Both parents must pass on the gene for the child to be affected; one in four will have the disease, two in four will be carriers, and one in four will be free of the disease. Hemophilia is an example of an X-linked recessive disease. More males than females are affected by X-linked recessive disease, and males can't pass them on the sons.

Checking out common and not so common genetic diseases

Some genetic diseases are fairly common, such as the tendency toward heart disease, diabetes, and certain types of cancer. Others are rare, with only a few known cases in the world. Genes can spontaneously mutate, so a genetic disease can show up in a family without a previous history of that disease.

Race and genetic diseases

Some diseases are more likely to be found in persons of a certain race: African Americans are more likely to carry the sickle cell anemia gene, for example, and cystic fibrosis is found more frequently in Caucasians.

Ethnicity and genetic diseases

Populations that have intermarried more often over the years are more prone to carrying certain genes. One such well documented group is the Ashkenazi Jewish population, which consists of Jews from central and Eastern Europe. Around 80 percent of American Jews are of Ashkenazi descent. Two well known examples of genes carried by people of this descent are:

- ✔ Tay-Sachs Disease: 1 in 31 Ashkenazi Jews is a carrier.
- ✔ Gaucher Disease: 1 in 10 is a carrier.

Another example is the Pakistani community in the United Kingdom, in which:

- ✔ Between 20 and 88 percent of the population are related to one another
- ✔ One out of every one hundred babies dies from life-threatening malformations
- ✔ Nonlethal malformations are four times more likely to occur than in the general population

Testing for abnormalities

If you have a known hereditary disease in your family or are experiencing recurrent pregnancy loss, you may want to know more about your individual genes because knowing what genes you carry can predict whether or not your future child will inherit certain diseases. If you've had recurrent loss, genetic testing may be able to tell you whether you have a chromosomal abnormality that's causing pregnancy loss.

Chromosomal testing is done by different techniques, depending on what you're looking for. Chromosomal tests look only at the number and shape of chromosomes. It doesn't evaluate the genes found on the chromosomes. Many genetic abnormalities are found by chromosome testing because the diseases are caused by extra chromosomes or too few chromosomes. Down syndrome, or trisomy 21, for example, is caused by an extra copy of chromosome 21.

Genetic testing can also be done if you're looking for a specific known gene. Changes in that specific gene can be evaluated for presence of disease. All that's needed for testing is a blood sample.

Chapter 3

Practicing Positive Behaviors — Before Conception

In This Chapter

▶ Changing your lifestyle for conception

▶ Eating properly

▶ Avoiding bad habits

▶ Treating sexually transmitted diseases

*E*ven though you're probably anxious to get started on baby making, take a little time to make sure that you're in the best possible condition for conceiving a healthy baby. This means making sure that you're not carrying an infection that could harm you or your baby and taking a look at your lifestyle habits, good and bad. In this chapter, we tell you how to get in shape physically if you're trying to get pregnant and discuss some behavior that could be decreasing your odds of getting pregnant. We also take a look at how what you eat could influence your chance of conceiving.

Making Healthy Lifestyle Changes

"Everything in moderation" is certainly a good motto for habits, good and bad. Too much exercise can have a less than desirable effect, while coffee, drunk in moderation, can be benign. But, before you say yes to things that are better left in the no category, consider that some things are best eliminated entirely, particularly when you're trying to conceive.

Giving up smoking

Smoking is bad for you. You all know it. Yet 30 percent of women in the United States still smoke. Need some good reasons to quit? Here are a few:

- Smokers are 50 percent more likely to miscarry.

- Smokers are two to four times more likely to have an *ectopic* pregnancy (one that implants in the fallopian tube rather than in the uterus, a topic we discuss in detail in Chapter 6).

- Smokers go through menopause earlier, decreasing the number of years pregnancy can occur.

- Smokers' eggs have more genetic abnormalities.

- Smokers' eggs are prone to *polyspermy,* where two or more sperm enter an egg. The embryos that result are chromosomally abnormal and will not grow.

If you've quit but your partner hasn't, he may want to consider the following:

- Men who smoke have a lower sperm count.

- Men who smoke have a 20 percent decrease in sperm motility.

- Smokers' sperm have more abnormal shapes. Abnormally shaped sperm have a higher rate of chromosomal abnormalities.

Eliminating alcohol

Studies show that heavy drinkers (more than three drinks a day) have more trouble getting pregnant. Continuing to drink while pregnant increases the chance for miscarriage and can also cause fetal alcohol syndrome (FAS). FAS babies have learning and behavioral problems and typically have small heads, a flat midface, small eye slits, and a low nasal ridge.

In addition, drinking heavily can cause menstrual irregularities, and can also make you forget about trying to get pregnant!

What about an occasional drink on a special holiday or on New Year's Eve? It's best to follow your own doctor's recommendation on alcohol and to remember that an *occasional* glass means just that — occasional, not every day!

Saying no to drugs

Undoubtedly you know that illegal drugs are taboo when trying to become pregnant! Here are the problems that some common drugs can cause when you're trying to get pregnant.

Cocaine

Cocaine causes constriction of the blood vessels, which can result in early miscarriage, preterm delivery, and problems with the *placenta,* the organ that nourishes the baby. In addition, cocaine can cause menstrual irregularities, possibly making it harder for you to become pregnant.

Marijuana

Marijuana lowers sperm count, decreases sperm's motility or ability to move forward, lowers the amount of testosterone in males, and results in an increased number of abnormal eggs and sperm.

Avoiding anabolic steroids

Some studies show that as many as 6 to 7 percent of all males have used anabolic steroids before age 18 to build muscle mass. Anabolic steroids suppress the body's ability to make testosterone, which is necessary for normal sperm production. This damage can be permanent, so stay away from the steroids.

Eating Well When Trying to Conceive

Because the best parents generally practice what they preach, setting up some good habits even *before* conception occurs is as good a start as any! Good nutrition is important at every stage of your life, but particularly when you're trying to conceive and maintain a pregnancy and ultimately deliver a healthy child. Although a perfectly tuned body isn't a necessity for having children, it certainly provides an ideal starting point. Nurturing your mind and heart is equally important. The following sections offer some tips on keeping your entire self in tiptop baby-making shape.

Obtaining the proper nutrition

Although vitamins provide good supplementation, get as many nutrients and minerals as possible from the food you eat. So before ingesting supplements ranging from vitamin A to zinc, start instead with your diet. Eating three square meals a day, plus a snack, is a good place to begin. What should those meals be made of? If you consider chocolate a food group, read on.

Getting in the right shape — nutritionally

Look at your fertility diet in the shape of a pregnant woman's body. See Figure 3-1 for a visual of a pregnant you as a food chart. At the top, the smallest spot (your head) should be reserved for fats, oils, and sweets. This category includes jam, mayonnaise, margarine, candy, and so on. Use these foods sparingly.

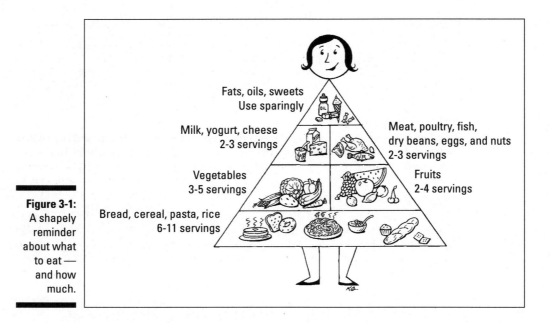

The next step down on the chart consists of two slightly larger categories: the milk, yogurt, and cheese group and the group that includes meat, poultry, fish, dry beans, eggs, and nuts. It is recommended that you consume two to three servings from the milk, yogurt, and cheese group. In this category, a serving is considered 1 cup of milk or yogurt or 2 ounces of processed cheese. Two to three servings (ounces) are recommended in the group that includes lean meat, poultry, fish, eggs, dry beans, and nuts. This level provides you with calcium, riboflavin, protein, iron, and B vitamins.

The next level calls for three to five servings of vegetables and two to four servings of fruit. A serving size of vegetables consists of 1 cup of raw leafy vegetables, ½ cup of cooked vegetables, or ¾ cup of vegetable juice, and a serving size of fruits consists of one medium apple, banana, or orange, ½ cup of chopped cooked or canned fruit, or ¾ cup of fruit juice. Notice that the recommended servings have increased from the higher level of this food chart. Pay attention to this recommendation. Vegetables and fruits are your most important source for fiber, vitamin A, vitamin C, and carbohydrates.

At the bottom of the pregnant woman food chart, you find the largest food group, which contains bread, cereal, rice, and pasta. Consider this the abdomen! The recommendation is that you eat six to eleven servings of this group per day. But before you wolf down a plate of pasta, remember your serving sizes. A serving in this group consists of one slice of bread, half a bagel, 1 ounce of ready-to-eat cereal, ½ cup of cooked rice or pasta, three to four small, plain crackers, or one 4-inch pancake.

If this seems like any other food plan you've ever seen, there's a reason for it — it is! Healthy eating is a standard practice. There are few tricks to eating healthy. When trying to conceive, eat enough but not too much and use your calories for healthy foods and not empty ones (such as chocolate). If you're not lactose intolerant, you may want to up your dairy intake; if you're *lactose intolerant,* which means that you can't properly digest milk products, you can get calcium from oral supplements.

Be careful of health foods such as soy, sunflower seeds, or herbs such as Vitex that promise to raise your estrogen level. (You can read more about herbs in Chapter 5.) Your body — more specifically, your ovaries — should be producing estrogen. By introducing an exogenous (outside) source, you're not assisting your body in manufacturing its own supply; you're only supplementing it artificially. This addition does not change the quality of your eggs or their output of estrogen. It only confuses any measurement of estrogen, as it's impossible to distinguish what your body makes on its own from that which you gain from outside sources. Skip any supplement or food that claims to increase your estrogen level.

Weighty warnings

Another practice to avoid is dieting, particularly fad diets. Conception is an act of incredible balance and timing. You don't want to throw your body off with the latest diet that promises to help you lose five pounds fast. More than likely, such a diet is a method that probably won't help your weight or your health any more than it will help your fertility.

If you're significantly overweight or underweight, you may want to consult your physician first (an OB/GYN will do). Either extreme can cause problems in fertility, particularly if your weight is symptomatic of another condition such as diabetes, polycystic ovary syndrome (PCOS), or amenorrhea. Twelve percent of all infertility is a result of weighing either too much or too little. The good news is that 70 percent of all women diagnosed with infertility related to being overweight or underweight conceive spontaneously when their weight normalizes.

If weight loss or weight gain is in order, consider addressing this matter before trying to conceive. Check with your physician and ask for a healthy diet and exercise plan. If you must embark on a weight adjustment program simultaneously with your baby-making efforts, make sure that your physician is aware of *both* goals.

In an Australian study of 3,500 women, very obese women were half as likely to conceive when compared to their healthier peer group. The researchers also concluded that it was no good being underweight either: Women who were below moderate weight also had less of a chance of becoming pregnant.

Ways in which extremes of weight can affect fertility include menstrual disturbance, disturbance to the lining of the uterus, inability to ovulate (*anovulation*), and increased risk of miscarriage.

Taking vitamins

Multivitamins are a good way to supplement your diet, but they're not a substitute for good nutrition. While you're trying to conceive and when you get pregnant, you need both. Much has been written about the importance of folic acid in early pregnancy. It has been shown to diminish certain birth defects, such as spina bifida.

Most garden-variety multivitamins contain adequate amounts of folic acid and suffice while you're trying to conceive. Your OB/GYN can switch you to prenatal vitamins as soon as you become pregnant.

Complicating Things through Common Infections

The onset of the sexual revolution in the 1960s caused a lot of fallout, and some of it fell on future fertility. Sexually transmitted diseases, or STDs, have increased dramatically in the last 20 years. More than 13 million Americans each year are affected, and many STDs pack a major anti-fertility wallop for both sexes. You may not even know that you have a sexually transmitted disease. Some STDs cause a vaginal or penile discharge, others cause itching or small sores, but some cause no symptoms at all. Most are easily treated with antibiotics. The problem is that many women don't realize they have an infection because most have no clear symptoms. The following sections describe a few of the most damaging STDs and provide some statistics about the diseases in the United States.

Chlamydia: The most common STD

Chlamydia is the most common sexually transmitted disease in the United States. The bacterium *Chlamydia trachomatis* is responsible for the infection. Both men and women can be infected, and both male and female fertility can be damaged. Chlamydia is easily tested by swabbing the penis or vagina and sending the swab to a lab for testing. A new test using urine is also being developed. Chlamydia is easily treated with antibiotics.

Here are some facts about the disease:

- About 4 million new cases of chlamydia are diagnosed every year.
- Approximately one in ten sexually active adolescents has been exposed to chlamydia.
- Women with untreated chlamydia have a 40 percent chance of developing pelvic inflammatory disease (PID), a major cause of damaged fallopian tubes.
- Women with PID are seven to ten times more likely to have an ectopic pregnancy, a pregnancy that grows outside the uterus, usually in the tubes. (For more about ectopic pregnancies, see Chapter 6.)
- Most women (75 percent) have no symptoms of infection; symptoms include lower abdominal pain, burning with urination, and vaginal irritation.
- Twenty-five percent of men have no symptoms from chlamydia; seventy-five percent have a discharge from the urethra, or pain and burning on urination.
- Men with untreated chlamydia can develop *epididymitis,* an infection in the testicles, where sperm are developed. This condition can lead to low sperm counts.
- Each year, 100,000 women become infertile from chlamydia. With a first infection, 12 percent of women become infertile; a second case increases infertility to 40 percent. Eighty percent of women who have had chlamydia three or more times are infertile.
- Untreated chlamydia when you're pregnant can lead to blindness in your child.

Gonorrhea

Gonorrhea is caused by the bacterium *Neisseria gonorrhoeae,* which can infect the genital tract, mouth, or rectum. It can be carried by males and females and can be cured with antibiotics. Here are some other facts about gonorrhea:

- Each year, 650,000 new cases of gonorrhea are diagnosed.
- Gonorrhea is diagnosed second only in frequency to chlamydia.
- Like chlamydia, gonorrhea in women can cause PID, leading to tubal damage. Most doctors test for gonorrhea and chlamydia before doing common fertility tests such as a *hysterosalpingogram* (HSG), in which dye is injected into the uterus and fallopian tubes to see whether there

are any irregularities. (We discuss HSGs in more detail in Chapter 11.) If you have gonorrhea or chlamydia and push dye into the tubes and uterus, you may push the infection up also and end up with more tube or uterine damage than you had to begin with.

✔ Men with gonorrhea usually have a discharge from the penis and a burning sensation; women may have no symptoms.

Syphilis

Syphilis is caused by the bacterium *Treponema pallidum*. The bacterium can be transmitted through genital, oral, or anal contact. Syphilis is easily cured with penicillin. Contrary to folklore, syphilis can't be caught from a toilet seat. But consider the following:

✔ Syphilis can cause stillbirth, blindness, mental retardation, or chronic syphilis in your unborn child if you have this disease while pregnant. Syphilis is treated with antibiotics.

✔ Lest you think syphilis is a thing of the past, 35,000 cases were reported in the United States in 1999, with 556 cases of congenital syphilis in newborns.

Genital herpes

Genital herpes is caused by the herpes simplex type 2 virus. The cold sores some people are prone to on their lips are caused by the herpes simplex type 1 virus (although you can get genital herpes with type 1 and cold sores with type 2, STD's don't always play by the rules!). Scientists are working on a vaccine against herpes, which would work only for those not already infected with the virus. Here's some more information:

✔ Sixty million Americans are infected with genital herpes, with 500,000 new cases diagnosed each year.

✔ If you have an outbreak of genital herpes at the time your baby is ready to be delivered, you'll need to have a cesarean section; if you deliver vaginally without treatment, your baby may suffer from mental retardation or may die.

✔ Herpes can't be cured; outbreaks are treated with antiviral medications.

HIV

Human immunodeficiency virus (HIV) causes the disease AIDS (acquired immune deficiency syndrome). At present, there is no cure for AIDS, although antiviral medications may keep the disease under control for some time.

Check out the following facts about HIV and pregnancy:

- ✔ Women with HIV can become pregnant and carry the pregnancy to term, but they risk transmitting HIV to the baby.

- ✔ The risk of transmission is about 25 percent if you're untreated but may be reduced dramatically if you receive AZT, an antiviral drug, while you're pregnant.

- ✔ Some doctors believe that the stress of pregnancy may cause your symptoms to worsen.

- ✔ You may reduce the risk of transmission of the disease to your baby if you have a cesarean section rather than a vaginal delivery.

- ✔ You must wait 3 to 18 months after delivery to find out whether your baby is HIV positive, because during pregnancy your antibodies are passed to the baby. This means that all babies of HIV-infected moms will test positive at birth. It can take as long as 18 months for all your antibodies to disappear from your baby's blood. After your antibodies are all gone, if the baby tests positive, it means he or she is infected with the virus.

You can be tested for sexually transmitted diseases, including HIV, before trying to conceive. If you suspect that you may have an STD, or have been exposed to one, you need to rule out this potential danger to your fertility and your unborn child.

Ureaplasma and mycoplasma

Ureaplasma and mycoplasma are microorganisms that can affect different parts of the body, depending on the strain. The genital tracts of both sexes can carry mycoplasma or ureaplasma. The following list gives some other information about the diseases:

- ✔ As many as 40 percent of women and men are carriers of bacteria called *ureaplasma* or *mycoplasma*.

- ✔ Some controversy exists about whether certain strains of ureaplasma and mycoplasma cause problems in getting pregnant; some studies show that they increase the incidence of miscarriage and/or problems with the embryo implanting in the uterus. This seems to be related to either partner having the infection, which is easily passed between partners.

- ✔ There's no scientific data to prove that either ureaplasma or mycoplasma reduces fertility.

- ✔ As with other STDs, both partners are easily treated with a 14-day course of an antibiotic, such as doxycycline. Both partners must take the drug, or they'll probably continue to reinfect each other.

Looking at Everyday Lifestyle Issues

Most everyone knows about drinking, smoking, and drugs being bad for you when you're trying to get pregnant. In this section, we talk about a few things that affect getting pregnant of which you might not be aware.

Cutting back on caffeine

Caffeine is controversial, but several studies have suggested that drinking several cups of coffee a day may increase the risk of developing difficulty becoming pregnant and early miscarriage. A cup of coffee contains twice the caffeine of one can of soda. Limit caffeine to less than 300 mg, which is three cups of coffee, or, better yet, cut it out completely! Teas also contain caffeine, but much less than coffee — 12 to 100 mg per cup.

Staying out of the hot tub

Anything that raises the temperature of a man's testicles can decrease sperm production and motility. Hot tubs, saunas, steam rooms, and tight underwear are out for men! And in case you're thinking of jumping in the tub without him, high temperatures have also been associated with egg damage and miscarriage. Find another way to relax when you're pregnant or trying to be.

Exercising with caution

So your partner decided to work out stress by bicycling or playing rugby. This exercise should be a good thing, right? Wrong! Prolonged cycling can cause damage to the groin from constant pressure of the bike seat, and contact sports can lead to injury to the testicles and can damage sperm production.

Women who exercise heavily may find that their periods have stopped. This condition is called *amenorrhea* and is common among women who are very thin and exercise daily. Obviously, you can't get pregnant if you're not having periods; you're not making any eggs. So what can you both do to reduce stress that won't cause fertility problems? Knitting is nice. If knitting isn't enough for you, exercise in moderation is fine — for both of you!

Dumping the douche

Douching is a bad idea whether you're trying to get pregnant or not. Women who douche regularly have a 73 percent increase in pelvic inflammatory disease (PID), which can cause damage to the fallopian tubes and uterus. The ectopic pregnancy rate is about 75 percent higher in women who douche regularly. Thirty-seven percent of women between the ages of 15 and 44 douche, and their risk of developing cervical cancer is about 80 percent higher than those who don't. Dump the douche!

Checking prescription medications

Have you overlooked something that could be interfering with your getting pregnant? Think back a few months, especially when thinking about sperm production; the sperm being ejaculated today have been over two months in the making, so anything your partner was taking a few months ago could be affecting his sperm count today. Ask yourself the following questions about a few possible deterrents you may not have thought about:

- ✔ Has your partner taken antibiotics, such as erythromycin or gentamycin, or antifungal medications, such as ketoconazole, or been treated for psoriasis with methotrexate? Has he been on anabolic steroids? These medicines can all affect sperm production.

- ✔ Does your partner take medication for high blood pressure? Sometimes, when you've been taking a medication for a long time, you almost forget that it can have serious side effects. Men who take certain types of antihypertensives called calcium channel blockers may produce sperm that can't penetrate eggs well; other high blood pressure medications may cause *retrograde ejaculation,* a condition in which the semen is pushed backwards into the bladder instead of being ejaculated out; or may cause an inability to get and sustain an erection. Other antihypertensive drugs are available that don't have these effects. Suggest that your partner talk to his doctor about switching medications if possible.

- ✔ Are you using a lubricant for sex? Lubricants are helpful because inadequate lubrication during sex can cause vaginal abrasions, and can lead to yeast infections. There are lubricants specifically manufactured for couples trying to conceive, which are supposed to be less likely to slow sperm down in their race to the egg.

Avoiding toxins in the workplace

Changing your job isn't always easy, but you do need to consider potential exposure to dangerous substances and take steps to protect yourself from them. Here are some examples:

- ✔ Think about substances that you're exposed to at work. For instance, if you're a home remodeler, bridge painter, welder, or solderer, you may be exposed to large amounts of lead. You run the same risk if you're remodeling an old house and scraping old paint off the walls. Lead exposure in men has been linked to low sperm count and decreased motility of sperm. In women, lead exposure may cause low birth weight in babies, high blood pressure during pregnancy, damage to the baby's nervous system, and developmental delays.

- ✔ Healthcare workers are exposed to a number of potentially dangerous drugs, as are pharmacists; exposure to chemotherapy drugs, radiation from X-rays, or inhaled anesthetics used in the operating room all can contribute to infertility.

Reducing stress

Can stress keep you from getting pregnant? Severe stress can change your menstrual cycle, even make you skip a few cycles. Every cycle you skip means one less chance to get pregnant, since you're not making an egg that month.

What can you do to reduce stress? We talk more about stress reducing techniques in Chapter 8, but in general:

- ✔ **Talk it out.** Stress increases when you hold everything in.

- ✔ **Try to focus on the "big picture."** When you're trying to get pregnant, every failed month seems like a year — or the end of the world. When you finally do get pregnant, it won't matter whether you got pregnant in November or January. Remember that the odds are on your side, in most cases, and that you *will* get pregnant.

- ✔ **Don't lose sight of the rest of your life.** While trying to have a baby may be a big part of your life at this moment, it's not the only thing you have going on in your life. Make time for your family, your partner, your friends, your hobbies — and anything else that helps you remember that you had a life before you started thinking about pregnancy, and you still do!

Getting Checked Out From Top to Bottom

Having a checkup even before you try to get pregnant is always a good idea, and it's essential if you've been trying for a few months and still getting "not pregnant" results on the home pregnancy tests. Sometimes simple imbalances in your thyroid levels, or other levels easily checked by a simple blood test, can be keeping you from getting pregnant.

Having a full physical

You can see either your primary care physician (PCP) or your gynecologist for a check up — or both! Your PCP looks at the "big picture" while your GYN looks mainly at your reproductive issues. Either one can order blood work and do a physical exam. (See Chapter 8 for more on choosing a doctor to help you get pregnant.)

Do you need to book a full body MRI or CT scan to find out if you're in shape to get pregnant? No, a half hour with your doctor should do the trick. If you're putting off a visit because you're afraid of being "yelled at" because you're overweight, have bad habits you know you'll be lectured about, or are terrified of having blood drawn, now is the time to put those fears aside.

A simple checkup by your gynecologist or family doctor may be all you need to help you get pregnant; for example, your doctor can look at the following possible pregnancy stumbling blocks:

- ✔ **Your weight:** Are you underweight or overweight? Being either over- or underweight may interfere with pregnancy.
- ✔ **Your sexual practices:** Are you missing the big day each month because you've been misinformed about when you ovulate?
- ✔ **Your sexual history:** Do you have a sexually transmitted infection (STD) that could be preventing pregnancy? (See the section, "Complicating Things through Common Infections" for more on STDs.)
- ✔ **Your habits:** Do you douche right after sex? You may be washing some of the best swimmers away!
- ✔ **Your blood pressure:** Women with high blood pressure may be prone to developing serious hypertensive disease during pregnancy.

Checking your blood levels

The good thing about having blood drawn is that a single specimen can be used to test for many different health conditions, including some that can interfere with getting pregnant; we look at a few in the next sections.

Looking at your thyroid function

Women who have an underactive or overactive thyroid may have trouble getting pregnant. Thyroid abnormalities can cause anovulation (no egg is released) irregular menstrual cycles or short menstrual cycles. (See Chapter 2 for more about menstrual dysfunction).

Hypothyroid, or low thyroid levels, can raise your prolactin level (*prolactin* is a hormone that helps control milk production in breastfeeding women). High prolactin levels can prevent ovulation; prolactin levels can be diagnosed with a blood test.

Running a chemistry panel

A chemistry panel tests your blood sugar to show if you have diabetes; it also tests your liver and kidney functions. Many health problems that can impact on pregnancy can be found through a chemistry panel.

Checking your blood count

A complete blood count, or CBC, tests your hemoglobin, which shows if you're anemic. It also tests your white blood count, which can show chronic infection.

Deciding if you need a mammogram

It's not essential to have a mammogram before getting pregnant, but it can't hurt, especially if you're over the age of 40 or if you have a family history of breast cancer.

During the time of your pregnancy (10 months), along with the time you plan to breastfeed, mammograms will not be a good option. This could be one to two years, depending on how long you choose to nurse. Talk to your OB/GYN about this before you get pregnant, as he/she may elect to do a baseline mammogram prior to conceiving.

Chapter 4

Struggling with Secondary Infertility

*I*n the immortal words of Baseball's Yogi Berra "It's Déjà vu all over again!" For many, Yogi's words perfectly describe the struggle with secondary infertility, or difficulty getting pregnant a second time . . . or a third.

Although exact numbers are difficult to pin down, experts estimate that in 2005 about 3 million people suffer from secondary infertility (less than half the number that suffers from primary infertility). According to Resolve, a national infertility organization, that figure represents an increase from an estimated 1.8 million in 1995. In this chapter, we define secondary infertility and then take a closer look at its emotional impact, as well as what you can do to deal with the merry-go-round of infertility — take two.

Defining Secondary Infertility

Secondary infertility is defined as the condition where a woman is unable to get pregnant or carry a pregnancy to term after already having had one or more children. Some experts put the added caveat of "after 12 months of trying to conceive naturally on their own," to better qualify the term. Some experts define secondary infertility as occurring anytime after a previous conception, whether that conception ended in a birth or a miscarriage.

Secondary infertility can occur whether the first conception was difficult or easy. It can be due to female issues, male issues, or a combination of both.

Whatever the exact nature of the definition, few disagree that secondary infertility, whether an adjunct to primary infertility or a new challenge all its own, can be a confounding and painful experience that seems to prevent many from creating the complete family of their dreams.

Facing Secondary Infertility

Knowing *what* you're dealing with, particularly if it is secondary infertility, doesn't make it any easier. Often, if a woman had little to no problem conceiving a first or second child, the diagnosis of secondary infertility can be confusing. If there were problems the first time around, facing them again can be too much to bear. In the following sections, we discuss some of the different challenges that secondary infertility can present.

Will it feel as bad as it did the first time?

Secondary infertility can be as bad or worse as dealing with infertility the first time around. Coping with secondary infertility after the pain of infertility sometimes seems unbearable. Perhaps you thought that despite the five years of trying to conceive baby number 1, baby number 2 would just miraculously appear one day. Sometimes that is the case and conceiving and giving birth to number 1 seems to open the floodgates. More often than not, however, patterns tend to repeat themselves, including the 'pattern' of primary infertility.

The obvious answer is to try the exact same plan that worked for you the first time. If you want to try on your own, hoping for the possible reprieve from Infertility, Part 2, go ahead. But, for your peace of mind and for the sake of giving yourself the best opportunity within a reasonable amount of time, set some parameters. If you haven't conceived naturally within 6 months to a year (less time if you're over 40), consider going back to the drawing board and/or the original "architect," whether that be your primary physician, OB/GYN, or reproductive endocrinologist.

Until you've given the tried and tested method another go-round, this probably isn't the time to switch doctors, switch protocols, or go out on a brand new limb. Give the old method at least a few tries before discussing moving to different options with your physician or before you discuss moving to a different physician with your partner.

But it worked before . . .

Perhaps one of the most confusing physiological and psychological dilemmas occurs when something worked before and suddenly, apparently without reason, ceases to be effective.

Those struggling with secondary infertility commonly lament:

> "We conceived the first month we tried."

> "All my husband had to do was look at me and we got pregnant with our first two."

> "Conceiving a child was never the problem with us."

Sometimes secondary infertility seems to defy proper or satisfying explanations; other than being a year or two older than you were the last time you had a baby, nothing seems to have changed. Other times, getting to baby number one might have been a challenge, and the fact that it's not going to be easier the second time around is disappointing, but not unexpected.

Some healthcare providers deny the existence of secondary infertility, claiming that it is actually primarily infertility where the patient "got lucky" the first time around. From an emotional standpoint, that line of reasoning is akin to telling a victim of a disease that his or her condition is not valid.

One thing that can be taken from this line of thinking, however, is a careful review of your first successful go-round. Ask yourself the following:

- Was it as easy as it seemed the first time or is that merely in comparison to the current struggle of secondary infertility?

- Did you miscarry two or more times on the way to a healthy baby? Were these miscarriages investigated and found to be due to chromosomal abnormalities, which increase with age?

- Was it ever suggested, prior to conception, that there might be issues that *could* cause a problem in conceiving or carrying a child (for example, abnormal hormonal levels; structural issues in the uterus, ovaries, or fallopian tubes; a family history of infertility; and so on)?

It's not uncommon to disregard a previous observation, even if it was made by a medical professional, particularly if their diagnosis proved to be wrong, and the proof is now pulling all the pots and pans out of your cabinet and trying to flush them down the toilet. It's even more common to ignore a family member's recollection of history (for example, every woman on your mother's side went into menopause at the age of 35) if you seem to be the exception.

Conduct your own investigation if you feel that you might have overlooked a comment or a speculation the first time around. Ask your partner if you can't remember correctly or check with whatever physician whose care you were under prior to the conception of your first child. You may also see this as an opportunity to open or re-open discussion with family members to get an accurate picture of your genetic history when it comes to reproduction. You may well end up finding out that you do indeed have a clean bill of health, but you may also uncover information that could help you get to the bottom of secondary infertility.

Looking for What's Different This Time Around

So the reproductive system isn't working like it used to — what could be the problem? Similar to primary infertility, the answer to secondary infertility could take awhile and fill up at least an entire book such as this one. But, for the sake of getting to the point, we list some quick and perhaps not so obvious possibilities.

Changes in age

Unless (or even if) your last child was born six weeks ago, time does march on! And from an infertility point of view, that's never a good thing. One of the primary reasons for secondary infertility is the age of the mother. Age-related male infertility can also be a consideration, although Father Time does seem to be a bit more forgiving when it comes to the dads. Regardless of whose age we're discussing, by definition, both you and your partner (should both parties remain the same!) will be older when you try to conceive your next child. As we have seen in preceding chapters, fertility declines throughout the years, so the baby that popped up so easily in your 20s, might not be as forthcoming in your 30s or 40s. The longer the interval between children, the more likely that time is not on your side. The fact that you have conceived, carried, and delivered a baby are certainly positive predictors of your ability to do so, but realize that many cite the age of the mother as the primary reason for reproductive success. Is this true? Only time will tell.

Remember, your age isn't an admonishment. Family planning is all about the spacing of children to fit with your lifestyle, finances and capabilities. Having children back to back is not necessarily the best thing to do, for your health and well being and that of your family. Most physicians recommend a minimum of one year in between pregnancies in order to allow your body to heal. Considering that sex is a no-no for the first six weeks after delivering, those that have a 10-month difference in the age of their children are ignoring *someone's* advice. While age is certainly a large factor in planning your family, it can't be the *only* thing.

So what now? You're older and having problems. As with primary infertility, if you are over the age of 35 and have not conceived after trying naturally for six months, it might be time to visit your primary care physician, OB/GYN, or reproductive endocrinologist. They will likely run the same battery of tests on you that they would on a patient that presented with primary infertility. Be patient. You want a thorough report, not a speedy one. The difference in two weeks will not a difference make!

Changes in health

As with primary infertility, your overall health does make a difference. While you may still be living the clean life, it doesn't mean that your body hasn't undergone changes all its own. Have you had an increase or decrease in your weight? As we discuss in previous chapters, BMI (body mass index) can certainly play a part in your fertility or lack thereof. Have you suddenly become a marathon or long-distance runner? This too can affect your metabolism and your body's responses, including the reproductive ones. While these can be positive health changes, they can also upset the delicate balance to which your body may be clinging. Take a look at any lifestyle changes, good or bad, and discuss them with your physician to see if therein lies the culprit.

Occult, or not yet uncovered, chronic or acute illness can also play a role in reversing your fertility. Diabetes, autoimmune disease such as lupus, thyroid problems, and a host of other issues, large and small, can also affect your ability to conceive and could be brewing without your knowledge. If you haven't had a complete physical workup, as well as a gynecological one, now would be the time.

Are you fresh from your first, or last, pregnancy? Still breastfeeding? Or burning the midnight oil trying to rock Junior to sleep? Again, even subtle changes such as a shift in your sleep patterns can wreak havoc on your system, which can leave your fertility in less than fighting shape. Another thing to consider and discuss with your OB/GYN is any lasting effects from your previous pregnancy(ies). Could you have developed adhesions as a result of a caesarian section? Did you have problems with excessive bleeding that might indicate unresolved issues? Make sure that you check out as normal from your last foray into baby making before jumping into the next.

The other large category of problems in secondary infertility is the status of the pelvic organs: Are you having abnormal bleeding (especially between periods) that might be indicative of a fibroid or a polyp in your uterus? Have you had any kind of abdominal surgery since your last delivery (appendectomy, gall bladder surgery, ovarian cyst removal)? All surgery is associated with a risk of scarring (adhesions), which may either block the fallopian tubes or pull them away from the ovaries so that they cannot pick up the ovulated eggs. The good news is that all of these conditions can be identified with the use of appropriate diagnostic tests that your doctor can order.

Throughout the process of secondary infertility, make it a point to take optimal care of *yourself* through nutrition, rest, and exercise. You will need to be in tiptop shape to handle children in multiple forms; this would be a good time to start the process.

Changes in partners

No, we're not suggesting you go out and look for a new partner if you're not getting pregnant the second time. But you may be focusing on the wrong part of the equation, if you're only thinking about what's different with *you* this time around. Remember, primary infertility is split fairly evenly between women's issues, men's issues, and those issues that are shared by both. If you have changed partners since your last child, perhaps the problem lies with your other half. Has he recently taken up running marathons? Has he developed a passion for spending hours in the Jacuzzi? Has he built a Finnish spa in the backyard and loves to sit in it and read "War and Peace"?

Even if you're with the same partner, once again, age can play a factor with men as well. More recent studies have shown that men over 40 have a decrease in the motility and morphology of sperm, reducing their fertile potential. In addition, DNA changes that come with age can also negatively impact a man's sperm, making it abnormal and less likely to fertilize an egg.

And, just as with you, your partner's health status can change over time as well, having a less-than-desirable effect on his contribution to the baby mix. If you've been checked out in all areas, maybe it's time to check, or re-check, dear old dad.

Hurting Just As Much: The Emotional Pain

"I'll be happy when . . ."

It's easy to place caveats on joy, particularly when it comes to getting what you want. Remember when you thought/said/prayed/swore that if you could only conceive this one child, you would never ask for anything again? Like many "foxhole prayers," it's easy to forget previous promises. It's human nature.

While some couples are more relaxed the second time around, others bring the same intensity to conceiving number 2 (or number 3!). As with everything in life, it's how you see the situation . . . is the cradle half empty or half full?

Longing for another child

"Another child is a bonus," a friend once said in describing her desire to have another child. Her belief is that she and husband are forever grateful for their beautiful daughter, and their one and only has given them their dream and a wonderful life to go along with it. This friend has not conceived again since her four-year-old daughter was born, but she has stood by her promise. While she may occasionally dream of giving her child a sibling, she is ultimately happy and satisfied.

While this mindset may be an ideal, it is certainly not shared by most and more often forgotten by many. Secondary infertility can, and often is, every bit as painful as the first go-round. Some friends have said that it can be even more difficult. Suddenly, you are thrust into the world of children where everything seems to come in pairs, if not higher multiples. The "lonely only" child is regarded by many in the child-abundant world as somehow missing out, whether it be in social interaction or family dynamics.

You can't miss out on what you don't have. Children without siblings tend to be higher achievers, quite social, and often leaders in society. And you can certainly have spoiled, lonely, or maladjusted children, even amongst large sibling groups. "I don't want my only child to grow up spoiled," whine many parents. Yet, upon having baby number 2, many of these families find that indeed they don't have one spoiled child anymore, they now have two! Remember, history repeats itself. Don't assume that another child will miraculously convert you . . . or your parenting skills. That's a job that YOU have to do, whether with one child or twenty.

Losing support the second time

Another emotional dilemma of secondary infertility can be the lack of support by those who once mopped your tears. "Be thankful for the child you have," family and friends may snap at you impatiently. It's hard to explain that you're immensely grateful and through the joy of conceiving, delivering, and raising your first son or daughter, you have awakened your own inner parent, one that dreams of adding to the flock.

You can't quantify pain, particularly not that of another. Many women grieve as much for the inability to have child number 3 as others do for number 1. Dreams are highly personal and don't generally adjust themselves too easily to life's ups and downs. But, explaining that to family and friends who don't understand can be as challenging as any other aspect of secondary infertility. Even "classic" forms of support, including the internet, often disregard those suffering from secondary infertility, claiming that at "least" they have a child.

You are not alone. Look for specific friends and organizations, whether online or in person, that address some of the issues of secondary infertility. You may be surprised, upon getting to know other parents in your child's playgroup, to find that others have or are dealing with the same issues.

After a particularly painful second-trimester loss of a second child, Jackie was swinging her daughter Ava in the park one day in between two pregnant mothers (just for the record, Jackie was there first!). As Jackie quietly bemoaned her fate, feeling sorry for herself and simultaneously jealous of these strangers, she found herself eavesdropping on their conversation. One of the mothers was sharing how she was just approaching the "critical" point of her pregnancy. As she appeared to be ready to pop, Jackie was a bit confused and continued her nosy vigil. Apparently, she had prematurely delivered her last child at seven months and the baby had not made it. This woman, who Jackie saw as filled with baby and with hope, had endured an even greater tragedy than Jackie had. This is a good reminder to not measure your insides against another's outsides.

Wanting an Heir and a Spare?

"I want another child," Jackie cried out, only weeks after her long-awaited daughter was born (following a three-and-a-half year battle with primary infertility). "That's because you haven't spent enough time caring for the one you have yet," laughed Sharon, "Wait a year." Sharon was right. Those first few weeks of babydom were filled with all of the promised dreams of baby food commercials everywhere. Jackie and her husband often looked down upon their (then) sleeping baby and commented that if only they "could," they'd have many more. And then the long-awaited daughter came to.

Seriously, the next few months were consumed with feeding issues, sleeping issues, adjustment issues, family issues, and so on. We could barely imagine how we could care for the child we had, let alone another. In case you're wondering the same thing, we give you some good reasons to not rush into trying for another child:

✔ **Underestimating the responsibility and work of a new baby:** Perhaps this is one of the reasons why sex is forbidden in the six weeks following delivery. If it wasn't, maybe in that pink (or blue) cloud of new parenting, second babies would be sprouting up everywhere!

✔ **Wanting to have a spare:** As a friend of multiples pointed out, doubling your child load doesn't "halve" your fears of bad things happening. It actually doubles your fears, since it doubles your love.

✔ **Trying for that elusive son or daughter:** Trying again just for another gender is a sure way to set yourself up for disappointment. You need look only as far as Jackie's poor grandmother who birthed *seven* daughters prior to finally producing a male heir. Jackie's uncle didn't marry until much later in life and then decided to limit himself to one child who he adores — who is a daughter and who will *not* continue the family name anyway!

✔ **Giving your child a playmate:** As an only child myself, I (co-author Jackie) always imagined the "luxury" of having a sibling to share my joys and the responsibilities of dealing with my parents as time went on. All I needed to clear up that misconception was time and eyesight. For as many inseparable siblings that exist, so do those that never speak at all. Biology is no guarantee of love or friendship. Nor is it a promise of commitment. Most families that I have encountered are made up of one child that bears many of the family burdens, including mending fences, dealing with aging relatives and facilitating communication throughout the flock. Seldom are those responsibilities equally divided. The other lack of equality is in perception. I often wished for a sibling to share my views on my parents, our home and life itself. Yet, it seems that there are as many different views of a family as there are members. Being raised together and/or in the exact same way does not guarantee a shared vision.

Ideally, the parents of multiple children truly enjoy the experience of raising each child as an individual as well as part of a family. Giving your child a playmate is an added bonus to having more than one child, but not a reason in and of itself. Wanting to share your love again and again is cause for trying again, whatever the process of again might entail.

So, if siblings and families bring no promise of inherited closeness through thick and thin, then what *are* the reasons to duplicate or triplicate your efforts in the area of reproduction? We give you some good reasons in the list that follows:

✔ **There is a joy and warmth that *can* come in larger and extended families.** If having a houseful of people around all the time makes you happy, a houseful of kids will guarantee it — at least until they grow up and leave the nest.

- ✔ **Siblings take off the pressure that only children are sometimes subject to** — the pressure to be all things to their parents, the total fulfillment of every pre-parent dream.

- ✔ **Siblings can teach each other valuable life lessons** — as well as some not so valuable ones. Sibling influence isn't always beneficial!

- ✔ **You just want another baby.** There's nothing wrong with that, as long as you remember that a new baby will, like the first, grow into an individual person with quirks and characteristics that may have you wondering why you thought this was a good idea in the first place!

Part II

Stepping Up
Your Efforts

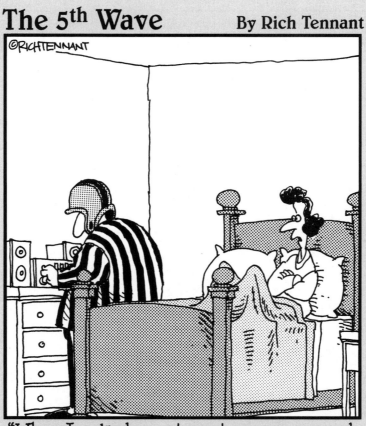

The 5th Wave

By Rich Tennant

©RICHTENNANT

"When I asked you to put on some mood
music, 'On Wisconsin' wasn't the mood
I was going for."

In this part . . .

This part helps you fine-tune your conception efforts by using methods to predict ovulation, and helps you understand how complicated getting pregnant, whether infertility is involved . . . or not, really is. We also guide you through your initial gynecology visits for simple infertility treatment. Next we take a look at some alternative approaches to pregnancy, from herbs to acupuncture, discuss the special issue of secondary infertility, and last but not least, help you avoid the emotional pitfalls that can be the most painful part of infertility.

Chapter 5

Trying Simple Techniques in Not-So-Simple Situations

*A*fter you start trying to get pregnant, you expect results — that's human nature. But Mother Nature isn't always on your timetable, and you may find yourself still trying after a few months, and anxious to step up the pace a bit with some scientific aids. In this chapter, you can find out about some low-tech but helpful methods of trying to pin down an elusive positive pregnancy test.

Many women can read their bodies' signals well enough to pinpoint ovulation almost to the minute; others need scientific aids to help pin down exactly when they're ovulating. We discuss both the simple and the scientific in this chapter.

We also look at how all this planning may affect the romance in your relationship and give you some ideas for keeping the spark alive. In addition, we help you avoid sparks in your relationships with family and friends when you're under stress, and give advice about living through major stressors like the holidays — or your friends' baby showers.

Ovulation is the monthly release of an egg from your ovary. Ovulation is the one time during the month that you can actually get pregnant. Your window of opportunity is approximately two to three days.

Reading Your Body's Signals and Signs

Sharon had a patient tell her that the patient's family doctor told her just to have sex on day 14 of her cycle if she wanted to get pregnant. While this advice might work for some women, it was a complete bust for Sharon's patient, who ovulated around day 10, because she had short menstrual cycles. (See Chapter 2 for a thorough discussion of menstrual cycles and their variations.)

Despite popular belief, not all women ovulate on day 14 of their cycles. And knowing when you ovulate is crucial to your success in getting pregnant because sperm and egg can only get together if they're both in the same place at the same time. Having sex too early — or as little as one day too late — can reduce your chance of success.

This doesn't mean you have to have sex at a precise instance, or even a precise day, to get pregnant. Pregnancy rates are the same whether couples have sex on the day of ovulation, the day before, or two days before, so you have a window of several days on which to have sex. We hope this will take some "performance anxiety" off both of you!

Planning with "natural" methods — get out the calendar

Some women can chart their periods back for years; they religiously mark an "X" on the calendar when their period starts, and they always know exactly when their next period is due. Others are always surprised when their periods start, either because their cycles are irregular or because they never mark anything down on the calendar.

If you're the regular, record-keeping type, it will be easy for you to figure out when you're ovulating. If you're irregular and/or disorganized, it may take you a month or two to determine when you're ovulating. Never fear, though; your body has ways of telling you when ovulation is approaching, and we can help even the most irregular/disorganized women figure it out.

Counting the days — correctly

Most women ovulate 14 days before the start of a new menstrual cycle. So if your cycles are 28 days apart, you ovulate on or about day 14; if your cycles are 25 days long, you ovulate earlier, around day 11. If your cycles are long, like 33 days, you don't ovulate until day 19. This is why it's so easy to miss the right day for conception; most women don't have on-the-dot, regular-as-clockwork periods, and may ovulate on a different day each month.

To figure out when you're most likely to be ovulating, you need to keep track of your menstrual cycles each month. This will give you an idea of when you're most likely to ovulate. This, combined with simple observation of your fertility signs, can result in success if you've just been missing the mark every month.

Determining the shelf life of eggs and sperm

Do you have to have sex at the exact moment of ovulation to get pregnant? No, thank goodness, or getting pregnant would be much harder than it already is! Fortunately both sperm and egg have a lifespan that, although short, allows them to stick around long enough to meet even if your timing isn't perfect.

Sperm live longer than eggs; in the proper cervical mucus (we talk about cervical mucus more in the section "Observing cervical mucus"), sperm can live as long as five days, although two to three days is a more average lifespan for sperm. So you can have sex up to a few days before ovulation and have sperm ready and waiting for an egg to appear.

Eggs, on the other hand, go bad fast; after ovulation, eggs live only 24 hours or so. That means that if you have sex more than a few hours after ovulation, there won't be time for sperm to reach the egg before it disintegrates.

Timing is everything — but don't make it too complicated!

The proper timing is necessary to get pregnant, but you don't have to have sex at the exact moment of ovulation to improve your chances. Pregnancy rates are the same whether couples have sex on the day of ovulation, the day before, or two days before. In contrast, having sex just one day too late (after ovulation) results in no pregnancies.

It's better (and probably less nerve wracking) to have sperm waiting for the egg by having sex every other day around the time you're expecting to ovulate, or even all month, if you're feeling that energetic! There's no evidence that having sex too often decreases the chances for pregnancy, although it does decrease the sperm count.

The point is that although timing is essential, you don't need to spend the whole month on pins and needles, wondering if now is the right time for conception. Predicting ovulation is a matter of watching the calendar and having a rough idea when you might be ovulating and observing your body's natural signals that precede ovulation.

Observing your body's natural signals

So what are all these signals that your body puts out before ovulation? Don't worry — they're not a secret, and you can easily learn to watch for them.

Most occur a day or so before ovulation, so you have plenty of warning before the big day (or night).

Taking your morning temperature

Recording your basal body temperature (BBT) is one of the oldest methods of predicting ovulation. Sharon remembers doing this before getting pregnant with her son, who is now over 30 years old! A basal body temperature is just a long-winded way of saying your individual normal temperature. You use the same type of thermometer you do whenever you take your temperature to find out whether you have a fever when you're not feeling well.

This method of predicting ovulation is simple but requires a certain amount of determination and a good memory. You need to remember to take your temperature every morning *before* you get up. Most doctors recommend that you not get up, eat, drink, or smoke before taking your temperature because any activity at all will raise your temperature, and eating or drinking will raise or lower it, depending on what you had.

Some doctors also recommend buying a special BBT thermometer, which has larger numbers and reads only up to 100 degrees or so. Each one-tenth of a degree is much easier to read on this type of thermometer. You don't need a BBT thermometer, but it's nice to have if your temperature doesn't fluctuate much or if your eyesight is going.

Many charts are available to help you chart your temperature (you can just use the one we've provided in the front of this book!), but you can easily make one yourself. Here's what you do:

1. **Draw a graph.** You can use graph paper or just draw the lines yourself; you're not going to be graded on neatness!

2. **Mark off spaces for 30 days.** Use more if your periods run longer. Mark these spaces on the bottom of the page (horizontal).

3. **Mark off spaces for temperature readings from between 97 degrees and 99.5 degrees in 1/10th increments down the side of the paper (vertically).**

4. **Take your temperature before getting out of bed in the morning, or before performing any other activities.**

5. **Mark down your morning temperature to the exact one-tenth of a degree.**

6. **Connect the "dots."** You'll notice that your temperature is lowest when your period first starts.

7. **Have sex every other day, to cover all the bases.**

8. **Look for a subtle drop in temperature, followed by a sustained rise in temperature, meaning a rise for more than three days.** Your temperature should rise at least 0.5 degrees and remain elevated. The drop

occurs around ovulation, and the rise indicates an increase in your progesterone levels.

9. **If you're having sex every other day, you should be "covered" at the time of ovulation by having waiting sperm ready for the released egg.** If you've been a little lax in this, make sure you have sex the day of your temperature drop.

Even though progesterone increases only after you've ovulated, several studies have found that most women ovulate after the temperature has risen. So don't stop trying until the temperature has been high for at least two days.

This method has a few drawbacks:

- ✓ **You need to be scrupulous about taking your temperature and recording it so that you don't forget it.**

- ✓ **You have to keep your chart for the whole month.** If you're the type who loses things easily, keep a few copies of the chart around in case you lose one.

- ✓ **Your temperature can be influenced by factors other than hormones.** If you're sick, even small temperature fluctuations may make your chart inaccurate, and you'll think you've ovulated when you actually have the flu. Alcohol, too little or too much sleep, and subtle illnesses can all change your temperature.

Your BBT can also give you an idea of whether you're pregnant. If your temperature stays elevated more than 15 days, there's a good chance that you're pregnant — unless, of course, you have the flu. If your temperature starts to drop after ten days or so, you may have a *luteal phase defect,* which means that your progesterone may be too low to sustain a pregnancy.

If you're prone to losing paper charts, you may be interested in a digital thermometer that stores your previous temperature. This device is handy in case you forget to write your temperature down one morning. Digital thermometers are a little more expensive than glass ones, but not more than $7 or $8 for a good one. Or you can "store" your last temperature even with a glass thermometer by *not* shaking it down immediately after using it. This tip is especially convenient if you don't have time to record your temperature right away. The mercury will stay at your temperature point until it's shaken down.

Observing cervical mucus

Cervical mucus changes consistency around the time of ovulation. Right after your period stops, cervical mucus is very thick, which makes it difficult for sperm to penetrate. Cervical mucus is normally thick (viscous) because it protects the uterus from invading bacteria from the vagina.

As you get closer to ovulation, cervical mucus becomes thinner, more slippery, and stretchy, and more copious, all of which helps sperm get through it into the uterus. In addition, all the lubrication makes it easier to have sex — ingenious, isn't it?

In addition to becoming thinner and stretchy, cervical mucus becomes more alkaline, because sperm live longer in an alkaline environment. You can check the acidity or alkalinity of cervical mucus with an over-the-counter product called TesTape, which comes in a long thin roll of yellow paper. You tear off a small piece of the yellow paper and wrap it around the end of your finger. Next, you reach into your vagina and touch the paper to the end of your cervix. Then you bring out the piece of paper see whether it turns color. It will first turn an olive color a few days before ovulation and then turn dark green or blue when your cervical mucus is alkaline, as it is right before you ovulate.

After ovulation, cervical mucus again becomes thick, cloudy or white in color, and scant.

Feeling your cervix

If you have no idea how to find your cervix, it's pretty easy. You just *carefully* insert your clean finger into your vagina until you feel a firm bump that feels somewhat like the end of your nose. That's your cervix.

You'll notice that your cervix itself also changes at different times of the month; around ovulation, it becomes softer, feeling more like your lips in firmness, and feels slightly open in the center. You'll also feel an increase in moisture. All these changes, like the changes in cervical mucus, help the sperm get through the cervix.

The cervix also moves to a lower and more central position, so it's easier to find with your finger, which means it's also in a more direct line with ejaculated sperm.

Ouch! I think I ovulated

About 20 percent of women have pain called *mittelschmerz* (German for "middle pain") when they ovulate. The pain seems to be caused by blood and fluid irritating the tissues around the ovary after it releases from the follicle. Sometimes a small amount of vaginal bleeding occurs with ovulation, too.

Mittelschmerz can be a very precise way of pinpointing exactly when you ovulate; the only downside of using mittelschmerz to help you conceive is that it usually occurs at the time of ovulation. In other words, once you've ovulated, the clock is ticking and your egg is on a countdown with destruction within 24 hours or so, so you've got to have sex pretty quickly.

Even though your egg hangs around for 24 hours after ovulation, you can't wait that long to have sex and get pregnant, because it takes a little time — possibly only 15 minutes or so, but still time — for sperm to meet up with the egg. It's better to have sex a few hours or a day before ovulation, so the sperm are ready and waiting.

Keeping a Fertility Chart

Although a fertility chart sounds exotic and complicated, it's nothing more than a record of observation of your body's natural fertility signals: your temperature, your cervical mucus and changes in your cervix itself. You can make a simple chart yourself, recording your daily temperature on a graph with cervical changes and mucus written in underneath, or you can download one of the many fertility charts found on the internet. One place to download a fertility chart and get some useful information as well is www.ovulation-calculator.com/fertility-chart.htm

Maybe you write everything down on little pieces of paper and keep losing them and think you'd do better to keep track of your data on your computer. There are programs you can download to allow you to keep everything organized online — just don't let your boss see you poring over your "data" at work!

Two software titles available on the Internet are TCOYF (Taking Charge of Your Fertility) Software found at www.tcoyf.com, www.fertilityfriend.com, and CycleWatch, found at www.cyclewatch.com. All let you download software to chart your basal body temperature, cervical mucus, and cervix changes to let you know that you should "have sex now," as the software puts it. If you have an OvaCue II saliva tester (see "Just spit here – the saliva test" for details on saliva testing), you can buy software to use with it that will let you download your information, chart it, graph it, and print it out.

Predicting Ovulation: Kits, Sticks, and Software

Maybe a month of trying to get pregnant has gone by — or maybe two, three, or four months — and you're beginning to feel frustrated and even a little scared that you're never going to get pregnant. Go back and read the statistics in Chapter 1 to remind yourself that nature is inefficient, and remember that everyone in your family took six months to get pregnant. You may be thinking, "That's all well and good to read about," but you want to do something *now*. There must be something more scientific and more successful that you can do. You thought that you hit all the "right" days to have sex for the last few months, but maybe you're still missing the right day or misinterpreting your body's ovulation signs. This section covers a few ways to monitor your ovulation cycle that are more "scientific" than stretching cervical mucus and counting calendar days. Hopefully, one will work for you!

Using an ovulation predictor kit

Ovulation predictor kits (OPKs) are a popular way to test if and when you ovulate. The tests measure the amount of LH (luteinizing hormone) found in your urine. LH generally rises 24 to 36 hours before ovulation; the rise of LH is called your *LH surge*. You should have sex the day or two before ovulation and the day of ovulation to improve your chances of getting pregnant.

OPKs are easy to find; every drugstore carries them. They use your urine, a cheap and abundant substance, to test for ovulation. The sticks are small enough to carry around with you.

The OPKs, or "pee sticks" as they're called, have some drawbacks. Certain women, such as women with polycystic ovaries (see Chapter 7), may have a high LH all the time, so the kits will always be positive. Women over 40 or those in premature ovarian failure (POF) may also have a higher than normal LH, because LH and FSH (follicle-stimulating hormone) both rise in POF. Some tests are also difficult to read, require several steps that need to be carefully done for good results, or start to show positive only when the LH reaches 40mIU/ml, the International Standard for an LH surge.

Some women may not have a surge that registers as high as 40mIU/ml; look for kits that register positive at 20mIU/ml.

Most kits show a positive as a line as dark as or darker than the control line. Read the test at exactly the time indicated; sometimes the lines darken over a few hours, but that doesn't mean you're having a surge.

For many, reading an OPK can be a frustrating test of judgment and trial and error. Is the test line lighter than the control line? By how much? Is it darker today than it was yesterday? What about in bright light? All of these may seem like legitimate questions when determining the right time of ovulation, but keep in mind that the best indication of a surge is a test line that is *as dark as or darker* than the control line. Just like in horseshoes, "almost," doesn't really count.

The kits are harder to use if you don't have regular cycles; unless you know approximately when you ovulate each month, you may use up a lot of sticks trying to figure out when your surge starts. If you have regular cycles, you can start testing about 16 days before you expect your next period, but if your cycles are irregular, you need to start testing earlier to make sure that you don't miss the big-O day. Table 5-1 can help you determine when to start testing.

Table 5-1 Counting Days, Saving Sticks	
Length of Normal Cycle	*Start Testing This Many Days After Your Last Period*
40	23
39	22
38	21
37	20
36	19
35	18
34	17
33	16
32	15
31	14
30	13
29	12
28	11
27	10
26	9
25	8
24	7
23	6
22	5
21	4

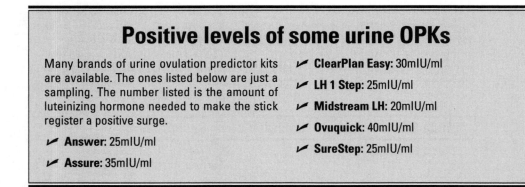

Positive levels of some urine OPKs

Many brands of urine ovulation predictor kits are available. The ones listed below are just a sampling. The number listed is the amount of luteinizing hormone needed to make the stick register a positive surge.

✔ **Answer:** 25mIU/ml

✔ **Assure:** 35mIU/ml

✔ **ClearPlan Easy:** 30mIU/ml

✔ **LH 1 Step:** 25mIU/ml

✔ **Midstream LH:** 20mIU/ml

✔ **Ovuquick:** 40mIU/ml

✔ **SureStep:** 25mIU/ml

OPKs aren't cheap; they cost about $14 for five sticks. You'll use one stick each time you test, and you need to test every 12 to 24 hours around the time of ovulation to accurately "catch" your surge. Resist the urge to buy the cheaper kits. They may not register lower LH levels, and they may be much harder to read. As a result, you use up more sticks because you're showing all your friends and asking their opinion on which line is darker. In addition to using up a lot of sticks, you may use up a lot of friends, too!

OPKs register only when your surge has begun, so you won't be able to time sex as accurately for the two days immediately before ovulation. Also, the strips must be stored at temperatures between 59 and 86 degrees F to ensure their accuracy, so carrying them around in a purse can be problematic unless you live in a totally climate-controlled world.

Also remember that the test measures a concentration of LH in the urine. This means that if the urine is too concentrated (like first morning urine, which looks dark), the test may show a false positive even if you are not surging. Along the same line, if your urine is too diluted (looks clear and not yellow, like if you just finished a 32-ounce soda), it won't show a positive test, even if you're ovulating. A good rule to follow is to do the test about two hours after eating, after you haven't had anything to drink for an hour or so, and the urine should look yellow, but not too dark.

Adding computer power with a fertility monitor

If you want to go a little higher tech than the OPKs, you may be interested in a fertility monitor. A fertility monitor works a little differently than the standard OPK. These devices are actually small computers that store data about your cycle to tell you when you're going to ovulate. They're more labor intensive; you need to start testing the first day of your period and test every day around the same time. Morning is recommended as the best time to test. Because they test both estrogen and LH levels, fertility monitors can better predict ovulation about five days before it occurs, giving you a better chance to have sex two days before ovulation.

The fertility monitor can be used if you're taking fertility medications, unlike some of the one-use OPK urine tests. It also "sets" itself to your cycle if you're somewhat irregular.

These monitors are expensive — about $200 — and you also need to buy the sticks. Like the less expensive kits, they may not be accurate if you are menopausal or breastfeeding, have polycystic ovaries (see Chapter 7) and a normally higher than normal LH level, or are taking tetracycline antibiotics, which means they won't be able to tell if you've released an egg.

Just spit here — the saliva test

This is one of the newest and most interesting ovulation prediction tests out there; it tests your saliva for a rise in salt content, which rises as your estrogen rises. This method has several advantages:

- ✔ **Carrying this around isn't too conspicuous.** The tube that holds the lens you place saliva on and the tiny lighted microscope you look through are all contained in what looks like a tube of lipstick.
- ✔ **Because the lens can be washed and reused, this is a one-time purchase.**
- ✔ **According to the U.S. Food and Drug Administration, this method is about 98 percent accurate.**
- ✔ **Unlike ovulation kits, which use urine, these can be used any old time, not just when your bladder is full.** Peeing on demand can be hard, but you always have saliva. Plus, you can use the saliva kit on the bus, which is out of the question with urine-based OPKs!

Disadvantages to this method include the following:

- ✔ **It's fairly expensive, about $60.**
- ✔ **It's slightly more complicated to use.** You have to take the lens out and put it back properly or you won't read it correctly. You also risk the possibility of breaking or scratching the lens.
- ✔ **Also, as with OPKs and TesTape, this tells you only when you're about to ovulate.** It won't confirm that you did actually release an egg.

The saliva test can be done every day starting at day one of your cycle; at first you'll see only little dots (of salt) when you look through the viewing piece. As ovulation gets closer, you'll see what look like ferns (see Figure 5-1); when the ferns cover the whole slide, you're about to ovulate. It takes about five minutes for the slide to dry so you can accurately read it.

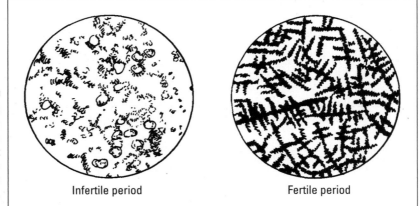

Figure 5-1:
Ferning appears on a saliva test when you're close to ovulation.

Infertile period   Fertile period

The saliva tests have an advantage over urine-based OPKs, which will only give you a yes or no answer as to whether you're ready to ovulate. The saliva test gives you more advance warning that ovulation is coming. With the saliva test, you can also avoid some of the false positives from LH kits and the fluctuations in temperature that can throw off results of the basal body temperature method (see "Taking your morning temperature," earlier in this chapter).

Even though the saliva test is initially expensive, it may be cheaper than buying ovulation predictor kits every month. And if you do get pregnant, you can use it after you deliver to *prevent* pregnancy until you want another baby! This method of birth control is approved by the Catholic Church and in some cases is thought to be more accurate than the rhythm method of counting days to avoid pregnancy.

Saliva monitors that store and analyze data, just like the urine monitors, are now available. These are quite expensive, however — over $200.

If you already have a microscope and slides hanging around the house from a leftover science project or something, you can test saliva at home without any of the expensive packaged equipment. Put some saliva on a slide and take a look! You should also know that most doctors prefer the urine LH tests for accuracy.

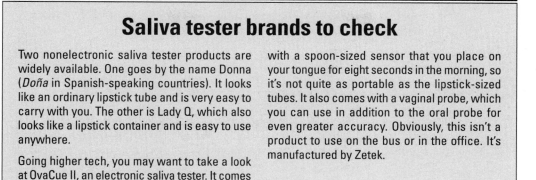

Saliva tester brands to check

Two nonelectronic saliva tester products are widely available. One goes by the name Donna (*Doña* in Spanish-speaking countries). It looks like an ordinary lipstick tube and is very easy to carry with you. The other is Lady Q, which also looks like a lipstick container and is easy to use anywhere.

Going higher tech, you may want to take a look at OvaCue II, an electronic saliva tester. It comes with a spoon-sized sensor that you place on your tongue for eight seconds in the morning, so it's not quite as portable as the lipstick-sized tubes. It also comes with a vaginal probe, which you can use in addition to the oral probe for even greater accuracy. Obviously, this isn't a product to use on the bus or in the office. It's manufactured by Zetek.

Sperm testing at home

While you're doing all this home testing on yourself, it might seem like a good idea to get your partner in on the act with a little home testing of his own.

It's now possible to do a very rudimentary semen analysis at home; this method won't give you detailed information, but it will let you check out two semen samples to see whether the concentration of sperm meets the accepted fertility level of 20 million/ml. The brand name is FertilMARQ. You can purchase this product online and have it sent directly to your home, to avoid an embarrassing trip to the drugstore. Two Web sites that sell the sperm test are www.babyhopes.com and www.completefertility.com; both also sell basal digital thermometers, home pregnancy tests, and OPKs.

Hoping for a Boy or Girl: Will Timing Help?

You may wonder if you're equally likely to have a boy or girl. As far as conception goes, more boy babies are conceived than girl babies by a ratio of 130:100, but by the time of birth, this ratio drops to 105:100, signifying the higher rate of miscarriage for baby boys. Are you really, really hoping for a child of one sex or another, and looking for ways to maximize your chances of buying pink or blue? One theory is that boy sperm (those that carry the Y chromosome, which, combined with the woman's X chromosome, creates a boy baby) are shorter lived but faster swimmers; girl sperm (those that carry the X chromosome to create a girl) live longer but are slower. So if you want a girl, have sex two days before ovulation; if you want a boy, try to hit the day of ovulation straight on. Is there any real proof that this works? Not really! (We discuss high tech sex selection further in Chapter 21.)

Getting through the Two-Week Wait

The *two-week wait* (2WW) is the time between ovulation and your next expected period, when you're on pins and needles waiting for enough time to pass to be able to look for pregnancy symptoms or to buy the ever popular home pregnancy test.

You, like many women before you, may spend this time analyzing every possible pregnancy symptom — "Are my breasts tender?" "Am I peeing more?" "Was that a twinge of nausea?" — looking for something — anything! — that indicates success in the pregnancy department.

The 2WW may seem like 1,000 years, and it's not likely that much will divert you from constantly thinking about pregnancy. If it's possible, putting pregnancy completely out of your mind may help you maintain your sanity; staying busy at work, going on vacation, taking up a new and incredibly complex hobby, or cleaning your house from top to bottom may help keep you occupied and away from the home pregnancy tests until two weeks have passed.

Looking for a Positive — Home Pregnancy Tests

If you think that you used a lot of ovulation predictor sticks, wait until you start using the home pregnancy tests (HPTs)! They're widely advertised on TV, depicting a couple excitedly waiting for the good news or a tense woman alone hoping for the happy news that she's *not* pregnant. The sections that follow give you all you need to know about HPTs.

Getting to know HPTs

The first home tests were available in the 1970s, and everyone probably would have been a little more squeamish about leaving them in the fridge next to the milk if they had known that they contained prepackaged red blood cells. These tests were very sensitive to movement, so you had to put them someplace quiet and leave them alone for a few hours. When you finally peeked into the fridge, you looked for the dark ring at the bottom of the tube — that's what appeared if you were pregnant. The clumping together of red blood cells if you were pregnant is what formed the ring.

All the tests, from the 1920s on, measured hCG (human chorionic gonado-tropin), the hormone released by the implantation of the embryo and the growing placenta. The newest tests are very sensitive; the most sensitive tests of the 30 or so brands on the market claim to detect concentrations of 25mIU/ml, which usually occur about ten days after ovulation, or about four days prior to the time you would miss your first period. Others don't test positive until the hCG level is 50 or even 100mIU/ml, so read the box before you buy. Even though most tests are accurate a few days *before* your period is due, a negative test at that time may not be accurate. You may have had a late implantation, or you may have ovulated a day or two after you thought you did. Another test should be done a few days later if your period still hasn't started.

The average level of hCG 10 days post ovulation is 25mIU/ml; it is 50mIU/ml 12 days post ovulation, and 100mIU/ml 14 days after you ovulate. Keep in mind that these numbers are averages; your number may be higher or lower and still be perfectly normal. Also, as with LH kits, the concentration of the urine can play a large role in whether or not the test turns positive. Because any positive value is important, using first morning (most concentrated) urine is a good idea.

Blood tests can also measure hCG, detecting concentrations less than 5mIU/ml. (We talk about pregnancy blood tests more in Chapter 15.)

Using HPTs

Home pregnancy tests are available in every drugstore, so if you're buying in bulk because you're a compulsive tester, you can hit every grocery store and drugstore in town, and no one will know that you're compulsive — er, anxious to know! These tests give fast results, usually in two to five minutes. Most tell you to not urinate for four hours before you test so the concentration of the hormone will be high. Some kits suggest that you urinate in a cup and dip the wand into it, and other kits suggest peeing directly on the stick. Some show a positive as a little plus sign; others want you to drag all your friends back in to the bathroom (if you still have any friends left after ovulation) and have them compare the control line to the test line to see whether they match. Usually a positive is indicated by a test line that's as dark as or darker than the control, and many women drive themselves mad staring at the line trying to determine its exact shade of purple. Some tests now eliminate the "match game" by spelling out, "Yes, you're pregnant" or some variation if your test is positive.

Don't let the test sit around before looking at it, as some test results will change after an hour or two and will not be accurate. See Figure 5-2 for positive and negative results on a home pregnancy test.

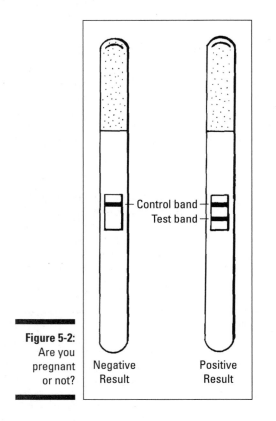

Figure 5-2: Are you pregnant or not?

Negative Result

Positive Result

Control band

Test band

Table 5-2 lists the common brands of home pregnancy tests and the lowest number they claim will register a positive result. Sensitivity is measured in units called *mIU,* which means milli-International Units per milliliter.

Table 5-2	Home Pregnancy Test Sensitivity Levels
Home pregnancy test	*Lowest sensitivity level*
AimStick Pregnancy Test Strip	20 mIU
AccuHome Midstream Pregnancy Test	25 mIU
Answer Early Result Pregnancy Test	25 mIU
Answer Pregnancy Test (Cup)	25 mIU

Home pregnancy test	*Lowest sensitivity level*
Clearblue +/-	25 mIU
Confirm 1-Step Pregnancy Test	25 mIU
Equate Pregnancy Test	25 mIU
First Response Early Result Pregnancy Test	25 mIU
One Step Be Sure Pregnancy Test	25 mIU
Walgreen Digital	25 mIU
e.p.t. Home Pregnancy Test (one line = not pregnant; two lines = pregnant)	40 mIU
e.p.t. Certainty Digital Test	40 mIU
Fact Plus Pregnancy Test	40 mIU
Clearblue Digital	50 mIU
CVS Cartridge Pregnancy Test	50 mIU
CVS Midstream Pregnancy Test	50 mIU
Drug Emporium Brand Pregnancy Test	50 mIU
e.p.t. + / - Test	50 mIU
early Pregnancy test	50 mIU
RiteAid Brand Pregnancy Test	50 mIU
Target Brand Pregnancy Test	50 mIU
Wal-Mart Brand Pregnancy Test	50 mIU
Walgreens Pregnancy Test	100 mIU

Understanding false positives

False positive results are rare in home pregnancy tests. You may have a false positive if

- You're taking injections of the hormone hCG to induce ovulation or for any other reason; it takes 14 days for 10,000U of hCG (a standard dose) to completely clear your system.

- You recently had a miscarriage or ectopic pregnancy, and the hCG levels have not dropped to a negative range yet. (This can take up to 4 weeks.)

✔ You have developed a rare cancer called a choriocarcinoma. This cancer usually follows a full-term birth, miscarriage, or other pregnancy loss. This is a fast-growing cancer, so if you recently had a pregnancy loss of any kind and have a positive home pregnancy test and heavy bleeding, you *must* see a doctor immediately

Including OPKs, sperm tests, and pregnancy tests in one kit

Some enterprising manufacturers have marketed kits containing about seven ovulation predictor sticks and one or two HPTs, plus a sperm kit for your partner! Of course these are more expensive than buying just the home pregnancy tests, but it certainly cuts down on all those embarrassing trips to the drugstore.

✔ **First Response Pregnancy Planning Kit:** This kit contains seven ovulation predictors, one HPT, and some Tums antacids! We guess this process is *supposed* to give you acid indigestion!

✔ **Baby Start:** This kit contains six ovulation predictor sticks and a sperm testing kit good for two uses. They should put an HPT in there, too.

✔ **Web Womb:** This Web site (www.webwomb.com) sells a kit with 12 spreadsheets to chart your BBT, and also a home pregnancy test.

Dealing With Buttinskis (Also Known As Friends and Relatives)

There's no question that dealing with infertility is a strain, and it's a strain that can turn into a major emotional drain when friends and relatives decide to involve themselves in your situation.

You can try, nicely but firmly and, one hopes, unemotionally, to let relatives know that their concern is welcome but their advice and opinions are not. Most often, you'll find they don't really want to know all the details. They just want to feel like they're an important part of your life and that you care enough about them to include them in what's going on.

Jackie told each and every one of her family and friends that she would let them know as soon as she actually became pregnant and that they didn't need to ask her on the hour. More friends than relatives got the hint, but certain situations, such as holidays, baby showers, or lunch time, seemed to bring out the nosiest in everyone. In the sections that follow, we give you some tips on how to cope with these situations and people that try your patience.

Remembering that you need your friends and family — even if they drive you up a wall!

You may be faring pretty well and your partner may be a rock, but your mother, sister, or best friend may be a royal pain in the proverbial you-know-what, wanting to know all the details of how things are going, how you're feeling, how your partner is reacting, and so on.

The obvious way to handle this situation is to just tell everyone to stay out of your business, but as you well know, this is much easier said than done. Like it or not, these people are usually important to you or you wouldn't let them interfere in your lives this way, and you *do* want your potential child to have a grandma, aunt, or godmother some day.

Some families consider this sort of interference as sort of a family right. Inquiring into your reproductive plans may have started the minute your relationship with your partner began. A polite "I'd rather not discuss it" isn't going to work in this kind of family. Before you know it, the whispering has begun, and the word is out in the family that something is wrong with you.

How much you tell is up to you and your partner. Usually your partner isn't as eager to blab the details to one and all as you may be, but you may want to consider that even the most prying parents and friends may turn out to be a real source of support after they know what you're going through.

Surviving the holidays

Holidays bring their own special challenges to almost everyone, but those trying to conceive may be particularly affected. The summer holidays always seem to be the perfect setting for family picnics, reunions, and other get-togethers where carefree children frolic and nosy relatives coyly ask when you will be eating for two. Winter provides little relief as Thanksgiving, Hanukkah, Christmas, and Kwanzaa all seem to focus on extended family, talk of Santa, the latest children's toys, and holiday newsletters that share every painstaking family detail, from birth to potty training to Junior's first car accident.

Some of this family updating is normal, but you may be especially sensitive to the topic while you're trying to conceive yourself. Try as best you can to determine whether the conversation is the speaker's way of trying to connect or reconnect with family and friends or whether you're face to face with an insufferable boor. If you discover it's the latter, realize that you can't do much to guard against people like this, whether they're related to you or not. Even when you do have children of your own, they're little protection in this situation. Those who want to prattle on endlessly about themselves and their families will do so anyway, with little notice given to whether you're with child or without. In such situations, the art of the smile, the nod, and the hasty exit will serve you well.

If you plan on spending extended time with your extended family, consider cluing in a few folks about your situation. They can be helpful in deflecting family or friends who are notorious for ill-timed comments. Arriving late and/or leaving early is another way to minimize your contact with difficult people and situations. You may want to plan something special for you and your partner or a friend after your family affair. This activity will give you something to look forward to throughout the family function.

Everybody else is doing it! Comparing and contrasting

When Jackie's college friend, Leslie, got married at 39 and began planning her family, Jackie was still on the infertility treadmill that had taken up three years of her life. The friends had discussed fertility at great length. They were the same age, and Jackie anticipated that her friend would also be faced with the same uphill battle. Jackie walked her through the ovulation predictor kit and the tale of the little purple line. Two months later, after recounting their latest high-tech fertility strategy, Jackie asked her friend Leslie how her low-tech attempts were faring. "Jackie," she said, her voice breaking, "I'm pregnant." Jackie couldn't believe it. Hadn't she gotten married only 15 minutes ago? Jackie managed to blurt out, "When?" struggling with the conflicting emotions of wanting to congratulate her and wanting to cry. "I'm six weeks along," she replied. "It happened the second month." Thank God for call waiting. When the other call beeped in, Jackie quickly wished her all the love and luck in the world and cut the conversation short. That poor telemarketer. Talk about making the wrong call at the wrong time.

Jackie loves her friends and wishes them the best. And despite this, Leslie's success seemed to be Jackie's failure, even more so than the unsuccessful years of trying. Luckily, Jackie had her network in place. A call to her friend Susan, who was also experiencing infertility, quickly salved Jackie's wounds, at least temporarily. "Don't you hate it when that happens?" Susan said with a sigh. She proceeded to share her stories of a sister-in-law who conceived every time her husband walked in the room. Susan, on the other hand, had spent the last five years in low-, medium-, and high-tech fertility treatments with no baby to show for it (although she has since given birth to a healthy baby girl, who came about in a completely unplanned, nontechnological way!). Susan's ability to immediately understand helped Jackie to begin to put the situation in perspective. Sharing with the newly pregnant Leslie that she (Jackie) felt happy for her *and* jealous also eased the pain. Jackie remembered how difficult it was when *she* had lost friends who couldn't deal with the fact that Jackie was getting married while they remained single. Jackie knew she didn't want to give up her friendship no matter how difficult it felt. Instead, Jackie committed to working through it by continuing to communicate with the same honesty and sensitivity that she was seeking. When all else fails, try to see another's pregnancy as a chance to observe just what you're getting yourself into! Perhaps you can put this more intimate knowledge of the pros and cons of being pregnant to good use in the future.

Jackie was certain that, after attending family functions solo for years, her discomfort would end if and when she was married. How was she supposed to know that there was still another hoop to jump through? What she did learn was that there will *always* be another obstacle, if she allows it. Even if Jackie were to arrive with her perfect family in tow, some new challenge would always await. Holidays can become a time for comparison rather than a time for joy, if you choose to compete. Instead, consider meeting those ill-timed comments and people with a hug and an expression of good wishes. Your grace may just stop the others in their tracks.

For those who are truly interested in you and your life, share some of the positive things from the past year. They may truly appreciate the chance to connect, much more so than a bouncing baby story.

Rather than ignore the children playing with their new toys, get in there and play with them. Doing so is wonderful practice for the future. And in the meantime, you may just discover some of the fun of being with children and sharing their joy, before giving them back to their rightful owner after the excitement wears off! Consider this your gift of the holiday season.

Declining invitations

If a family member or friend is expecting, you may find it difficult to attend any gathering that this pregnant woman attends. Don't chide yourself for your absence. A little denial can go a long way toward helping you gracefully deal with a painful situation. You may decide to bow out of a family dinner or two or 'fess up with the truth and count on the understanding of those who love you. Either way, you'll preserve your integrity and that of your family relationships by not forcing yourself to handle even one bit more than you think you can. This too shall pass.

Forecast: Baby showers likely

Definition of a baby shower: A seemingly benign tradition that can wreak havoc in the hearts of infertile women everywhere (many men claim this as well, no matter what the circumstances). Here's some advice on the topic:

✔ **If you choose to attend (and remember you don't *have* to), don't go it alone.** Sometimes that may mean sharing your situation with the pregnant guest of honor. Although it is *her* day, a little bit of knowledge goes a long way toward sensitivity.

✔ **If you don't choose to confide in the lady of the hour, hang with a friend.** Face it: Baby showers can be very emotional, but they can also be very, very humorous, particularly when shared with someone who understands your situation and can help you see the (inevitable) comedy of errors that often surrounds the pregnant population. This tactic can help you to laugh your way through situations that you may have spent months dreading. Remember though, be nice — isn't that how you want to be treated when you're pregnant?

✔ **If no allies are in attendance, the telephone can be a wonderful thing.** Try to make a difficult situation tolerable by calling a trusted friend before, after, and sometimes during (that's what bathrooms are for!) the event. Cellular phones are wonderful for this purpose and have helped many a pregnant woman through a tough spot. Consider turning down the ringer and/or putting your phone on vibrator mode if you expect a "cavalry call" to help you through. This way, you can get the support you need and not disrupt the party.

✔ **If you're going solo to the shower, you can always use the bathroom, the porch, or your car for temporary refuge . . . or for a good cry if you need it.**

✔ **You don't have to stay until the last present is unwrapped either.** Making an appearance is sufficient, particularly when you're under pressure. You can be the life of the party another time. Your friends will understand.

Chapter 6

Considering Special Circumstances

In This Chapter

▶ Age before baby . . . what difference does it really make?

▶ Diseases that affect and/or complicate fertility

▶ Is reversing a tubal ligation worth it?

▶ Beating cancer . . . and infertility

Going through infertility treatments is generally about as "special" as one wants to be, but you may have other problems that make it harder than usual to get pregnant. Do you have issues? We have answers! In this chapter, we talk about the effects of age on getting pregnant and look at some diseases that can make getting pregnant a challenge. We also help you decide what to do if you had a tubal ligation in the past and want to get pregnant now.

Are You an "Older Mom?" Calculating Your Fertility Odds at Different Ages

More and more women and men are delaying childbirth until later years. In fact, over 20 percent of new mothers are now over the age of 35, and the average age for women to have their first baby is now over 25.

Checking out the statistics

But Mother Nature is apparently not one for statistics (see Table 6-1). For women, optimum fertility occurs when you're about 18 years old. It stays pretty constant in the early part of your 20s and then begins a gradual downward turn at about the age of 30. By the time you turn 35, the process has accelerated. When you hit 40, the slide becomes even more dramatic; 33 percent of women over 35 have some difficulty getting pregnant, and 66 percent of women over 40 have infertility issues.

Table 6-1	Statistics for Age versus Infertility, Miscarriage, and Chromosomal Abnormalities				
Age	*Under 30*	*30–35*	*36–40*	*41–45*	*Over 45*
Percentage of women who have difficulty conceiving (trying to conceive naturally for one year without success)	20%	20%	33%	66%	95%
Miscarriage rate	15%	15%	17%	34%	53%
Rate of chromosomal abnormalities	1 in 526	1 in 385	1 in 192	1 in 66	1 in 21

Why the decrease in pregnancy and rise in miscarriage as you get older? It's because of the increase in chromosomal abnormalities in your eggs as they age. At age 20, your chance of having a baby with a chromosomal abnormality such as Down syndrome (also called trisomy 21), or trisomy 13 or 18 (these usually result in newborn death shortly after delivery), is 1 in 526. By age 30, the risk is 1 in 385; by age 35, 1 in 192; by age 40, 1 in 66; and by age 45, 1 in 21. And this is just the tip of the proverbial iceberg. Information from pre-implantation genetic diagnosis (PGD) strongly indicates that the majority of embryos in women over 40 are chromosomally abnormal. Of course, most of these don't implant, and those that do are usually miscarried. That's why the miscarriage rate increases with age.

Men have it a little easier (don't they always?). Their peak fertility generally remains constant throughout their 30s. It does begin to decline over time, but at a slower pace than their female counterparts. Recent studies, however, do show a rise in chromosomal abnormalities in men over 35, and by age 50, most men show a 33 percent decrease in the number of sperm produced. So although their problems may be less obvious when it comes to conceiving, the effects of age may play a significant role down the road.

A new study on autism, a spectrum communication disorder which can range from mild to severe, suggests that the age of the father plays a significant role as well. Fathers over 40 are six times more likely to produce a child with autism as those under 40. Autism spectrum disorder has been on the rise over the past few decades with some experts pointing at environmental factors as well as possible links to preservatives used in vaccines. The "age" issue is an interesting correlation as the age of the average father, like that of the mother, has also risen over the years, which could be another explanation for the rise in the disorder.

Being an "older" mom — Jackie's personal opinion!

Under the category of "things I didn't expect in life," having children in my 40's was certainly one of them! Infertility was another one. On the upside, I always hoped but never dreamed that I would find a partner as wonderful as my husband. And *he* was worth waiting for! That all said, I am the proud "older" mom of a beautiful 3½-year-old girl, and I wouldn't change a thing.

Being an older mom certainly has its downsides, primarily if you "aged" while waiting to conceive! But, for me, and many of my "older mom" friends, we see the glass as more than half full. As an older mom, we may lack a bit in energy (although truth be told, I'm in better cardiovascular shape than I was in my 20s), but I believe that many of us more than make up for this when it comes to maturity and stability.

I often said that I could barely figure out what I wanted to wear when I was in my peak reproductive years (generally classified as younger than 27 years old), let alone raise a child or two. While others in their 20s may certainly possess a more grownup attitude than I did, most young women go through extraordinary changes at this time of their life, centering on self discovery, life's goals and their own place in the world. In my not-so-humble opinion, this process is best conducted solo, without partner or child, in order to truly understand what you want out of life and how to get it. (Co-author Sharon, who had children in her early twenties, doesn't necessarily agree!)

Financial, educational, and career stability is also often lacking in these younger years. While plenty of women choose to have children first and complete their education later, many will also tell you that going back to school, changing careers, and so on can be far more difficult at a later age, particularly with family in tow. Statisticians have also cited the higher level of divorce amongst couples who marry in their early 20s, due in great part to the changes that both partners will inevitably go through as they "grow up."

For young marrieds, I believe there is a crucial and wonderful period of time, the "honeymoon" phase of discovering one another, that is best done as a couple without a couple of children in the mix.

All this said, most people are secure enough in themselves, their relationships, and their careers by their late 20s or early 30s, which is certainly an excellent time to plan (and have!) a family. Unfortunately, also falling in the category of "Things we don't expect, plan for, and can't control," many women and men do not meet their partners on nature's timetable. At the end of the day, we all do the best we can with what we have and what we "got" and being an Older Mom is a pretty amazing gift.

Understanding how much age itself matters

We say this often throughout this book: Human reproduction is a very inefficient process *at any age*. When a woman is 35, one out of four embryos is abnormal; this number increases to one out of two at age 40, and five out of six at age 45. Although these statistics certainly show that age is a factor in conceiving, remember that you're an individual, not a statistic, and your odds may be better or worse than the statistics.

And remember, once you are pregnant, advanced maternal age (a lovely medical term!) will contribute to an increased risk of chromosomal defects, of which Down syndrome is one.

Consider Table 6-1 to give you a better picture of how age affects not only fertility but the risk of birth defects.

As with everything, there's good news and bad news to being an older mom . . . or dad. The best we can tell you is to use age as a suggested guideline. Fertility, most often, decreases *over time*. You will not become infertile overnight. Indeed, studies have shown that many women experience *perimenopause* (the stage prior to menopause, which can last up to ten years) and subfertility for as long as five to seven years before the onset of actual menopause (which *generally* signifies the end of your reproductive years).

The average age of menopause is 51. You can still become pregnant during perimenopause, although it may be more difficult and/or require medical intervention because you ovulate less frequently and the quality of your remaining eggs is not as good as it once was. That's not to say you should purposely delay childbirth until your "golden years". Common sense, and knowledge of the facts, will help you make the best decision for you and your family.

What's "older" these days?

We read a lot of ink on how 50 is the new 40 and 40 is the new 30. That's all well and good, but someone forgot to tell our ovaries, or for that matter, any other part of our body that is busy adjusting itself to our chronological age, regardless of what ages our faces, figures, or fantasies place us.

In all fairness, however, we are seeing an extraordinary rise of pregnant women and mommies over 40, 50, and sometimes even 60. This isn't a reflection of the end of menopause as we know it, but rather the new technologies such as donor egg, sperm, and embryo, which allow women and men to bear children much later in life.

You can't pick up *People* magazine or turn on *Oprah* without hearing it: the great fertility debate over what age is appropriate when it comes to conception. Unfortunately, much of the *information* in magazines is inappropriate and just plain inaccurate. Recent statistics report an approximate 5 percent chance in a given month for a woman over 40 to conceive. This number sounds frighteningly low, until you compare it with the statistic that shows that a healthy couple in their 20s has only a 20 percent chance of success during any given month. This comparison is seldom brought up because the one isolated, surprising statistic often sells better than the facts. Our advice: Be a skeptic when it comes to supermarket medical opinions.

Over time, most people become fairly desensitized to the latest surefire cures or health warnings used to sell everything from the scientific to the supernatural. Apply the same approach when weeding through the information on fertility. You wouldn't take medical advice from your car mechanic, so don't just assume that everyone who offers up an opinion, even a public one, knows anything more. Instead, ask your doctor, ask your nurse, or read a book (like this one) written by someone actually in the field. Although the media may provide you with a source of information, make sure that you qualify that source. More often than not, you'll find that the information presented has a mere modicum of truth in it surrounded by a lot of hype designed to get your attention. Ignore the hype. The next big story will take its place in no time.

But I don't look my age!

Whether you're dealing with fertility or fitness, age *does* play a role. Whether you *feel* like you're 15 or 50, whether you look your age or not, your body knows how old you are, and your ovaries do too.

In truth, there is only *one* answer to how old you are . . . and it can be found on your birth certificate.

You can keep yourself in better baby-making shape (and better overall health) through good self-care, including nutrition and exercise. These measures will make a difference in your overall health, and may actually improve your health during pregnancy, even decrease the risk of obstetrical complications (for example, losing weight may decrease the risk of gestational diabetes). We touch on these topics in Chapter 3. But ultimately, you can't fool Mother Nature. In other words, there is no known way to reverse the aging of the eggs.

Putting age in its (proper) place

Reversing the aging process is not an option, and if it you've found a way to do so, we recommend writing a book . . . and a movie! But when it comes to conceiving at a later age, there are a few things that you can do to help the odds:

✔ **Keep yourself in the best health, and baby-making shape, possible; regular checkups, good nutrition, plenty of sleep and exercise.**

✔ **Consult with a physician, be it OB/GYN or reproductive endocrinologist, who has experience in working with older wannabe moms.** Not all fertility doctors specialize in advanced maternal age, or want to for that matter. Ask around and/or check with RESOLVE or online resources to find a doctor who will have the latest and best information to help you address your individual issues. (If you're over 35, you should seriously start with a reproductive endocrinologist.)

✓ **Don't compare yourself to younger women suffering from infertility, or any other woman for that matter.** Your issues may be entirely different and call for a completely different approach. Just because your friend's sister-in-law was successful with a high stimulation protocol at the age of 32, doesn't mean that this will work for you at the age of 39. It's important to work with a physician, and a plan, tailored to *your* needs.

✓ **Jackie was convinced that high-tech IVF with lots of drugs was the only thing that would work for her.** Luckily, Jackie's physician believed differently. Even so, it took Jackie quite a few months to believe him! After trying his lower tech, low-dose medication protocol for a while, lo and behold, Jackie ended up with a bouncing baby girl. Being wrong was one of the few right things that she did in trying to conceive!

✓ **Surround yourself with a good support team.** Whether it be friends, family, clergy or professional help, this is not a battle that you want to fight alone. Your support team can help keep you sane and realistic.

✓ **Consider your options.** Would you be willing to adopt? Use third-party reproduction (for example, donor eggs, sperm, embryo)? A surrogate? Success can often be found in Plan B, C, and so on down the line.

✓ **Set a timetable.** You don't want to make baby making a midlife project or crisis. Decide how long you want to spend trying and stick to it as best you can. Knowing that there's an end in sight can relieve a great deal of pressure.

✓ **Investigate alternative treatment if you're interested.** Some women swear by acupuncture, naturopathy, or massage. Certainly, these are easier alternatives for your mind and body and just might deliver your baby to you as well. These measures are excellent for decreasing stress and helping you tune into your body's own signals. Just remember that alternative treatments can't reverse ovarian aging any more than "traditional" medications.

✓ **Be patient.** Even at a young age, consider trying to conceive as a marathon, not a sprint. With each passing year, the time that this could take you is likely to be longer and the effort more intense. Don't set yourself up by expecting success the first month around ... or the second. If this does happen, you'll be pleasantly surprised, and extraordinarily lucky!

Living with Diseases That Affect Fertility

Just a few generations ago, systemic diseases such as diabetes or lupus ruled out the possibility of having a baby. Now, pregnancies in patients with systemic disease are commonplace, and obstetricians or perinatologists who specialize in high-risk patients guide women with a history of cancer, kidney problems, heart problems, or just about any other health condition through successful pregnancies. Discuss the potential problems of pregnancy with your doctor beforehand so that you can be prepared for the problems you may face getting pregnant or carrying a pregnancy to term.

Polycystic ovaries

Polycystic ovarian syndrome, sometimes called PCO or PCOS, although in medicalese it's known as Stein-Leventhal Syndrome, is the most common hormonal problem in women of childbearing age, affecting between 5 and 10 percent of women. PCOS is often associated with infertility, but affects women in many other ways as well.

PCOS can be diagnosed by physical exam, including pelvic ultrasound, which may show polycystic ovaries, or ovaries which contain many small cysts. Blood tests may show an abnormal luteinizing hormone (LH) to follicle-stimulating hormone (FSH) ratio. Normally, the ratio between these two hormone levels is 1:1, but in PCOS patients, the LH is elevated, with a ratio of about 2:1 or higher. Insulin levels, free testosterone (a male hormone), and glucose may be high, and thyroid levels may be low.

The official definition of PCOS as determined by a workshop sponsored by ESHRE/ASRM (the European and American conferences on reproductive endocrinology) in 2003 is that PCOS is present if 2 of the 3 following criteria are met:

✔ Anovulation (no ovulation) or oligoulvation (ovulating only occasionally rather than every month)

✔ Excess androgen activity

✔ Polycystic ovaries diagnosed by ultrasound and not related to any other cause

It's difficult to say what causes PCOS; some women, but not all (about 50 percent), with PCOS are overweight, which can be related to the body's ability to make insulin, a hormone that regulates the body's use of starches and sugars. This is why one of the treatments for PCOS is Metformin (Glucophage), a medication that is most commonly used for Type 2 (adult-onset, noninsulin-dependent) diabetes. The unanswered question is, which came first, *being overweight or the PCOS?* Most doctors today think that the PCOS is the cause of being overweight rather than the other way around. There may be a genetic component to PCOS.

The overabundance of insulin production in women with PCOS may lead to the ovaries making too many androgens, or male hormones. The excess of androgens leads to many of the symptoms associated with PCOS, which include the following:

- Discoloration of the skin under the arms, breasts and around the groin (*acanthosis nigricans*)
- Excess facial hair
- Acne
- Thinning hair or male pattern baldness
- Excess weight

PCOS can also affect women systemically, outside of the reproductive system, causing:

- Type 2 (adult onset) diabetes
- Heart disease
- High blood pressure
- High cholesterol levels
- Sleep apnea

Women with PCOS may start to develop follicles, but because of the imbalance between FSH and LH, they don't mature and don't ovulate. Instead, the follicles get "stuck" in the surface of the ovary in a state that can best be described as "suspended animation." Because there is no ovulation, there's no monthly period. Periods become irregular and, when they do occur, they may be quite heavy because the uterine lining has become thickened as a result of not shedding on a regular basis.

This lack of regular shedding and thickening of the uterine lining can eventually lead to a risk of hyperplasia (a pre-cancerous thickening of the uterine lining) which can, if left untreated, lead to uterine cancer. If you have PCOS and don't ovulate regularly, your doctor may recommend doing endometrial biopsies (a small piece of the uterine lining is scraped off and sent to pathology to be tested for abnormal cells) to check for cancer cells.

Women with PCOS may also have a higher rate of miscarriage, and are more likely to develop gestational diabetes during pregnancy. Some women have an easier time conceiving if they take insulin-lowering medication; it's not yet clear if these same medications can also lower the risk of miscarriage in women with PCOS.

If you have PCOS, you may need to see a fertility specialist to get pregnant. There are treatments that can help you get pregnant; the most common are:

- Medications like Clomiphene Citrate and gonadotropins (see Chapter 22 for a description of different fertility medications) to induce ovulation.

✔ Medications to lower insulin resistance; these medications, Glucophage and Avandia, are also taken by people with diabetes.

✔ Ovarian drilling: A number of small punctures are made in the ovary using a laser during a laparoscopy, resulting in a lowering of male hormones.

✔ Weight loss; the catch-22 is that women with PCOS have a harder time losing weight.

Endometriosis

Endometriosis is the growth of pieces of endometrial tissue (the inner lining of the uterus) outside the uterus. Endometriosis is commonly found in fallopian tubes, ovaries, bladder, and sometimes even outside the pelvic cavity, in the abdomen. In rare cases, it has been found in the lungs, and even under the skin or in the brain! How does it manage to leave the uterus and travel to all these places?

There are many theories about how endometriosis travels; the most common are that endometriosis travels along with menstrual blood that flows "backwards" out of the uterus and into the fallopian tubes, ovary, pelvis, bladder, and abdomen. This theory doesn't explain how endometriosis ends up far from the pelvis; theories for how this happens range from travel through the lymph system to a theory that endometrial tissue doesn't travel to these places, but is present in these locations from birth (pick up a copy of *Endometriosis for Dummies,* [Wiley 2006] for all you ever wanted to know about endometriosis).

Endometriosis is a big player on the infertility field; around 30 percent of women suffering from infertility have endometriosis. Conversely, if you have endometriosis, you have around a 40 percent chance of having some degree of infertility. In addition, more than 30 percent of laparoscopic surgeries for unexplained infertility result in a diagnosis of endometriosis.

Endometriosis may affect fertility in a number of ways, including the following:

✔ Blocking fallopian tubes so the ovulated egg can't reach the uterus

✔ Destroying the fimbriae, the hair-like projections on the end of the fallopian tubes that guide the released egg into the fallopian tube

✔ Causing cysts that may interfere with the release of eggs from the ovary

✔ Creating an immune response in the pelvis that interferes with fertilization

✔ Partially blocking fallopian tubes, so the embryo is more likely to implant in the tube (ectopic pregnancy)

Does all this mean you should throw in the towel on having a baby if you have endometriosis? Not at all! As many as 70 percent of women with minimal or mild endometriosis and infertility do conceive within three years of trying without any therapy.

However, you may not want to wait three years to get pregnant. And if you have moderate to severe endometriosis, your chances of pregnancy may be significantly lower without medical intervention. The good news is that surgical treatment of minimal or mild endometriosis increases pregnancy rates; in one study, more than 40 percent of women with moderate or severe endometriosis became pregnant after surgery.

In vitro fertilization (IVF) has helped many women with endometriosis conceive, even in previously "hopeless" cases. (Check out Chapter 15 for more info about IVF.) In spite of its other effects on natural conception, endometriosis does not diminish IVF success rates.

Diabetes: More than a "sugar" problem

Diabetes affects about 17 million Americans, or approximately 6 percent of the population. There are actually several different types of diabetes, including the following:

- ✔ **Type 1 diabetes,** which used to be called juvenile diabetes, usually develops before puberty, but can develop at any age. Five to ten percent of diabetics have Type 1 diabetes, which is an autoimmune disease. In Type 1 diabetes, the beta cells of the pancreas stop making insulin altogether, so people with this problem must take injections of insulin every day.

- ✔ **Type 2 diabetes** usually develops in people over 40, but it can develop earlier. It is often associated with being overweight; 80 percent of Type 2 diabetics are overweight. It develops more slowly than Type 1 and can possibly be controlled with diet and pills rather than injections.

Diabetes leads to problems with blood vessels, circulation, and nerve function. Therefore, men with diabetes often have problems with erection and ejaculation; some male diabetics have retrograde ejaculation, a condition in which sperm back up into the bladder.

Women with diabetes need to have well-controlled blood sugar levels during pregnancy. Even with good control, the rate of birth defects in women with diabetes is two to three times the normal rate. Women with polycystic ovary syndrome may develop Type 2 diabetes later in life.

Diabetics tend to have large babies, which can create problems at the time of delivery.

Lupus: Not just a rash

Systemic lupus erythematosus, commonly called lupus, is primarily a disease of women, although a small percentage of men also develop it. One of the outward symptoms of lupus is a facial rash, but lupus can affect every organ in your body. A few generations ago, women with lupus were advised not to have children, because it was felt that pregnancy worsens the disease. More recent studies have shown this belief not to be true, although one-third of pregnant lupus patients have "flares," or increases in disease activity. About 10 percent of pregnant lupus patients find that their symptoms actually improve.

Fifty percent of women with lupus have normal pregnancies and normal deliveries; about 25 percent deliver prematurely, and another 25 percent experience miscarriage or stillbirth.

Miscarriage may be related to antibodies called antiphospholipid antibodies (discussed earlier in this chapter) found in some lupus patients. These antibodies cause clotting and interfere with the growth of the placenta. Baby aspirin and/or heparin may be given in pregnancy to help blood flow to the placenta.

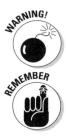

About 20 percent of lupus patients develop *toxemia,* a condition that results in high blood pressure, liver and kidney malfunctions, and premature delivery and can lead to eclampsia, which can cause maternal seizures and death.

If you have lupus, you need to be followed carefully by an obstetrician who specializes in high-risk patients.

Cancer and Fertility: The News Is Cautiously Optimistic

Just a few years ago, having cancer meant that you would probably not be able to conceive and carry a child. Surgery, radiation, and chemotherapy, the mainstay treatments of most cancers, could destroy ovaries and sperm cells as well as your hope of having a child.

Today, however, new advances have made it possible for cancer survivors to become parents, and the really good news is that more advances are being made all the time. The information of today may be obsolete soon, and the chances for parenthood will hopefully be better than ever. The good news even today is that there's no evidence that your baby will have a higher risk of birth defects or childhood cancer if you become pregnant after cancer treatment.

For women . . .

Because women are involved not only in the production of gametes but also for carrying a baby to term, cancer in women who want to be parents can be more complicated than cancer in men. In the next sections, we look at different types of cancer that can impact future motherhood.

Beating breast cancer

Breast cancer survivors are now being told that pregnancy after treatment is possible, as long as their ovaries are intact and haven't been irradiated. Many doctors encourage patients to wait two years after treatment before trying to get pregnant. Pregnancy doesn't increase the chance of cancer recurrence, according to most recent studies, but doctors want to make sure that the cancer doesn't recur on its own.

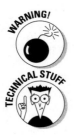

If you do have a recurrence of cancer while pregnant and require chemotherapy, you need to be aware that chemo in the first trimester may cause fetal malformation, while waiting till the second or third trimester may result in preterm labor or fetal loss.

At the time of this writing, a study showed that breast cancer patients trying to get pregnant through in vitro fertilization made more eggs when given tamoxifen.

Battling ovarian cancer

If you've been treated for ovarian cancer with radiation or ovarian ablation, your ovaries will not be functioning, and you'll need to use donor eggs to become pregnant. If you were treated with multiple-agent chemotherapy, there's a good chance you'll go into premature ovarian failure. One-third of women under age 30 and two-thirds of those over 30 go into POF.

It's sometimes possible to remove only one ovary or move the ovary not affected by cancer out of the way (surgically lift the ovary out of the pelvis), so it won't be affected by radiation treatment.

Fighting uterine cancer

The treatment for uterine cancer is usually removal of the uterus; this means you won't be able to carry a pregnancy, although if your ovaries are not removed, you can produce eggs that can be fertilized and implanted into a gestational carrier.

New therapy for very early endometrial (the lining of the uterus is called the endometrium) cancers involves treating patients with the hormone medroxyprogesterone and also performing repeated dilatation and curettage, scraping the uterine lining until it's free of cancerous cells. This method can be used only in cancer cases that are discovered very early and confined to the endometrium. Because the cancer can return, very close follow up is required.

Coping with cervical cancer

Early stage cervical cancer can be effectively treated by the removal of only part of the cervix; this process is called cervical conization. It may also be possible to remove the cervix while leaving the uterus intact when treating cervical cancer (this is called a *trachelectomy*).

For men . . .

Although testicular cancer is rare, making up only 1 percent of all cancer, it's the most common cancer found in men between the ages of 20 and 34, with 7,000 new cases diagnosed each year. It is four times more common among Caucasian men than African American men.

If only one testicle is removed surgically, the remaining testicle will produce enough sperm so that fertility won't be damaged. If both testicles need to be removed, several semen samples can be frozen before surgery and used for insemination later on. If only one testicle is affected, the man has a 2 to 5 percent chance of developing cancer in the other testicle.

Some chemotherapy treatment causes temporary loss of fertility, but sperm counts may return to an acceptable level after two to three years. Radiation may also cause temporary infertility, but some men regain adequate sperm counts within a short time.

If certain lymph nodes are removed, the nerves that control ejaculation may be affected, although the sperm count may be normal. This condition may require sperm aspiration with ICSI and IVF to achieve a pregnancy.

Turning Around a Tubal Ligation

Nearly 40 percent of American women of childbearing age have been surgically sterilized. (See Chapter 12 for info on reversing a vasectomy, the male sterilization procedure.) Unfortunately, at least 10 percent regret their decision down the road. Can tubal ligation be reversed? The answer is yes, no, and maybe, depending on when the surgery was done and what kind of surgery it was.

Surgical sterilization is very common in the United States. A 1995 study showed that 41 percent of ever-married women ages 15 to 44 were surgically sterile. About 1 million women have their tubes tied, a procedure known as *tubal ligation,* each year. Human nature being what it is, at least 10,000 of these women regret their decision and want to have another baby.

If you want a tubal reversal, look for a surgeon skilled in microsurgery (find them through the Society for Reproductive Surgeons website at www.asrm. org, the website of the American Society for Reproductive Medicine.). Depending on the surgeon and type of surgery done, your surgery can take up to four hours to perform and may require several weeks of recovery. However, most surgeons only require only a one-night hospital stay.

Risks after surgery include scar tissue formation, infection, and increased risk of ectopic pregnancy. If the fimbriated end of the tube (the part that the egg enters from the ovary) is intact and your doctor believes that you have enough tube left to reconnect, your pregnancy chances after reanastomosis can be higher than IVF success rates. This is because with repaired fallopian tubes, the couple can "try at home" every month, whereas IVF is a one-shot deal.

A *tubal reanastomosis,* or tubal reversal, has some drawbacks. For one thing, it's expensive — around $10,000, about the same as an IVF cycle — and insurance usually doesn't cover the cost. For another, the success rate depends on how long ago your tubes were tied and how they were tied. Success rates can be anywhere from 20 to 70 percent, depending upon your individual situation.

Before you decide to have your tubal ligation reversed, consider these factors:

- ✔ **Your age:** Are you in your late thirties or younger? If you're over 40, you may have other fertility problems related to age, and in vitro fertilization (IVF) may be a better option for you.

- ✔ **Your partner:** If your partner has sperm problems, you may also be better off doing IVF rather than reversing your tubal ligation.

- ✔ **How your tubes were tied:** If your tubes were blocked off or clamped with clips or rings instead of being cauterized or having a large section removed, your chance of success is higher. Studies show that you need at least 4 cm (about an inch and a half) of healthy tube to successfully conceive after having the tubes reconnected (the average length of fallopian tubes before sterilization is about 10 cm, or about 4 inches).

Chapter 7

Seeing a Doctor — and Keeping Your Cool

In This Chapter

▶ Finding a doctor to help you get pregnant

▶ Working with your doctor

▶ Locating a specialist

*T*wo classic Norman Rockwell drawings show a family on vacation in the station wagon. In the first scene, everyone is in clean new outfits and wearing big smiles. The second scene shows the return from vacation — everyone is dirty, bedraggled, and grumpy, and Dad looks like he's ready to drive the whole group over a cliff.

You may have started toward pregnancy in the "starting vacation" mode, thinking "I can't wait to do the nursery," "What kind of maternity clothes should I get?" and "I wonder who'll give me a baby shower?" After a few months with no pregnancy, you may resemble the return group, worn out and testy, ready to slap the next person who asks when you're going to have a baby. It's time to get some help — from your doctor.

In this chapter, we explain the ins and outs of finding a doctor who can help when you're not getting pregnant on your own, help you decide when to see a specialist, and give you an idea of what to expect at your first visit.

Deciding When You Should Make an Appointment with Dr. Basic

Conventional medical opinion says that you should consult a physician if you haven't gotten pregnant in one year if you're under age 35, or six months if you're over 35. These guidelines must have been written for very patient people. If you're under 35 and patient enough to wait for a year — a *year* — before talking to a doctor about getting pregnant, let's just say you have the patience to make a very good parent!

Seeking professional help is a big step. Here you always thought you were an average sort of person, and now you find yourself part of the 20 percent of women who don't get pregnant in a year of trying. For the first few months, you could pretend it wasn't a big deal, but now, well, open the phone book. It's time to call Dr. Basic. Who's Dr. Basic? He can be your primary care physician or your regular GYN (gynecologist). In most cases of infertility, Dr. Basic is the only doctor you'll need to get pregnant.

When not to wait — even a few months

Sometimes even conventional wisdom, that conservative soul, says not to wait six months or a year before seeing a doctor about not getting pregnant. For example, see your doctor before even trying to get pregnant if:

- ✔ **You're over age 38.** You may want to do more thorough testing before trying because your aging ovaries are making fewer good eggs.
- ✔ **You've had a previous ectopic pregnancy or have pelvic inflammatory disease.** You may have damage to your fallopian tubes, which may make surgery necessary.
- ✔ **You're not getting your period, or you're getting it very irregularly.** You may need help regulating your cycles so that you produce an egg every month.
- ✔ **You have very painful periods.** You may have endometriosis (see Chapter 6 for more discussion of this condition) and may need treatment to get pregnant.

You may want to have your partner do a semen analysis early on if he:

- ✔ Has a history of trauma to the testicles
- ✔ Had undescended testicles
- ✔ Had mumps as a child

Any of these conditions may have caused damage to his sperm; he may need to see a urologist (a doctor that specializes in the urinary-genital tract).

If you've had your tubes tied or if your partner had a vasectomy, you need to see a specialist to discuss either reversal of the surgery (see Chapter 11) or in vitro fertilization (which we discuss in detail in Part IV).

Choosing between a family doctor and an OB/GYN

So who *is* Dr. Basic when you're trying to get pregnant? The average doctor has about nine initials after his name, so how are you supposed to know which one you should see when you're trying to get pregnant? Some of the more common abbreviations you may see include the following:

- **M.D.:** Medical doctor trained in traditional medicine with four years of medical school after college and a residency length varying with specialty. After that, residency can be from two to ten years, depending on the specialty.

- **D.O.:** Doctor of osteopathy. These doctors used to be more trained in manipulation and homeopathic methods, but today's osteopaths train in programs virtually identical to traditional medical schools.

- **OB:** Obstetrician. This specialist is trained to take care of pregnant women and handle labor and delivery. OBs are also gynecologists but may specialize in pregnancy.

- **GYN:** Gynecologist. This physician is trained to take care of women's health. Obstetricians and gynecologists all start with the same four-year residency training after medical school, but they may choose to specialize in one area of the specialty.

- **RE:** Reproductive endocrinologist. This doctor is a graduate of an OB/GYN program who has chosen to specialize in infertility. After medical school, these doctors complete three years of additional training, called a fellowship, to take tests to become certified for this sub-specialty.

- **FP:** Family practitioner. These doctors have chosen to specialize in the health of the entire family. In some parts of the country they, rather than OBs, handle many women's health problems, including pregnancy and deliveries.

- **FACOG:** Fellow of the American College of Obstetricians and Gynecologists. A doctor who has FACOG after his name is board certified in Obstetrics and Gynecology and is a member of this national society.

You may also come across these terms when doctor-shopping:

- **Board eligible:** These doctors have completed the education in their specialty and can now take the tests to become board certified.

- **Board certified:** These doctors have practiced their specialty for two years, taken the tests necessary to be certified, and have passed them.

If you live in a remote area, you may need to start with your family doctor because specialists may not have offices in your area. Also, you may feel more comfortable starting with a doctor who already knows you, such as your OB/GYN or family doctor. If your doctor believes that your case is more complex than he is qualified to treat, he'll probably refer you to someone more experienced in your particular situation.

The "top of the heap" in fertility specialists are board-certified reproductive endocrinologists, doctors who have completed an additional three years of fellowship in Reproductive Endocrinology and Infertility after becoming OB/GYNs.

Bringing your partner to the OB/GYN office

Back in the olden days of gynecology, say before the 1960s, you *never* saw a man in the OB/GYN waiting room. Today, however, the situation is different; some men accompany their partners to every OB/GYN visit. Many doctors even specifically request that you bring your partner to a visit so that you can all get to know each other.

So should you encourage your partner to attend your first why-aren't-we-pregnant visit? That depends on a few things:

✔ Will he feel horribly out of place, not pay attention, or say something you'd rather he didn't?

Some men don't like to go to the doctor, ever, for anything. Whether it's the loss of control, the digging into what they consider their personal business, or just discomfort in the face of an authority figure, many men are not assets at the doctor's office. You probably know by now whether your partner will do well at the doctor's office. If you're going to sit there (half naked, no less) worrying about what embarrassing thing he might say or do, go by yourself.

On the other hand, if your partner is the person in your twosome who remembers details, writes things down correctly, asks sensible questions, and provides moral support, by all means, take him to your first doctor visit. If you don't get pregnant right away, he'll probably need to have his own testing done, so he may as well get familiar with the doctor right from the start.

✔ Are you going to have to impart information that you don't want your partner to know?

For example, did you have an abortion, give a child up for adoption, have a sexually transmitted disease, or do any other thing you'd rather your partner didn't know about? Then go to the first visit by yourself, frankly explain the situation to your doctor, and take your partner to the *next* visit. (Do *not* write confidential information down, as medical records have a way of getting copied and sent from office to office. Instead, tell the doctor, and explain that this information is confidential; he or she should not write it down, either.)

✔ Are you going to be embarrassed about undergoing an examination with your partner there?

Even today, in this let-it-all-hang-out age, some of you aren't comfortable having other people, even your partner, present for a gynecological exam. If this situation is going to make you uneasy, maybe your partner can wait in the waiting room until the exam is over and then come in when you're dressed.

Making a list of questions for your first visit

Whether you go alone or as a team to your doctor's appointment, prepare a list of questions ahead of time so that you won't forget anything. Here's a starter list. You'll probably have other questions specific to your own situation.

✔ Do you treat many patients trying to get pregnant?

Obviously, you don't want a doctor taking on your case whose practice mostly consists of gynecological surgery on women over age 50.

✔ Will you do any testing before we start treatment?

Some doctors just start you on medication for a few months before putting you through more invasive testing. Other doctors do blood work, semen analysis, and ultrasounds before starting you on medicine.

✔ Will my insurance cover any testing?

✔ What do you think my chance for success will be?

Obviously, your doctor doesn't have a crystal ball, but he should have some general idea, based on your age and history, what your chance of getting pregnant is.

✔ How long should we try this before we do further testing?

If your doctor shrugs and gives you the impression that she would do simple methods forever, you may want to find another doctor, especially if you're over age 35.

Answering Dr. Basic's Questions

Dr. Basic is going to have some questions for you, too. He'll want to know the following, so come prepared with the answers:

- ✔ How long have you been trying to get pregnant?
- ✔ How often do you have sex?
- ✔ Do you use any lubricants?
- ✔ How do you time intercourse (what days of the month)?
- ✔ How long do your periods last?
- ✔ How long are your cycles from day one of one cycle to day one of the next?
- ✔ What was the first day of your last period?
- ✔ Are your periods painful?
- ✔ Are your periods heavy?
- ✔ How many pads or tampons do you use a day?
- ✔ Do any sisters or other close relatives have children?
- ✔ Are there any known genetic factors in your family?
- ✔ Have you used ovulation predictor kits; if so, what have they shown?

Dr. Basic may also have questions aimed specifically at you. If you're heavy and have adult acne or facial hair, he may wonder if you have polycystic ovary syndrome (PCOS). PCOS patients often don't ovulate on their own. If you're very thin, he may be concerned about you not getting periods due to overexercising, anorexia, or poor nutrition.

Understanding What Your Doctor Says

Doctors and nurses aren't *really* trying to confuse you when they spew forth a list of initials or shortcut terms. But when your doctor says something like "Get an HSG and a sono, and then if your APA and FSH come back okay, we'll start the stims," your immediate reaction may be "Huh?"

Whenever you don't understand what the doctor or nurse just said, ask the person to stop and explain. Don't write it down, thinking that you'll look it up later, or nod just to look like you know what they're talking about.

You may find it necessary to take notes on what your doctor is saying. Some choose to tape record their conversations with their doctor. Any type of note taking can be a helpful tool in relaying this information to your partner or to your cousin who's a doctor. Always ask your doctor if doing so is okay, particularly when it comes to taping your discussions. Most doctors have no problem with this; it's better than a return phone call because you can't remember what was said. However, most *people* (including doctors) become a bit unhinged if they find out that they were being taped secretly.

A second set of ears is helpful as well. This can be a perfect spot for your partner to participate! Fertility is an emotional subject. Especially if the doctor is addressing problems that *you* have, you may be too close to the situation to hear and understand all the options that are available. Your partner or a friend may be a bit more detached and better able to comprehend and communicate the information to you. Many fertility patients view themselves (incorrectly!) in a battle against their doctors. In this case, you may be more open to your partner's interpretation of what the doctor has said. Either way, try to remember that your doctor *is* on your side. Your doctor is your advocate, and part of that duty involves giving you the complete picture, good and bad.

Keeping Your Own (Hit) Records

Fertility is certainly a project that can generate a lot of paperwork.

After initially relying on only her doctor's records, Jackie eventually discovered the need to keep her own records as well. The process was simple, but the organization was not. After every doctor's appointment, monitoring visit, or blood test, she asked for a copy of her records from that day. Jackie's records often consisted of nothing more than her notations from the day's blood work results, which she would date and keep in a separate folder. Her records proved invaluable during the course of her treatment. Seldom did Jackie have a question that couldn't be answered by reviewing her own information. She was able to compare her results from different cycles to see how she was faring in a historical sense. And, when the time came to switch doctors, Jackie had her own history to present to her new doctor at the first visit.

Keeping your own records certainly provides you with a point of reference as you go through your treatment. Doing so also allows you to double-check doctor's instructions and test results if the communication with your clinic is less than perfect.

As a cautionary note (from one who knows!), try to avoid making your records nighttime reading. If you bring this paperwork to bed with you, you may be becoming a wee bit obsessive about the process. This type of behavior will not help your cause or your sleeping patterns. A lighthearted magazine or book that has nothing to do with fertility is a better sleep aid.

Reviewing your information periodically and having an extra set of records for your files are very helpful to your treatment. Trying to diagnose yourself based on your past performance is a job better left to the pros. Your records are your backup. Your doctors are still the front line.

Moving Up to Dr. Specialist

After seeing Dr. Basic for a few months, you may have a better idea of what your fertility problems are, and you may decide that it's time to see a specialist. Or perhaps your testing hasn't shown any specific problems, and Dr. Basic has decided you should move on to a specialist in infertility.

Finding Dr. Specialist

Your family doctor or gynecologist may hand you a piece of paper with the name of an infertility specialist scribbled on it. "Go to this guy. He's the best," she may say, and you may do just that, without thinking a whole lot about alternative choices.

Before you set up your first appointment with Dr. Specialist, you may want to ask Dr. Basic *why* she thinks the person she has suggested is the best. Does the specialist have the best pregnancy rates, is he a prolific publisher in journals, or is he just a member of the same health organization?

Even worse, is he your doctor's golfing buddy? Many doctors refer patients to each other, and there's nothing wrong with the practice of referral. That system, however, doesn't ensure that you'll end up with the doctor best suited to you, either.

Although the name that Dr. Basic gives you is a starting point, you should check out other doctors, too, before making a final decision. At this point, you will probably be looking for a specialist in the field, such as a reproductive endocrinologist.

Start with the phone book (or the internet). No, you're not going to shut your eyes and blindly poke your finger at a name. You can use the phone book as a starting point, looking under the reproductive endocrinologists listing and accumulating the names of doctors in your area. This approach gives you a basic list from which to work and a starting point for some research.

Eliminate clinics that are too far away from you. "Too far away" is a subjective measure; if you work and have a very hectic lifestyle, more than 15 minutes away may be too far, and your options may be limited. If your schedule is more flexible, an hour or even two may seem reasonable. Remember that you may have to go in for blood and ultrasound monitoring several times a month and that some clinics do all their monitoring early in the morning. You may find that a clinic close to work is more convenient than one close to home. If you must work with a clinic that is quite far, ask if you can have some of the monitoring done in an office that is closer. Many RE's work with general OB/GYNs in your community who are perfectly adept at performing basic ultrasounds and blood tests. That way, you only travel far for the actual egg retrieval and/or embryo transfer.

Getting help from national organizations

If you have a core list of infertility clinics near you (if not, see the earlier section, "Finding Dr. Specialist" to find out how to make this list), you need to check each one out. You can visit each one, hanging around the waiting room and questioning people as they come out the door. Or you can call your local Resolve organization and see whether it has information on any of the offices you're considering. Resolve is the largest national organization dedicated to the treatment of infertility.

If you have Internet access, finding your local Resolve organization is easy; the Web site is `www.resolve.org`. Just click on the local chapter's hyperlink to find one near you. If you don't have computer access, check your local paper for listings of meetings or call Resolve's HelpLine at 1-888-623-0744.

The Resolve Web site contains clinic success rates published by the Centers for Disease Control (CDC). This information is compiled by the Society for Assisted Reproductive Technology (SART), which you can read more about in Chapter 10. These numbers give you some idea of your clinic's success rates, but keep in mind that these statistics are only for high-tech in vitro fertilization (IVF) treatment, not for medium-tech treatment such as IUI (intrauterine insemination). Keep in mind also that clinics that treat younger patients, or only those who have not failed previously, are more likely to have higher success rates. That's why the SART Web site has a disclaimer about over-interpreting success rates.

Local Resolve meetings will probably connect you with people who can give you the inside scoop on the local clinics, which may help narrow your search or at least give you some ideas about where you *don't* want to go!

The Resolve Web site contains a huge amount of information on insurance coverage for infertility, adoption options, and information on clinical trials and research studies being carried out around the country. Resolve is very vocal in lobbying for insurance coverage for infertility treatments. The Web site also has bulletin boards, lists of interesting meetings and events around the country, and a host of other information. Check it out!

Another patient advocacy group is the American Fertility Association (the AFA). Their website is www.theafa.org. This organization also has an active Web site with message boards, access to articles about infertility issues, a physician referral hotline, and more!

Your area may have other groups that meet to help you deal with infertility. Some are informal groups that started out as a few friends meeting to commiserate, and then grew into clubs with monthly meetings. You may also find local psychologists or therapists who have started groups for infertile patients.

All of these are good resources for information on who's good and who's not in your area. Always get more than one person's opinion on a clinic because each person may have a bias one way or the other, depending on her own outcome.

Going online for more resources and information

Resolve isn't the only information source online. In fact, after you start surfing the Net, your sources of information will be limited only by the amount of time you have to spend. Whether you're interested in reading scientific journals, chatting with new friends online, or checking out clinic Web sites, we guarantee that the Internet has enough stuff to keep you occupied until your children leave for college!

Chat rooms and bulletin boards

Perhaps one of the greatest sources of information and strength on the road to baby that Jackie found came from the countless women she encountered in cyberspace, some of whom became friends in real time as well. Jackie happened upon this wealth of relating and resources right after a failed in vitro fertilization attempt and a subsequent high FSH (follicle-stimulating hormone) reading, which, at the time, seemed a death knell to any future attempts.

After a good cry, Jackie logged on to www.google.com to see what she could find in reference to her new diagnosis of high FSH. Convinced that she was the only one to suffer from this odd disorder (actually a measure of diminished ovarian egg reserve), Jackie was surprised at how quickly Google returned a result listing over 38,000 Web pages on the topic. Okay, so maybe a few others out there had the same problem after all. The first listing, High FSH E-mail Group, connected her to a very lively, upbeat chat room. Through teary eyes, she asked one and all if she was doomed. Jackie logged off in despair and went to work her way through the other 37,999 sites. After visiting two more sites, she went back to the chat room and was amazed to find at least ten responses to her wail. She read each and every one, printed them all (and has saved them to this day), and spent until the wee hours of the morning reading every message of encouragement and every link to more information on high FSH, low FSH, infertility, and the best medical and nonmedical sources for help, including doctors, clinics, acupuncturists, and herbs.

Jackie never left that site through the remaining year of her fertility battle. From it, she garnered hope that she could conceive despite what her doctor had told her. She also found a new (and improved) doctor who (eventually) treated her successfully. Jackie also discovered insights on new treatments and medications and located a 24/7 support network that accompanied her through fertility, pregnancy, and all the stressors in between. She developed a core group of friends from all over the country who were the first ones she called when the pregnancy test came back negative and when it finally came back positive. She can honestly say that her high FSH diagnosis was a blessing, one that led her to a much greater place.

The beauty of the Internet is the availability of libraries full of information right at our fingertips. Bulletin boards help provide links to this information, along with the kinship so helpful in thriving through infertility. Man or woman, whatever problem that ails you, you can be almost certain that the Internet offers a chat room/bulletin board filled with others facing the same struggles.

Doctors' Web sites: Separating the glitter from the goods

When Sharon first started working for an infertility clinic, few infertility clinics had Web sites. Now it seems as if every infertility clinic has a Web site. Some are pretty basic, giving not much more than name, rank, and serial number, and others run a 24-hour-a-day media show, complete with question-and-answer sessions with the doctors, links to published articles, and testimonials from happy clients.

Some clinics list their Web site right next to their phone number in the phone book; others direct you to their Web site when you call the office. Some Web sites give detailed and frequently updated pregnancy rates. Other sites either don't supply or don't update statistics.

Here's what *not* to be impressed by when looking at clinic Web sites:

- ✔ **The way the doctor looks:** That picture may have been taken in 1963.

- ✔ **Testimonials from patients:** Unless you know the patients personally and can verify what they say, you have no way of knowing who wrote these glowing reports.

- ✔ **How many articles the doctor has had published:** Unless there's a listing of the articles, and you can see how long they were published and where. It's not hard these days to Google the journal and the article. But a simple listing of "50 articles" is not helpful.

- **Great graphics:** Splashy visuals may indicate that the doctor has a son or daughter who knows a lot about Web sites, but those graphics don't reveal anything about a doctor's medical ability.

- **Success rates:** Be careful, only those on the SART website are actually audited. Web site success rates are just an approximation of reality.

You can be impressed by the following Web site information:

- Clearly written, user-friendly information
- A list of clinic services
- Evidence that you will have access to the doctor or nurse with questions or problems — these *will* arise!
- The doctors' degrees and the schools from which they were obtained
- The doctor's board certifications and dates
- Lab certifications

Facing the Stranger in Your Sex Life — Treatment and Your Privacy

When going through fertility treatment, you open the door to your private life — yes, including your sex life — for all the medical world to see. This loss of privacy is bound to happen and takes some getting used to.

Talking sex

Your doctor (and his staff!) would rather discuss things other than your sex life (like their sex lives for instance!). They will not discuss your private life in their private lives. Their job, however, is to help you conceive a baby, and their inquiries are part of the process. Once again, consider this good training for pregnancy, when your body and your life will be oft-discussed topics with your physicians, your friends, and even your in-laws.

The frequency of intercourse, the quality of your menstrual cycles, and your past history of pregnancies, whether by hit or miss, are crucial bits of information in piecing together your reproductive profile. Offer information gladly because doing so only helps to educate your medical team. Feel free, however, to leave out the details that truly define intimacy. Remember that sexual intercourse is a biological process. Intimacy may occur in or out of the bedroom, and the specifics of that are all your own.

Discussing dollars with the doctor

When Jackie visited Dr. Badadventure for the first time, she was quickly whisked away to meet with Mr. Dollars and Sense, the finance guy. It should have been a warning. Needless to say, her fertility experience with Dr. Badadventure cost considerable dollars and yielded pennies in results.

We're not saying that you should turn tail and flee when the mention of payment comes up. Fertility doctors and clinics are for-profit institutions, so they're permitted and expected to make money from their patients. Most clinics ask for payment upfront for certain procedures, including extensive testing, surgery, and in vitro fertilization. Don't be offended. Because many insurers don't cover fertility, doctors do need to guarantee payment for their time, services, and staff. However, your initial health assessment and plan for treatment should come before you receive a price list for procedures. If you feel like you're getting a hard sell toward high-tech fertility from the finance guy (not the fertility doc), you probably are. If, however, your doctor determines, after careful review of you and your records, that high tech is the way to go, expect the issue of cost and payment to come up. You don't want to be surprised by a bill in the tens of thousands of dollars. For more information on dealing with the costs of fertility treatment, see Chapter 10.

Knowing When to Switch Doctors

So you've tried and tried and tried some more with your initial doctor of choice. Despite your efforts, he or she isn't sensitive to your needs, whether they're physical, emotional, or financial. Perhaps your doctor is stuck in a time warp of sorts, insisting that *eventually* you'll conceive naturally, or with minimal intervention, despite the fact that you've been trying for months or years with no success and a loudly ticking biological clock. Or else your doctor is pushing for expensive, invasive treatment for which you don't feel prepared. Your doctor may be the sort who travels from one office to another, meaning that he or she is virtually inaccessible, except for those occasional appointments.

Any of these reasons, or no particular reason at all, is perfectly understandable in your decision to switch doctors. The personalities of some patients and doctors just clash. For many, this alone can be a reason to run.

One thing to consider at any time during your treatment, (including before you begin, by the way) is getting a second opinion. Infertility treatment is not only very stressful, it can be extremely expensive. Before you plunk down $10,000, it might be worthwhile to invest another $200 to $300 for a consultation with another RE. It's a little-known fact that the initial consultation with a doctor is the biggest bargain at the infertility doctor's office! A whole hour alone with the doctor, reviewing records, making plans for the cost of what you'll end up paying for a single ultrasound which may take as little as 5 minutes! Your doctor should understand that you want to consult with someone else. If he or she doesn't, that's not a good sign. If you would rather not have to deal with the stress of telling him or her, keep a copy of all your medical records for yourself. That way, you not only know exactly what is going on, but are free at any time to have another specialist review that information and give you a "thumbs up" or "thumbs down" as the case may be about your treatment.

Chapter 8

Taking Supplemental Steps on the Road to Baby

*Y*ou're feeling tired. You've charted your ovulation, timed your sex life, and possibly even tried a few of the more basic fertility medicines. Nothing has worked so far, and your doctor may be suggesting stepping up the pace, as if the present pace isn't hard enough. His advice may involve injecting medications made from such odd ingredients as the urine of pregnant or menopausal women. "Wait a minute!" you cry out. "Isn't there another way?"

Yes, there are other ways, and you may have already tried one of them. In the first stages of trying to conceive, you may have been met with the well-intended, but unasked for, opinions of those who tell you to just relax and you'll get pregnant. Sometimes, this directive may actually work, but more often it doesn't. Now, as you prepare to move to the next level, the middle-tech road to baby, you'll more than likely hear of (and from!) others who swear by other, nontraditional ways of conceiving.

Alternative therapies, which can include everything from acupuncture to Traditional Chinese Medicine, from massage to meditation, have become a popular means of either supplementing or substituting for the standard "Western" approach to infertility (a.k.a. doctors, tests, and blood work).

Some clinics are offering alternative services to their patients through liaisons with providers. Others, while not adding to their staff, are allowing outside providers to come into their clinics and service patients upon request, such as acupuncture treatments before and after IVF embryo transfers.

In this chapter, we talk about those "other" ways to become pregnant, alternative measures from basic to beyond, and help you decide which ones are worth trying and which ones may just result in expensive urination.

Eating for Two? Sampling a Fertility Diet

Eat meat if you want to get pregnant with a boy, and eat sugar if you want a girl, an old wives' tale states. But what if you just want to have a baby — of *any* kind? When Jackie first ventured online to learn more about this road that had become a little longer than she had first anticipated, she found an entire civilization of people trying to conceive by using a variety of dietary means, claiming that diet changes put them in tiptop reproductive shape. These women (and men) had purged their diets of red meat, dairy products, white flour, sugar, and a host of other staples that she viewed as necessary. She was terrified. Their list of don'ts was Jackie's diet in a nutshell.

Some people swore by omega-3 fatty acids, found most commonly in salmon and other fish, as the magic potion for improving and/or restoring fertility. The only fish Jackie consumed were Goldfish (those popular snack crackers, that is). She thought she was in big trouble. The prospect of shots, whatever they were made of, seemed more attractive to her than a complete overhaul of her diet, but she didn't want to skip what could be a crucial step. But is your diet a factor when trying to get pregnant? A good rule of thumb is to treat your body as though you were already pregnant. That way, when you get there, you'll already be in tune with your new state!

Here's a brief look at some foods and our recommendations (our recommendations may not help, but they certainly won't hurt, and they do represent a "common sense" way of eating):

✔ **Red meat:** Studies show that red meat can neither help nor hurt your chances of getting pregnant. Trim all visible fat and cook the meat thoroughly.

WARNING!

Do not eat raw or undercooked fish, meat, or poultry when trying to get pregnant or during pregnancy. These products have a higher than normal chance of carrying listeria, a bacteria that may make a mom somewhat ill but wreak havoc on an unborn child's nervous system. Listeria has also been linked to an increased rate of spontaneous abortion.

Many pregnant women are also advised to heat up luncheon meats (sliced turkey, bologna, et al) which can also carry listeria. If you choose to do so, heat the meat in a microwave and eat it while it's still hot. Once it cools, the bacteria can reform.

✔ **Dairy:** Many women trying to conceive cut dairy products from their diet, but there's no conclusive medical or scientific data that supports the notion that dairy foods compromise fertility. Use organic products if possible. If you're lactose intolerant, dairy products can create havoc on your system, so be aware of your personal dietary needs.

✔ **White flour and processed sugar:** No studies have proven that refined sugar or processed flour decreases fertility. We recommend limiting their intake.

✔ **Artificial additives:** Despite hot debate, no definitive studies prove that additives such as aspartame and MSG are harmful. Limit or eliminate these additives from your diet if the controversy worries you.

✔ **Omega-3 fatty oils:** Studies are underway to evaluate the use of omega-3 oils in male infertility and in women with endometriosis. Omega-3 oils, present in fish, soybeans, flaxseed oil, canola oil, wheat germ, and walnuts, have been shown to reduce heart disease. We recommend (and the FDA/EPA guidelines also suggest) that you eat no more than 12 ounces of fish each week and limit canned tuna to an occasional serving. Avoid shark, swordfish, king mackerel, and tilefish (also called golden or white snapper), tuna steak (fresh or frozen), orange roughy, Spanish mackerel, marlin, and grouper because these fish are at the top of the food chain and contain the highest levels of mercury.

✔ **Soy:** Some studies have shown that a very high soy intake may decrease fertility, and soy may disturb thyroid function, decreasing fertility. The recommendation: Skip the soy or limit it severely.

Soy is a source of phytoestrogens, weak estrogens that can enhance or suppress natural estrogen production. Knowing whether you produce enough, or too much, estrogen on your own is a part of the diagnostic process in your fertility treatment. Confusing the matter with outside sources of estrogen will do just that — confuse the matter. Keep it simple.

Good nutrition is something that you should *not* ignore. Consider it common sense, as well as medical sense, that the healthier your body is, the healthier all its systems, including the reproductive system, are. Nutrition is part of the bigger picture that also includes such basics as getting enough sleep, exercising, and nourishing your body as well as your mind. Although good nutrition is rarely the sole factor that brings about a baby, it does help to better preserve your overall health so that you may enjoy your future child as well, and as long, as possible.

If you choose to opt for a complete nutritional overhaul, realize that this is a long-term commitment and is unlikely to produce a quick fix for your fertility issues. Books such as *The Infertility Diet: Get Pregnant and Prevent Miscarriage,* by Fern Reiss, can provide you with a menu plan of fertility foods if you want to try a complete dietary overhaul. For most people, this is a major lifestyle change and may lead to better overall health. On the fertility front, however, keep your expectations in check; diet changes alone are unlikely to get you pregnant. And conversely, it is unlikely that your dietary habits, whatever they are, are playing a large role in your infertility.

For those looking to take the more moderate road, consider planning your diet around the major food groups that we discuss in Chapter 2. You may also choose to consult a nutritionist to make sure that you get the proper balance of vitamins and minerals. A good diet is a good idea whether you're trying to conceive or not.

The Controversy over Estrogen

The debate over possible side effects from the use of estrogen supplementation in menopause and in birth control pills (estrogen is the main hormone responsible for female sex characteristics) has been raging since time began. (But, really, it only *seems* that way.) Estrogen comes in several different forms; the form most familiar to women is the synthetic estrogen called ethinyl estradiol, which is found in birth control pills and some forms of hormone replacement therapy.

In 2005, the National Institutes of Health released the results of a long-term study of more than 11,000 women on the effects of estrogen on post-menopausal women undergoing hormone replacement therapy to relieve common menopausal symptoms such as hot flashes, depression, and low libido. This double blind (neither doctor nor patient knew whether the "drug" was in fact estrogen or a placebo) study sought to determine whether the use of estrogen post menopause did in fact decrease the risk of heart disease and/or increase the risk of cancer, primarily of the breast.

The results showed that there was little decrease in the rate of heart disease and an actual increase in the rate of breast cancer. The study was halted immediately and women were advised to exercise caution in the use of hormone replacement therapy. It was suggested that this use be as short term as possible and to be determined through careful discussion between patient and physician as to the benefits and possible risks involved (These findings are still considered controversial and more data are being added. By the time you reach menopause, one hopes some of the controversy will have been resolved.)

However, menopausal estrogen therapy has very little to do with fertility therapy. After all, your ovaries make estrogen (in the form of estradiol), and this is a very important function. You look like a woman because of estradiol! And estradiol is necessary to develop a healthy egg, to thicken the endometrium to get it ready for embryo implantation, to change the cervical mucus to the thin "stretchy" kind, and so on, and so on!

So when your doctor prescribes estrogen to help the uterine lining, or to "support the luteal phase", or even to help women with POF to ovulate (see Chapter 6 for more on POF), this is the same estradiol that your ovaries would be making if everything were going well.

So why is there a warning on the estrogen pills you get from the store, saying you should not take them during pregnancy? Unfortunately, if women accidentally take birth control pills during early pregnancy, the hormones may have a bad effect on the fetus (girl fetuses can have changes in their genitals that make them look more "masculinized"). However, birth control pills contain not only synthetic estrogen in the form of ethinyl estradiol, but also a synthetic progestin (usually a derivative of testosterone), which has the ability to cross the placenta and have effects on the developing fetus. Even though this has nothing to do with natural estradiol, the drug companies are obliged to put a warning on all forms of estrogen.

Hormones are not necessarily bad; in fact, they are needed to make pregnancy happen. If in doubt, ask your doctor, and make sure that all the hormones you take are "natural" and not "synthetic."

Looking at Supplements — Vitamins, Minerals, Herbs, and More

Dietary supplements are very popular; one survey shows that over 40 percent of all Americans use some form of supplement. Dietary supplements include herbs, vitamins, minerals, amino acids, enzymes, and extracts. Because they're considered a dietary product rather than a medicinal product, they aren't regulated by the U.S. Food and Drug Administration the way prescription medications are. This lack of regulation means that the ingredient amount may vary from one pill to the next. Supplements have also been found to be contaminated with animal parts and toxic molds in some cases.

Because they're sold over the counter, without a prescription, supplements are often viewed as harmless. Studies have shown that many supplements are far from harmless. Some supplements, such as ephedra, have been implicated in causing death, and others, such as comfrey, can cause severe liver damage.

Yet many naturopaths, who believe that the body will heal itself if kept in proper balance, and herbalists tout supplements as a way to help get (and stay) pregnant. Internet sites abound with happy moms claiming that supplements were responsible for their pregnancies. So who do you believe, and are there any supplements that you absolutely should not take?

Herbs

Although herbs have been used for centuries, studies on their safety and benefits have been few. That's beginning to change, with the National Institutes of Health (NIH) now studying many herbs and other alternative medications. Herbs aren't always benign, and someone with some knowledge of their interactions should oversee their use. Practitioners in this area may include chiropractors, osteopaths, nutritionists, and naturopaths (those who employ a drugless approach to keep the body in balance).

Here's a look at some of the more popular herbs used in the treatment of infertility. This list represents a small sample of herbs that can be used and represents herbs that are both Western in origin as well as Chinese.

- ✔ **Black cohosh:** An herb with estrogenic qualities, black cohosh is often used to relieve the discomfort associated with menopause (hot flashes, for example). Studies have been mixed on whether black cohosh is effective. Black cohosh is also recommended to boost estrogen production, although there's no proof that this works. Side effects of black cohosh are dizziness, nausea, low pulse rate, and increased perspiration.

- ✔ **Dong quai:** Dubbed the "ultimate herb" for women, dong quai is used for everything from restoring menstrual regularity to treating menopausal symptoms. Dong quai is a blood thinner and should not be taken during an IVF cycle or by women who have very heavy periods.

- ✔ **False unicorn root:** Native Americans used this herb to improve menstrual irregularities and to alleviate problems associated with menopause and problems with infertility due to irregular follicular formation.

- ✔ **Nettle leaves:** This herb is considered to be an overall uterine tonic that better prepares the uterus for implantation of the embryo. (There is no scientific evidence for this.)

- ✔ **Primrose oil:** A fatty acid, primrose oil may increase cervical mucus to make it easier for sperm to get to the egg. An unwanted side effect of primrose oil may be thinning of the uterine lining, making implantation more difficult.

- ✔ **Red clover:** This herb is often used to boost estrogen in a women's body. This exogenous, or outside the body, form of estrogen may raise your estrogen levels artificially, which is meaningless if the rise isn't caused by the production of a mature egg.

✔ **Red raspberry leaves:** Another uterine toner, this herb reportedly increases the uterine lining thickness (in order to make the uterus more receptive to the embryo). Red raspberry causes uterine contractions and absolutely should not be used in early pregnancy.

✔ **Vitex:** Also known as chaste tree berry, this herb has been used by herbalists for many years to help regulate women's hormones. Some use Vitex to increase luteinizing hormone levels and help an egg release. According to others, Vitex can also increase progesterone levels and should be used only after you ovulate — not before. If taken earlier, it may keep you from releasing an egg. If taken in the luteal phase, after you ovulate, it may regulate and lengthen your cycle to give the embryo a chance to implant. Vitex is slow acting, so it may take several months for any effect to occur.

✔ **Wild yam:** In large doses, wild yam is used as a contraceptive; in smaller doses, it may promote progesterone production. Don't take wild yam until after ovulation occurs.

The following herbs stimulate the uterus so you absolutely should not take them after you get pregnant:

✔ Black cohosh

✔ Dong quai

✔ False unicorn root

✔ Feverfew

✔ Goldenseal

✔ Pennyroyal

In addition, avoid these drugs if you get pregnant:

✔ Blue cohosh: May cause fetal heart defects

✔ Mugwort: May cause fetal abnormalities

Herbal treatment of infertility is not a do-it-yourself approach! Let all your doctors know whether you're taking any kinds of herbs, whether they're the over-the-counter variety or prescribed to you by another source. Undesirable reactions may occur between one herb preparation and another. In addition, they may all cross-react with the drugs your reproductive endocrinologist is giving you. Deciding what to take on your own is complicated, because the same herb may be described as useful for two entirely opposing actions. Telling your doctor that you are taking supplements is the very least that you should do!

Lydia Pinkham's tonic

For half a century, Lydia Pinkham's Vegetable Compound was a best-selling "medicinal" used by women for a variety of female complaints, including problems with menstruation and symptoms of menopause. Whether the drug was so beloved because of its high black cohosh content or the 36-proof alcohol in the bottle is something we'll never know. But if you have an old bottle of this sitting around somewhere (it's still manufactured, but with different ingredients), don't dump it — antique collectors will be glad to take it off your hands!

Vitameatavegamin and all that jazz

A good multivitamin has the correct amounts of the vitamins you need, so rarely do you need to supplement with additional vitamins. Your body takes in only what it needs from water soluble vitamins (generally the maximum recommended daily dose found in most multivitamins) and urinates out the rest (talk about good money down the drain!). In addition, overdoing it on some vitamins can cause adverse reactions in your system. Excess amounts of fat soluble vitamins, such as vitamin A, are stored in your body instead of being excreted. Although adequate levels of vitamin A help to preserve your vision and immune system, an excess of vitamin A can result in liver disease and birth defects when taken by pregnant women. So, yes, you can really have too much of a good thing.

Overdosing on vitamins *through foods alone* is highly unlikely. Because most foods contain small amounts of any individual vitamin or nutrient, you would have to eat bushels of bananas, oranges, or spinach to get too much. Overdosage of any particular vitamin, mineral, or nutrient is generally only a danger if you consume it in a concentrated form, such as vitamin pills or powders.

Is taking a prenatal vitamin when trying to conceive premature? Not really. The primary difference between multivitamins and prenatal vitamins is the greater concentration of folic acid and iron in a prenatal vitamin. Folic acid is crucial in pregnancy to help prevent spinal and neural tube defects, while iron is often needed as a supplement for the loss of iron due to pregnancy. An excess of iron *can* result in constipation, which can be remedied through the introduction of additional fibers, fruits, and vegetables in your diet, a good thing no matter where you are on the baby-making quest.

Over-the-counter (OTC) prenatal vitamins may boast that they contain even higher levels of the necessary vitamins and nutrients. In order to achieve this, however, the OTC brand may require dosages up to three times a day while prescription prenatal vitamins pack their punch in one dose per day. If you're feeling childlike, even though you're not with child yet, you can also get the same ingredients of a prenatal vitamin by taking three Flintstones Complete vitamins per day.

If you're taking a standard multivitamin rather than prenatal vitamins while pregnant, make sure that it doesn't contain extra ingredients such as herbs. Many health food stores sell blends that contain herbs. Don't take these types of vitamins during pregnancy.

Are certain vitamins, taken in greater (or lesser) quantity, more likely to result in increased fertility? At the time of this writing, no direct evidence supports this. We advise you to stick with a standard multivitamin or prenatal vitamin. Your local pharmacist can recommend a good OTC brand, and your doctor can steer you toward a good prescription choice.

Some studies have shown that liquid prenatal vitamins are better absorbed than pills. They may also be less likely to make you nauseated after you become pregnant.

All the vitamins in the world won't get you pregnant, but they will help you keep your body in the best nutritional shape possible, along with proper diet, exercise, and general care. This balanced state is the best place for babies to come from!

Folic acid

Folic acid, a B vitamin, is essential when trying to get pregnant. Many studies have shown that 0.4 mg of folic acid a day cuts the chance of having a baby with neural tube defects by 50 percent. Neural tube defects occur in 6 of 10,000 births in the United States and include problems with the spine and brain. Neural tube defects develop very early in pregnancy, in the first four weeks, so taking a good multivitamin containing this amount while trying to get pregnant is essential. Many foods, including leafy green vegetables, fortified cereals, orange juice, and lean beef, contain folic acid, but overcooking can destroy folic acid, so take a vitamin even if you eat well.

Wheatgrass

For Jackie, it was a litmus test. When she dropped a wheatgrass pill on the floor, her basset hound (also known as the canine garbage disposal) raced toward it. Before she could grab it, he had it in his mouth. Then, to her disbelief, the dog, who has been known to view dead squirrel as a delicacy, dropped the wheatgrass pill and scurried away. It was not a testament to taste.

Despite Jackie's dog's opinion, many others claim that taking regular shots of wheatgrass (meaning a liquid taken in a shot *glass,* not through injection) or a daily handful of pills has lowered their FSH (follicle-stimulating hormone) levels, allowing for better egg production and/or egg quality.

Ann Wigmore, the mother of wheatgrass

Wheatgrass as a way to good health was popularized by Ann Wigmore (1909–1994), who immigrated to the United States at a young age from Eastern Europe. She believed that wheatgrass cured the insanity of King Nebuchadnezzar in the Old Testament after he was forced to live on grasses for seven years while wandering the fields. She also believed that the fact that animals ate grass when they were ill showed the value of eating various grasses. Her ideas became well known through her many books on the subject of raw diet and through her Hippocratic Health Institute. She was sued several times for claiming her elixir could cure AIDS or prevent cancer. Her institute is still active as the Wigmore Foundation. "Dr. Ann," as she was known, had no medical degree and was a self-taught naturopath. (Naturopaths believe that the body will heal itself if balance is maintained.)

What is wheatgrass anyway? Wheatgrass is a dark, leafy, green vegetable that can be harvested, dried, and bottled in pill form. Some people attest that the homegrown or fresh-grown variety is better and raise their own wheatgrass from seed, later shaving off the grass and blending it into a questionable-looking green froth. Many health food stores do this blending for you; however, *you* still must drink the stuff. In all honesty, wheatgrass juice is fairly flavorless, with a slightly sweet taste and an aroma similar to, well, freshly cut grass! You probably won't find a wheatgrass-flavored Blizzard at Dairy Queen anytime soon, however. Many people follow up a wheatgrass shot with a "chaser" of fresh vegetable juice.

Wheatgrass is an antioxidant, meaning that it can cleanse your body of impurities and toxins. It's also used to build hemoglobin (iron stores) in the blood, reduce blood pressure, and keep your hair from going gray.

Regarding the claims that wheatgrass lowers FSH levels and thus improves the number and/or quality of eggs, remember that you're born with a limited number of eggs that only decrease over time. There is virtually no way to increase that number or to change a bad egg into a good one. FSH is merely a measurement of ovarian reserve and is generally checked to determine the probable response to stimulation via fertility medicines.

L-arginine

L-arginine is another example of a product that has received cult status over the past few years for treating everything from immune disorders to sexual problems. L-arginine is a nonessential amino acid found in whole wheat, rice, nuts, seeds, corn, soy, grapes, carob, and other foods. Nonmedical individuals in the fertility community have used L-arginine (also known as arginine) in concentrated pill form during fertility cycles in efforts to improve egg quality. Some studies also show increased blood flow to the uterus. In males, some studies (but not all) have shown increased sperm motility and production when taking L-arginine.

A study published by the professional journal *Human Reproduction* pointed out a negative effect of L-arginine if you're taking fertility medications. The study showed that in a small test group, the use of L-arginine supplementation was detrimental to embryo quality and pregnancy rate during a sample cycle when the test also used fertility medicines.

If you're prone to cold sores, L-arginine may exacerbate them. Use with caution.

Like many supplements, L-arginine can cause adverse reactions at higher doses when taken in pill form as a supplement. It is virtually impossible to overdose on the amount of L-arginine found in foods, as even foods that contain it have it only in trace amounts. However, L-arginine can reach less than desirable levels when taken in more concentrated forms, such as pills. Pregnant women are advised not to use L-arginine.

Natural doesn't necessarily mean safe. If your fertility doctor prescribes any medication for you, let him or her know of any other herbs, pills, or treatments that you're already taking, in order to prevent a possible harmful drug interaction.

A walk down the aisle at a local "health food supplement" store to peruse the ingredients in all the bottles t may shock you! There are "natural" remedies that were made from animal thyroid glands, adrenal glands, and other parts of animals. Yet nowhere on the label does it warn the consumer that products made from animal thyroid glands contain thyroid hormone, which is identical to the one made by humans! This thyroid hormone is available without a prescription, in purity that could not be assessed and in doses that could not be determined! And products made from adrenal glands of course contain adrenal hormones, which include steroids (such as cortisol), adrenalin, and so on. All of these can and do have real physiologic effects on humans, and those trying to conceive are especially vulnerable.

Supplements for better sperm production

Fertility is not just a female issue. In fact, 40 percent of the time, male factor is responsible for a couple's failure to conceive.

So women aren't the only ones who may venture onto an alternative path for treating medical problems related to infertility. Keep in mind that studies have been mixed (at best) as to the efficacy of taking supplements. Also remember that in male problems where surgery is deemed necessary (to fix a varicocele or any other structural issue), diet and/or supplements won't do the trick. These tips, however, can benefit overall health, which can contribute to better reproductive health. A man produces new sperm every three months, so what you do today can theoretically affect conception down the line. The following supplements have been suggested to benefit sperm count and motility in some studies (but note that as with women, no conclusive evidence exists, and, just as with women, too much of a good thing can be quite toxic, never mind counterproductive):

- **Zinc:** Suggested to increase sperm motility and sperm count
- **Vitamin B12:** Suggested to increase sperm count
- **Vitamin C:** Suggested to increase sperm count
- **Vitamin E:** Suggested to increase sperm motility
- **Selenium:** Suggested to increase sperm motility
- **L-Carnitine:** Suggested to increase sperm motility and sperm count
- **L-arginine:** Suggested to increase sperm motility and sperm count
- **Folic acid:** Suggested to increase sperm motility and sperm count
- **CoQ10:** Suggested to increase sperm motility and sperm count

A good multivitamin will generally contain an adequate amount of all of the preceding.

Visiting a Traditional Chinese Medicine Practitioner

Traditional Chinese medicine (TCM), often referred to as Eastern medicine, works on a different set of principles and beliefs than Western medicine (that which is practiced in the United States and many other parts of the world). Traditional Chinese medicine views the individual as an integral mind/body organism and, in essence, believes that a delicate balance, the yin and yang, is necessary for optimal health and well-being. TCM divides the body into various *meridians,* or pathways, along which *qi,* or energy, flows. For example, fertility problems might be explained by liver qi stagnation, that is, congestion in the liver meridian. Primary treatment in TCM includes the administration of herbal formulas and acupuncture to clear the body passageways and restore normal function.

Although traditional Chinese medicine has been practiced since 204 B.C., only during the past two decades has it been recognized in the United States and other parts of the world. According to Western medicine, anecdotal evidence, as demonstrated in TCM, awaits confirmation in randomized clinical trials.

Despite this lack of scientific evidence, many patients, suffering from diseases ranging from cancer to chronic fatigue to infertility, have found a haven in the TCM community, which many times is warmer and fuzzier than the classic Western doctor/hospital setting. Some who have given up on Western medicine (or on whom Western medicine has given up) have found palliative relief, remission, and results under the guidance of a traditional Chinese medicine doctor.

Before you jump on the TCM bandwagon, check the credentials of the practitioner whom you select. TCM doctors must complete training, just as they do in Western medicine, and should be licensed or certified (if your state offers this). In addition, they should be nationally certified through the National Certification Commission for Acupuncture and Oriental Medicine. To confirm certification, visit the commission's Web site at www.nccaom.org.

Help from herbal formulas

Your TCM practitioner may prescribe an herbal formula containing up to ten different herbs. The combination of herbs to create a formula is one of the main differences between the Western and Eastern views. TCM relies on this ability to modify formulas in order to customize an individual approach based on a patient's needs. TCM herbal formulas are also available in pills that can be purchased from your TCM practitioner; however, they're considered to be less effective due to the extraction process necessary to convert them into this form.

Because there are over 6,000 herbs from which to choose, this formulation is a science in and of itself and, unlike the single-ingredient, Western herb approach, can't be self-administered.

Most TCM practitioners also use *moxibustion,* in which small mounds of herbs are burned over certain areas of the body, in the treatment of infertility. TCM practitioners also treat male infertility issues, so feel free to go as a couple.

Don't view traditional Chinese medicine as a shortcut. Nothing in medicine ever is. The treatments require consistency and commitment, but they may provide you with a more palatable process than Western treatments.

We also recommend that you "pick your poison," for lack of a better term. Whether your treatment is traditional Chinese medicine or Western medicine, don't try to combine the two. Many herbs, when taken with fertility medicines, can cause adverse reactions. Particularly when combined with treatments that involve surgical procedures, such as in vitro fertilization, the ingestion of herbs or other tonics can cause more severe problems, such as bleeding, or simply complicate matters. As a result, both your TCM doctor and your Western doctor may find it impossible to accurately define and treat your condition.

If you choose to try both TCM and Western medicine simultaneously (despite our suggestions to the contrary), make sure that all of your practitioners, doctors, and nurses, are aware of your protocol. Not revealing this information is an ideal way to confuse the people whose goals are to help you conceive.

On pins and needles — acupuncture for infertility

Perhaps one area of traditional Chinese medicine that has benefited the most from the recent interest on behalf of Western medicines is acupuncture. Acupuncture is based on the belief that a person's health is determined by a balanced flow of energy (qi) in the body. This 5,000-year-old practice is most often used to relieve chronic pain by inserting needles into a variety of pressure points on the head and body. Acupuncture is also used for treatments for everything from the common cold to drug addiction.

In April 2002, a study in the prestigious medical journal *Fertility and Sterility* cited evidence that acupuncture, when used in conjunction with in vitro fertilization, notably improved pregnancy rates. In the study involving 160 patients, acupuncture was performed just prior to the transfer of embryos into the uterus and again after the transfer took place. Needles were inserted along the spleen and stomach meridians, as well as other sites, in an effort to stimulate blood flow to the uterus. Of the acupuncture group, 42 percent got pregnant, compared to 26 percent of the nonacupuncture group. The sedative effect of acupuncture is also believed to assist in relaxing a woman, quieting her uterus, and making it more receptive to embryos.

Although this study will require additional follow-up to make sure that the previous results were not psychosomatic and are indeed repeatable, the findings were certainly of great interest to those in the fertility community.

Acupuncture has long been a popular alternative form of treatment for infertility. Many women have used this treatment in hopes of increasing blood flow to the uterus, thus helping to thicken the uterine lining. Other women have found that acupuncture has been crucial in helping them relax through the trials and tribulations of fertility treatment.

Whether its effects are actually physiological or not, acupuncture is an excellent adjunct to a fertility regimen. However, be sure that those performing the treatment are certified. Many fertility clinics work in conjunction with an acupuncturist and/or can recommend someone who specializes in fertility-based treatment.

Many states have their own acupuncture society, and some states have specific requirements that must be met. For example, in Indiana, people need a prescription from a physician in order to be treated by a certified acupuncturist. You can check online for your state's rules and regulations, as well as for acupuncture societies, which may also provide you with specific recommendations.

If you're scared of being stuck with acupuncture needles, take heart! The average acupuncture needle has the thickness of a human hair. You may feel a small stick, but it's far less discomfort than a blood test. But if you're still a bit apprehensive and too needle-phobic about the procedure, you may be better off skipping this particular form of treatment. Remember that the goal is to relax.

Bring along a favorite tape or CD to listen to during acupuncture treatment. Most acupuncture treatments require you to lie still with the needles in place for a short period of time, usually 20 minutes or less. This may also be a great time to use your visualization techniques (see "The Eyes Have It: Visualizing Your Baby," later in this chapter).

The Eyes Have It: Visualizing Your Baby

Have you ever come across an individual who appeared to set her mind on something and ultimately achieve it? Some credit this ability to positive thinking, while others say it's dumb luck.

Philosophers through the ages have said that if you change your mind, you change your life. Now, no amount of positive thinking will reverse uterine or tubal scarring that may be preventing conception, but your attitude can certainly help you walk whatever path you're on with greater ease and peace.

A study conducted by the American Society of Reproductive Medicine (ASRM, the medical organization for fertility professionals) saw a marked improvement in the response of in vitro fertilization patients who showed a more positive attitude going into the process. These findings were noted in the number of eggs produced, quality of eggs, and the overall pregnancy rate. Indeed, very few people doubt the negative impact of stress on all areas of your life and your health.

Visualizing your goal, whether it's to move peacefully through the process of fertility or to imagine the feeling of holding your own child, is a wonderful tool for both relaxation and focus. Legions have sworn by the teachings of Shakti Gawain, Deepak Chopra, and others whose books and tapes can lead you through the journey to your goals. Visualization can help you identify the skills (such as persistence, patience, or diligence) that can help you reach your goal and can also help you name and let go of those traits that may stand in your way.

How do you spell relief? R-e-l-a-x

Medical researchers have known for some time about what's called *relaxation response,* which is defined as a series of physiological changes that occur when a person blocks out intrusive thoughts by repeating a word, a sound, a phrase, or a prayer. Relaxation response can cause a decrease in metabolism, heart rate, rate of breathing, and brain wave activity.

When used in conjunction with nutrition and exercise, relaxation response has been proven to be effective therapy in treating a number of conditions, including cardiac disease, chronic pain, symptoms associated with cancer and HIV/AIDS, anxiety, mild and moderate depression, and the stress brought on by infertility and its treatments.

Some research says that infertile women are twice as likely to experience depressive symptoms as fertile women. No matter how large or small the effect may be, excessive stress and depression can certainly contribute to or exacerbate infertility.

Jackie participated in a six-week program that applied the techniques of relaxation response conducted by a nurse who worked for a local fertility clinic. Although she was initially skeptical about the benefits, she did find the relaxation techniques, nutritional information, open dialogue, and camaraderie to be helpful. Partners were invited to participate in the last class of the session, where everyone focused on communication skills to better express their individual problems and fears related to their infertility and treatment. She enjoyed this opportunity immensely, and her husband appreciated the refreshments.

To find out more about workshops in relaxation response in your area, ask your doctor (ideally your OB/GYN or a fertility specialist) or contact your local chapter of Resolve by visiting www.resolve.org.

Jackie found moments of peace, along with the occasional glide into a nap, while listening to Shakti Gawain's *Creative Visualization* tape. She listened to that tape on her personal tape player while waiting in many a fertility doctor's office and found that it helped her escape a difficult or painful situation by refocusing her thoughts. This consistent, positive reinforcement helped her to turn down the volume on the voices of naysayers, including herself.

Saying Om: Meditation and Yoga

For those who need a little more help than self-help, consider the structure of a class such as meditation or yoga. Although they're not cure-alls, these ancient arts can go a long way in easing your body and spirit.

Staying sane through the process is a goal that can carry you through your fertility rites. This goal is something you *can* control, and meditation or yoga can help. Check with your local gyms or wellness centers to see whether they have classes. Or ask your family or fertility doctor to recommend a particular class or instructor. You may be surprised at how many medical folks use the same techniques to bring peace to their own lives.

Both meditation and yoga can carry you through your pregnancy as well. Meditation can help relieve the discomfort and pain of everything from morning sickness to labor, and yoga can keep your gestating (or pregnant!) body fit and focused all the way through.

Massaging Away What Ails You

If you're more relaxed with a hands-on approach, consider massage. Although no evidence proves that regular massage improves fertility or increases the likelihood of pregnancy, few people question its ability to relax the body and mind. And although relaxation itself won't get you pregnant, it certainly makes the fertility process a little more tolerable.

Consider massage as a healthy, lowfat, guiltless way to reward yourself as you go through the fertility process (or any other stress-producing activity for that matter!). If the hormones, either naturally produced or artificially added, are getting you down, schedule a Swedish massage. Other, more vigorous forms of massage, such as shiatsu, may be useful in energizing your body. Some people believe that massage helps promote better blood flow.

Although massage can be very beneficial, make sure that your massage therapist knows that you're trying to conceive. Massaging certain areas can be harmful during pregnancy. Your massage therapist should be aware that you could be pregnant during this process, and she should be skilled in what areas to focus on and what areas to avoid.

A few clinics nationwide claim high success rates with the practice of deep muscle massage and internal massage to reduce or eliminate scar tissue such as endometriosis and other types of structural anomalies that might prevent pregnancy. Little proof supports these claims, as no one has shown that massaging away excess or scar tissue is possible. Take great care if pursuing this type of treatment. Internal massage can be detrimental, if not just painful, expensive, and altogether unnecessary.

Distinguishing the glitter from the goods

As with anything that involves entrusting your mind, body, or heart, it's important to know just WHO the trustworthy people and practices may be. As Alternative Medicine has grown, so have the resources that support it.

The National Institutes of Health (NIH), long considered the Gold Standard on determining protocol in the medical field, is now also dipping their feet in the water when it comes to alternative medicines and treatment. The National Center for Alternative and Complimentary Medicine is now a department of NIH, designed to investigate the efficacy, safety, and mechanisms of action of diverse complementary and alternative medicine (CAM) modalities. More definitive findings on many varieties of treatments will become available in the coming years. For now, you can check their Web site at nccam.nih.gov to keep up with the latest findings.

As we mentioned earlier, some clinics and physicians are working with one or more alternative providers in order to offer these options to patients. Ask your doctor or nurse if your facility works with anyone in particular (in whatever specialty area in which you're interested) or if they have recommendations for outside providers.

How about finding out the scoop on who the alternative practitioners in your area are? Services such as The Anji Connection (www.anjiconnection.com) offer a free and interactive Web site to locate alternative providers of all varieties in your city or town. You can use a resource such as this to read up on what different providers offer, charge, and who might best fit your needs. Ultimately, the proof is in the pudding and someone who looks great on paper may not work for you. Consider using resources such as this to narrow your search and then arrange time(s) to meet with the provider(s) by phone or in person to determine if you have the right match.

No one can or should guarantee you success! Physicians are prohibited from making promises due to their professional codes, rules, and regulations. This may not apply to alternative providers. If someone tries to promise you a pregnancy "if only you" (pick one): sign on the dotted line, write a check, make a long term commitment . . . *run!* Alternative medicine is another option for treatment, not a magic cure.

Seeking Help from On High

When you're caught up in the minutiae of fertility management (and there's plenty of minutiae!), you may have trouble seeing your daily struggles as part of a larger plan designed by a power greater than yourself. Whatever your faith, solace and relief are available to you.

Jackie has witnessed many women online and in person walking through the fertility process with confidence as they placed their fears and worries in the hands of their God, a special saint, or an icon. Many chat rooms started their own prayer group. And although many people claim to be disbelievers, the old adage "there are no atheists in foxholes" seems to be true. Online prayer groups grew at a lightning pace, bearing the names of those who were pious by nature, as well as those who just figured prayer couldn't hurt. And it can't.

Through the ages, certain groups have turned to the power of prayer for healing the sick and giving sight to the blind. A study was released in the United States in early 2002 that claimed that patients in a test group who were prayed for by outside individuals made a quicker and better recovery than those who weren't. Some physicians scoff at this notion. However, many people find credence in the idea that prayer helps patients relax and, in doing so, helps them to release whatever stranglehold they may have on their condition and to stop trying to force results. This type of help may make whatever road you travel a little less bumpy.

Individuals and couples may also benefit from the moderation of a third party, such as a priest, rabbi, or other religious figure. These professionals often act as counselors to help an individual or couple work through problems resulting from outside stressors, such as fertility. Religious leaders also respect your privacy and maintain confidences just as a therapist or doctor does. Their consideration of all things spiritual may also help to reveal another point of view or option. If nothing else, your local clergy can provide additional support, something that you can never get enough of, regardless of your situation.

Exercising without Overdoing It

Jackie found that one of the most difficult parts of infertility and its treatments was the loss of certain aspects of her life (for example, free time that she used to have was now spent running from one doctor appointment to another). As an avid runner, Jackie questioned her exercise routine and wondered whether the constant jarring might be preventing her from getting pregnant. She asked her doctor, who recommended moderate exercise. Jackie's not the type of person who understands the word *moderate,* regardless of its context. She decided not to take any chances and replaced running with a workout on a stair-climbing machine. After a few more months of failed attempts at pregnancy, she reevaluated the stair-climbing workout as well. And so it went until she was reduced to walking, which also became a personal no-no during the two-week wait after the time of ovulation. As the fertility bar seemed to get higher and higher, her stress management tools, such as exercise, had diminished to almost nothing. It was not a pretty sight.

Regular exercise is a good thing when trying to conceive, just as it is at almost any time in your life (except maybe when you're in traction). The key is to participate in moderate (there's that word again) activity that's consistent with your past routines. For example, if your previous exercise plan consisted of wind sprints to the refrigerator and back, training for your first marathon while trying to conceive isn't a wise idea. Some doctors recommend keeping your heart rate to a maximum of 140 beats per minute. You can use this as a guide to help build your exercise plan. When it comes to nonaerobic activity, the sky is (virtually) the limit. Again, use common sense when making your choices. Full-contact boxing may be a bit more precarious during this time (actually during any time!), but kickboxing for fitness could be a good compromise.

If you're someone who overexercises as a means to lose weight, your behavior could affect your fertility. Check with your doctor to make sure that you're within the proper weight limits. Carrying too little weight can affect your menstrual cycle as well as your hormones, therefore compromising your ability to conceive.

Above all, no matter what exercise in which you engage, stay well hydrated at all times. Doing so is especially important when trying to conceive and even more so while pregnant. Wear comfortable clothing and be aware of how you feel at all times. Exercise shouldn't be painful — ever! If it is, stop, rest, and consult a trainer or exercise physiologist before resuming your routine.

Ironically, after tiring of her lack of exercise and treating her body as though it was spun glass, Jackie began running again during her third year of trying to conceive. After one month of resuming her former exercise routine, she found out she was pregnant. Go figure.

Evaluating the Good and the Bad of Antidepressants

Few conditions seem to warrant the use of an antidepressant more than infertility. The insecurity brought on by the inability to conceive, the physical and psychological stress associated with treatment, and the repeated disappointments seem to be the perfect setup for creating a person in need of a little more help. Indeed, infertile women are twice as likely to experience depression as fertile women.

As with all things medical, refrain from diagnosing yourself. No matter how much your symptoms fit the latest commercial for Paxil, Prozac, or Zoloft, you still need to be evaluated by a psychiatrist (the only *mental health* professional who can prescribe medication).

Your fertility doctor can, and may, offer to put you on antidepressants to help you over the hump. Some doctors aren't sure of the long-term effects and may prefer to avoid them. Still other physicians use antidepressants as part of their fertility treatments (particularly when addressing immune issues). Be aware, however: Antidepressants aren't benign medications, and you shouldn't take them as such. You're better off being evaluated by a doctor who specializes in this area. Your fertility doctor, general practitioner, or therapist can certainly refer you to an appropriate specialist. You can also ask for recommendations from friends or family if you feel comfortable doing so, or you can contact your local mental health center and keep your request anonymous.

Don't start taking your sister's or your best friend's antidepressant prescription. These drugs are individually dosed, based on a person's needs, size, and medical history.

No significant long-term studies have been done on the effects of antidepressants on fertility. The jury is still out on these relatively new medications (which have been on the market 20 years or less), and no conclusive results of the effect of these medications on fertility may be available for many years.

Antidepressants, however, do have some side effects that may affect fertility. Decreased sexual desire is among the possible reactions, possibly opening the door to other reproductive interaction. Antidepressants can also dry up cervical mucus, which is crucial in transporting the sperm to the egg and in helping to build up the uterine lining. You and your fertility doctor are the best judge as to whether you're experiencing these side effects.

Ultimately, as with most medications, you must weigh the pros and cons when deciding whether to take antidepressants. Depression can be consuming and can affect your health, work, relationships, and, consequently, your fertility. If you're suffering through this, the uncertain risks of antidepressants may be far outweighed by your need for relief.

Taking a Break from Your Fertility "Job" — You Deserve It

When all else fails to help you relax, consider taking off, whether that's a break from your efforts or a real vacation!

Fertility often becomes a job with no benefits and dismal working conditions. Just like any job, time off is necessary in order to clean your mind, refresh your spirit, and come back to greet another day with your best efforts.

Many individuals and couples take anywhere from a few weeks to a few years off from the process of trying to conceive. This doesn't mean adhering to a celibate lifestyle. Instead, it's a reintroduction to sex sans schedule, trying to conceive a baby the old-fashioned way. Obviously, your age and condition are critical in determining just how much time away from fertility treatment you can spare, but a short respite will probably do nothing *but* refresh you. Try to avoid feeling guilty for needing the break. Actually, in giving your mind and body the time and space they need, you're taking the best possible care of yourself. And don't minimize your partner's need for a break either. He may need a respite from "performing" on demand, undergoing batteries of tests, or just providing you with the support you need, but he may not feel comfortable suggesting it.

Getting away from the daily grind also helps you to gain a better perspective and make decisions that best suit you, your partner, and your living style. Some people can do this by taking a fertility-free weekend that includes no discussion of anything to do with physicians, fertility, treatments, or future plans. Others find it necessary to truly get away from home. You'll be amazed by the perspective and peace that you can gain from a well-needed vacation. And although we don't advise planning a vacation with the hidden agenda of making this getaway the one that does the trick, perhaps it will! In the meantime, throw caution and your medical records to the wind and relax. Your baby will wait for you.

Chapter 9

Are We Having Fun Yet? Trying to Conceive and Your Relationship

● ●

In This Chapter

▶ Staying in touch with your partner's feelings — and your own

▶ Surviving the effects of stress on your relationship

▶ Seeing a counselor

● ●

"*W*hy oh why can't a 'growth experience' ever be fun?" lamented a popular sitcom character in a line that drew plenty of canned and real laughs. While making a baby certainly has all the right ingredients for a good time, once infertility is stirred into the pot, fun becomes a concept reserved for those for whom sex has remained — well, just sex.

In this chapter, we discuss how to traverse the lost and found sections of the couples fun department. While infertility certainly has its share of growth opportunities, which are anything but a good time, your relationship can actually grow in a positive manner, helping you and your partner learn ways to support and love one another through the rough spots. Consider all these learning experiences good practice for the many challenges that child rearing will offer you!

Navigating the Relationship Pitfalls of Infertility

Experiencing infertility can take your relationship to a whole new level—one you could probably live without. Human relationships are rarely improved by the addition of stress, frustration, anger and recriminations, at least not until the crisis is over and some perspective on the situation can be gained.

The potential loss of a dream as big as a family of your own can be devastating in a number of ways. The pitfalls you fall into while trying to navigate the uncharted waters of infertility will depend on your personalities, the way you relate to each other normally, and sometimes just on the time of day or the weather! In the next sections, we look at some of the common relationship challenges couples dealing with infertility may face.

This is easy! Early misconceptions about conception

Most couples start trying to get pregnant with barely a thought that success might not be immediate. Most couples are more afraid to start trying too soon, worrying more that they'll get pregnant the first month of trying. It usually comes as a complete shock to discover that pregnancy can, even under normal conditions, take up to six months or more to achieve.

A few months of negative pregnancy tests can be hard to process, intellectually and emotionally, when everyone else seems to be able to get pregnant so easily. "I never thought I'd be at this point," Jackie remembers lamenting to herself, and anyone else who would listen. Married at 34, she had been trying to conceive for two years to no avail. Her local doctor had been convinced, and convincing, that she would get her baby through the low-tech intrauterine insemination (IUI) procedures. "You have stingy ovaries," he would say with a wink. "We'll just push you a little harder and hope you don't end up with more than one."

After three failed attempts and increasingly higher doses of medication, that dialogue began to wear thin. Her faith in him and in herself had waned, and she was off to find a new doctor and a more direct line to baby. Now, here she stood contemplating in vitro fertilization (IVF), a $15,000-plus, two-month procedure for what she thought would have been accomplished in one night after a bottle of cheap wine. The mountain was indeed much higher than she thought.

Failing to get pregnant month after month can be especially difficult if one of you is still in the "No problem, we'll just keep trying, it'll happen eventually" mode while the other partner is ready to move on — to a new doctor, medical intervention, or a high tech procedure like IVF. If you're a couple with one laid-back partner and one gung ho partner, you probably know this already. How to cope with mismatched ideas of how to proceed when what seemed easy turns out to be really hard? Talk to each other! One of you may need to lighten up a little and the other may need to "get off the pot" so to speak, so you can proceed at a pace with which you're both comfortable.

It's not my fault — the blame game

Perhaps the most destructive force in any relationship is blame, whether it is deserved or not. All of us can take responsibility for our actions, but for the most part, our reproductive system is what it is, regardless of anything we did or didn't do. Remember, infertility is not punishment, it's biology.

There's almost a perfect balance between male factors and female factors as causes for infertility; 40 percent of the time the problem is due to male issues, 40 percent of infertility is due to female issues, and 20 percent is unexplained — or a combination of the two. With the scales so evenly balanced, there is no rational reason to play the blame game but inevitably, many couples end up in this no-win scenario.

The blame game is a diversion from the true problem of infertility. Consider other diversions instead. Playing cards can be just as competitive without the ill side effects on either one of your psyches.

We should have started sooner — more of the same game

Ah! Another one of those useless diversions . . . we should have known we would have had problems and started earlier! With such perfect 20/20 hind-sight, none of us would need gainful employment.

Waiting until age 50 to conceive might not be the brightest of ideas, unless of course, you are completely willing to use donor eggs, sperm, or both. But, other than an extreme case such as this, second guessing your decision to (pick one) 1. wait for the right person with whom to build your life, 2. put off having a baby to finish school, 3. become financially stable, or 4. improve a tumultuous relationship before bringing a child into it, is futile. These are probably all excellent reasons for putting the brakes on baby making.

Revisiting these choices when you encounter problems is similar to replaying an accident over in your mind, trying to imagine what might have happened had you taken another route. It's over, move on and make the next right decision. Don't waste your time and energy rethinking your motives. Resist the temptation to reinvent history. It doesn't work.

You just don't care! – When one partner seems more committed to conception

You probably won't be surprised to learn that people react to things differently. While one partner's emotions may often rise and fall with each test result, the other person's feelings may not.

One common view of some partners is that the proof is in the baby, not in the myriad details. He (often it's a "he" who has this behavior pattern) may not want to hear daily about your cervical mucus, your possible nausea, your maybe-slightly-a-little-bit-sore breasts, or your latest discussion with your mom about how long it took your cousin Susie to get pregnant. It's not that he doesn't want a baby, it's just that he doesn't want to hear about it ad infinitum. He'll be thrilled when you actually have the baby, but the details in getting the baby are more than he wants to hear.

If you're a micromanager (and many women are, especially when it comes to something as big as getting pregnant), this seeming nonchalance, if not out-right indifference, to the process of baby getting may infuriate you. You may goad your partner with "You just don't care" accusations, which probably aren't true and will probably provoke retaliation in kind, which isn't going to help either of you.

Some men want to talk about something once and then let it go until some-thing actually happens. Women, on the other hand, often want and need to talk things out — not just once, but daily, hourly, or sometimes even every few minutes. Many men seem better able to compartmentalize the things that are going on in their lives than women do, being able to put aside baby con-cerns when watching the Super Bowl, for example. You, on the other hand, may find the Super Bowl a perfect time to talk about baby names, or to wonder out loud if football players ever have infertility issues from wearing those tight pants or from being crushed at the bottom of a five-man pileup.

Once you've been assured — or reassured — once or twice by your partner that yes, he really wants a baby, and yes, he really does care about you and your future offspring, more than life itself, but could he just watch the Super Bowl now without thinking about how hard it must be for the player's wives to get pregnant when they're on the road all the time? Who knows? The score of the Super Bowl may actually have a greater impact on your life in the long run than the fact that your temperature chart looks totally different this month than it did last month. And even if it doesn't, your partner's extreme desire to talk about the game rather than your temperature chart when the game is in overtime is in no way a reflection of what kind of a dad he'll be.

If, on the other hand, you notice real foot dragging on your partner's part when it comes to matters of infertility, you may need to have a serious dis-cussion. Maybe he's got concerns he hasn't brought up; maybe he really isn't as committed to having a baby as you are. If that's the case, it's time to put on the brakes until you can talk things out and find out what each of you is really thinking. Having a baby when one partner isn't sure about the idea is rarely a good idea.

Fun and Games for Two – Remembering How to Enjoy Each Other Again

So sex isn't fun anymore. Dreaming about your family to be causes your eyes to mist up. So how do you bring the fun back into your relationship . . . and your life?

And you're not the only one. It may be hard to believe it, but it's the partner of the fertility patient who primarily faces the problem of loneliness resulting from the pursuit of a baby. While one partner is trying to cope with the possible loss of fertility, the other partner is dealing with a loss of a different sort: the loss of a partner immersed in the facts, figures, and minutiae that can become all-encompassing when trying to conceive. For the fertility patient, the struggle with fertility may bring a great deal of fear and pain, but it can also deliver new friends (real and cyber), enough reading and research to fill a lifetime, and a litany of emotions to sort through. A woman may find herself so busy with these activities that she doesn't even have time for a quiet night with her partner in front of the television.

To help solve this problem, we recommend "fertility-free zones," times and places where the subject is off-limits. Although detaching from what appears to be such a looming issue may be hard, the space created by these mini-vacations allows you to recharge yourselves as a couple and remember what brought you together in the first place.

Fighting with your fertility is a battle best won with kindness, toward yourself and your partner. Here are our suggestions for marking time:

✔ Take the time to appreciate good health; it's not a guarantee, whether you conceive or not.

✔ If you don't have a baby to love yet, direct that energy toward the children and adults who are in your life today. Doing so involves no risks, and the rewards will carry you through this difficult time.

✔ Are you angry? Makes sense to us. Perhaps you can channel that anger into a letter to your congressman lobbying for better healthcare coverage for fertility patients.

✔ Do you feel it's unfair that people you consider undeserving parents get to have the children that you dream of? Step up to the plate and volunteer to be a Big Sister or Big Brother for a child who will truly benefit from your good parenting skills.

✔ Pamper yourself and your body. Get a massage, enjoy fine (and healthy) dining, read a good book, go for a walk, or play with a puppy.

✔ Create a support network. While your old friends are like gold in getting you through this, no one can truly comfort and sustain you quite like another person experiencing the same thing. You'll find plenty of other women and men out there struggling with fertility.

To get pregnant is not a job, a cause, or a raison d'etre. It's a means to an end with the idea of creating a family as the goal. When your mind is too caught up with too many details concerning the problem, you have lost sight of your objective. Step back and let go. It's a great way to get some perspective and some space, for you and your partner.

Getting Some Professional Guidance

Everybody needs a shoulder to cry on from time to time. Those of you going through fertility treatments may need more than one person's shoulders.

Continued communication between you and your partner, devoid of blame and misdirected anger is key to working through the infertility battle as a team. But, sometimes, the hole feels a little too deep, and you may need further professional intervention.

Don't minimize the stress you're under. By acknowledging how difficult this may be for you, realizing that it may not be that difficult for your partner, and recognizing all points in between, you can define your starting point, a necessary step in determining your direction.

Although many of the more complex decisions in fertility treatment require medical guidance, you may find yourself getting stuck in areas that seem far simpler. Perhaps you're overwhelmed, a natural response when the path in front of you seems confusing. Talking about your options with your doctor is certainly one way to get clarity. A therapist, however, can help prevent you from getting bogged down with the small stuff and often help you to realize what's behind it all. Perhaps you're feeling the weight of the world on your shoulders in trying to conceive. Your partner's admonishment to "take it easy" may seem insensitive and unaware. It probably is.

Couples counseling is a great place to have your thoughts and feelings translated into a language that your partner might better understand. Do you find yourself snapping at every mail carrier and store clerk in town? Therapy may be a good place to unburden your frustrations before people scatter at the sight of you. Are you resentful of your or your partner's fertility problems?

Telling one another over dinner may exacerbate the problem, but the helpful mediation of a therapist can allow you to acknowledge your feelings and your partner's and move on.

Many fertility specialists advise the couples they treat to consult a counselor or psychologist, especially one that specializes in fertility. These counselors are particularly adept at dealing with differences in the way men and women deal with the stress of infertility. And because a counselor is not the physician treating you, he/she is often in a better position to offer objective advice about types of treatments, adoption, and so on.

There's an old saying that what doesn't kill you makes you stronger. Therapy is a good place to develop the mental muscle you need to succeed.

Throughout our many years of struggling to conceive their first and then second child, Jackie and her husband actually DID gain a deeper and more loving understanding with one another. As their marriage continued, they learned that life had even more ups and downs than trying to conceive. What they learned through the process of creating a child, however, made them better suited to face other challenges as well.

Part III
Asking for Directions: Finding the Problem

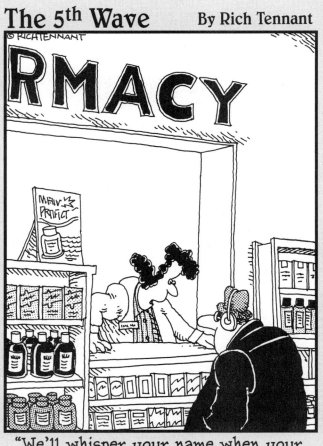

The 5th Wave   By Rich Tennant

"We'll whisper your name when your migraine medication is ready."

In this part . . .

This part explains the tests you may be doing to find out why you haven't gotten pregnant yet; we explain what the tests are and what the results may mean. We also give male factor issues a chapter of their own. We also give you information about miscarriage; why it occurs and what you can do emotionally and physically to overcome recurrent miscarriage.

Chapter 10

Finding the Problem: Testing 1, 2, 3

In This Chapter

▶ Poking and prodding: blood tests and more

▶ Taking a look inside

▶ Diagnosing problems with ovulation

*I*f you haven't gotten pregnant after several months to a year, it may be time to start doing some tests. Your doctor may suggest these tests to you, or you may suggest them to him or her if you feel that time is slipping away and you want to find out why you haven't gotten pregnant yet, or why you can't stay pregnant.

In this chapter, we give you a rundown of the tests that fertility doctors do on women most frequently, why they do them, and what you can expect to learn from the tests. If you're wondering why all the emphasis on you when there are two of you involved in the baby making process, never fear — we address male issues in Chapter 11.

For about 30 percent of couples trying to get pregnant, several problems contribute to infertility. This fact is especially important to remember if one of you has a known factor, such as previous tubal surgery or a known sperm problem. Many couples come to a clinic and tell the staff, "I don't need to do any testing — we already know the problem is him (or her)." You may think that you already know the problem, but keep in mind that for 30 percent of you, tests will reveal another problem, and pregnancy won't occur until both problems are addressed.

Understanding Female Structural Problems

Men's infertility issues seem simple at first because the problem all comes down to sperm: Are they produced, can they get out, and how do they look when they get there? Women's infertility issues can be more complex because so many different systems can be at fault. Is the problem uterine, tubal, hormonal, age related, or ovarian? Any one of these problems can cause enough trouble to prevent you from becoming and staying pregnant.

Looking in the uterus

Maybe you had an HSG to evaluate your fallopian tubes and uterus, which we discuss in the section "HSG (don't even try to spell out the word)," later in this chapter, or maybe you had a hysteroscopic surgery for an even closer look into the uterus. Looking at the uterus is an integral part of any fertility workup because the uterus nourishes and holds a baby for nine months.

Finding fibroids in the uterus

Fibroids, or benign tumors, are commonly found inside or on the outside of the uterus. They're extremely common, with 40 percent of women between the ages of 35 and 55 having at least one. Fibroids are even more common in African-American women, with 50 percent having at least one.

Fibroids can cause bowel or bladder problems, very heavy bleeding, or pain. Fibroids can be either inside or outside the uterine cavity; their location determines whether they cause a problem with your ability to get or stay pregnant. Fibroids completely outside the uterus, such as pedunculated fibroids, which are attached to the uterus by a stem, don't usually cause a problem with fertility.

Subserosal fibroids are located in the outer wall of the uterus and generally don't impinge on the cavity. *Intramural fibroids,* those within the wall of the uterus, can push the uterus in if they grow large enough. *Submucosal fibroids* grow through the lining of the inside wall and can make the cavity too small for a baby to gestate for nine months. In fact, 40 percent of pregnancies will miscarry if submucosal fibroids are present.

Fibroids can be surgically removed, a process called a *myomectomy.* A small fibroid inside the uterus can usually be removed by hysteroscopy, a procedure in which a thin telescope is inserted into the uterus through the vagina. This is outpatient surgery and is relatively atraumatic. In contrast, large intramural fibroids require an abdominal incision and a hospital stay. You generally need to deliver by cesarean section after an abdominal myomectomy.

Removing polyps

Polyps are small fleshy benign growths found on the surface of the endometrium. Very small polyps usually cause no problem with getting pregnant, but larger polyps or multiple polyps can interfere with conception.

Polyps can cause irregular bleeding; they can be diagnosed via sonohystero-gram or hysteroscopy and can be scraped off the endometrium. Polyp removal is called polypectomy.

Checking out the fallopian tubes

Most women have two fallopian tubes, one on each side of the uterus, next to the ovaries. Because these tubes are the transport path from the ovary to the uterus, a problem with one or both tubes can have a big impact on your baby-making ability.

Sometimes a tube is surgically removed after an ectopic pregnancy, a pregnancy that starts to grow in the tube rather than in the uterus. If this pregnancy is found early enough, it may be possible to dissolve the pregnancy with a chemotherapy agent called methotrexate. However, if the fetus grows large enough undetected in the tube, the tube can burst, causing life-threatening bleeding (we discuss this in Chapter 6). The only way to stop the bleeding is to remove the tube.

You can get pregnant with only one tube, but you must be aware that having one ectopic pregnancy leaves you at a higher risk to have another.

Investigating damaged tubes

Women who have only the left ovary and the right fallopian tube can get pregnant because the egg can "float" to the remaining tube. Of course, this also applies to women who have the left tube and the right ovary. (One study estimated that the egg gets picked up by the opposite tube about 30 percent of the time.) Sometimes fallopian tubes are seen to be enlarged on ultrasound or during an HSG. If the tubes are very swollen and dye doesn't flow through them, you may have a *hydrosalpinx,* the medical term for a chronically infected tube (see Figure 10-1). If both tubes are dilated, the condition is known as *hydrosalpinges.*

A hydrosalpinx interferes with pregnancy in two ways:

✔ The egg cannot be picked up by the dilated tube, whose fimbriae (the end) is blocked by scarring.

✔ The embryo, if it makes it to the uterus by traveling down the other tube, or perhaps even being placed there during IVF, may not be able to survive because the infected material from the tube drips down into the uterus, making an inhospitable environment for the embryo to grow.

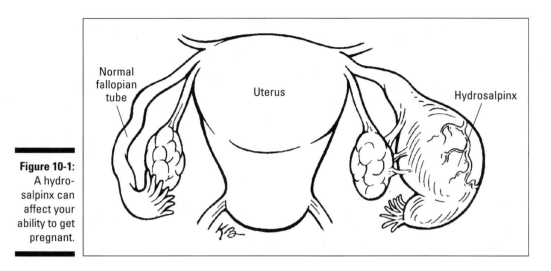

Normal
fallopian
tube

Uterus

Hydrosalpinx

Figure 10-1:
A hydro-
salpinx can
affect your
ability to get
pregnant.

The treatment for a hydrosalpinx is surgical. In mild cases, the end of the tube can be opened and the ends peeled back like a flower. However, in severe cases, the tube will not work even if it is opened. In these cases, the tube or tubes must be removed, and you need to have in vitro fertilization (IVF) to get pregnant because your eggs can no longer float down to the uterus. This diagnosis is a hard thing for many women to accept because it definitely ends any chance that they'll be able to get pregnant on their own.

In very rare cases, women can be born without any fallopian tubes; often the tubes are missing as part of a syndrome in which the external sex organs look normal, but the vagina, uterus, and fallopian tubes are missing. Of course, if you've had two ectopic pregnancies, you may have had both tubes surgically removed also.

Sometimes fallopian tubes look fine on an X-ray but may be surrounded by adhesions (scarring) that prevent them from picking up the egg. (See "Seeing the complications of scar tissue" for more about adhesions and infertility.) *Endometriosis,* tissue growths found anywhere in the pelvis, can grow in or around the fallopian tubes and is a common cause of adhesions around tubes. Normal tubes cannot be visualized by ultrasound.

Because the fallopian tubes play such a large role in getting pregnant, you'll probably need intervention, such as IVF, to get pregnant if a problem is discovered with them. Removal or absence of the tubes, or a blockage that can't be removed, makes IVF inevitable if you're trying to get pregnant.

Seeing the complications of scar tissue

In her years as a labor and delivery nurse, Sharon saw firsthand how scar tissue, or adhesions (as shown in Figure 10-2), can form in your reproductive system. Many women having a second or third cesarean section delivery or other surgery had scar tissue throughout the pelvis that needed to be cut away before the delivery team could get to the uterus.

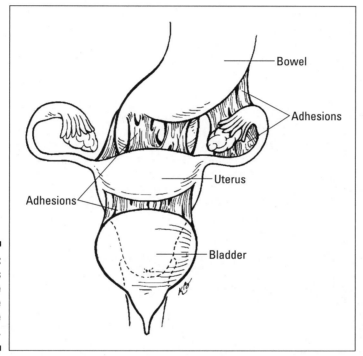

Figure 10-2:
Adhesions in the female reproductive system.

Adhesions form when blood and plasma from trauma such as surgery form fibrin deposits, which are threadlike strands that can bind one organ to another. They can be removed, but surgery to correct adhesions may result in — you guessed it — more adhesions.

Adhesions in the pelvis are common after a surgery, such as an appendectomy, tubal removal for an ectopic pregnancy, or fibroid removal. Between 60 and 90 percent of surgeries leave adhesions behind. Adhesions often cause pelvic pain; 30 to 40 percent of women with chronic pelvis pain have adhesions, and one out of seven women has chronic pelvic pain. Cesarean sections also commonly cause adhesions, but they tend to be anterior (or in front of) the uterus, and thus may cause difficulty during a subsequent C-section. However, C-sections don't usually cause problems with tubes (which tend to be behind the uterus), and thus don't usually cause infertility.

Your chances of getting pregnant after adhesion removal are highest in the first six months after surgery, before extensive adhesions form again. Some adhesions can't be removed without damaging the tubes or ovaries, and you may need in vitro fertilization to get pregnant.

If you have adhesions in the uterus itself, you may be diagnosed with Asherman's syndrome, also called uterine synechiae. With Asherman's, the adhesions crisscross the entire cavity and make it difficult, if not impossible, for a pregnancy to implant.

Asherman's can follow a dilation and curettage (D&C), an abortion, or a uterine infection. It can be diagnosed during an HSG but is best diagnosed with a hysteroscopy, where the inside of the uterus can be visualized. Asherman's is also suspected if you have scant or no menstrual flow or recurrent miscarriages following uterine trauma. If the mild to moderate adhesions are removed surgically, you have a good chance, probably 75 percent or better, of becoming pregnant and carrying to term. Severe adhesions may destroy nearly all the normal uterine lining, and pregnancy may not be possible.

Common Tests to Diagnose Structural Problems

Unfortunately, a quick exam isn't usually enough for your doctor to see that you have problems inside your reproductive organs that can prevent pregnancy. Fortunately, it's become much easier to diagnose tubal and uterine problems with new diagnostic tools, which we discuss in the nest sections.

HSG (don't even try to spell out the word)

An HSG, or *hysterosalpingogram,* is an X-ray that outlines the inside of your uterus and fallopian tubes to make it easy to see where abnormalities may be keeping you from getting pregnant. (See Figure 10-3.) Dye is injected through your cervix to make the uterus and tubes easy to see on an X-ray.

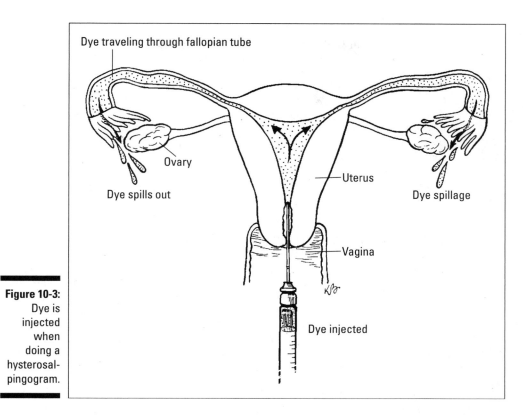

Dye traveling through fallopian tube

Ovary

Dye spills out

Uterus

Dye spillage

Vagina

Dye injected

Figure 10-3:
Dye is injected when doing a hysterosal-pingogram.

HSGs can be uncomfortable, causing mild to severe cramping, but they're a valuable tool in diagnosing fertility problems you can't see. Some of the problems that can be diagnosed with an HSG are fibroids in the uterus, large polyps in the uterus, an unusually shaped uterine cavity, a septum (a piece of tissue dividing your cavity), or adhesions (scar tissue) in the uterus. If you know that you have fibroids, an HSG can show whether they're intruding into the inside of the uterus, where they may prevent implantation of an embryo.

The dye also outlines the fallopian tubes, so your doctor can see whether your tubes are normally shaped and, most importantly, whether your tubes are open, which your doctor can tell by noticing whether the dye passes through the tubes and flows into the pelvis. The HSG is an important test because it lets you know that if your tubes are blocked in any way, or if they're very swollen, an egg or embryo won't be able to get through to the uterus. If dye does pass through easily, your HSG report will say that the fallopian tubes "filled and spilled," meaning that the dye passed easily up from the uterus, all the way up the tubes, and out the end of the tube into the pelvis.

How uncomfortable is an HSG? That depends on your own pain tolerance and whether your tubes are open. If the tubes are slightly blocked with debris, your doctor may need to push the dye more forcefully to clear the block, which may increase cramping. Most doctors tell you to take ibuprofen or a similar pain medication an hour or so before your test. Of course, it also depends on the skill (and "gentleness" of the doctor). Ask your fertility doctor if he or she is going to perform the injection or if they refer patients to the radiologist. If a radiologist is going to do the dye injection, ask who has the most experience. This may be one time when you should ask for a woman radiologist if one is available!

Schedule your test for the early part of your menstrual cycle, usually before day 12 (before you ovulate), because both the dye and the pelvic X-rays can be harmful if you're pregnant.

Many doctors also do cervical cultures for gonorrhea and chlamydia before doing an HSG because pushing dye through the uterus and fallopian tubes can spread the infection and cause serious complications. Your doctor may also prescribe antibiotics for you to take starting a few days before your HSG because between 1 and 3 percent of women experience some type of infection after the procedure.

If you're allergic to contrast dye or shellfish, you may not be able to have the test done. Contrast dye and shellfish both contain iodine, and some doctors believe an allergy to shellfish means you have a higher chance of having an allergic reaction to the dye.

After the test, a small amount of bleeding is normal; you'll also leak a small amount of dye (which is clear, not colored) over the next day or so. You may be crampy for a few hours after the procedure as well. Take someone with you so that you don't have to drive yourself home.

Hysteroscopy

Sometimes smaller polyps and fibroids are hard to see on an HSG. For a close-up look at the inside of the uterus, your doctor may want to do a hysteroscopy.

A diagnostic *hysteroscopy,* often done in the doctor's office, is a procedure in which a small tube is guided through the cervix into the uterus. The uterus is distended, usually with carbon dioxide, so that your doctor can clearly see the entire area, including any small polyps, adhesions, or fibroids. You may be given local anesthesia, such as a cervical block, or mild sedation, such as Valium, for the procedure.

If the procedure detects polyps, scar tissue, or small fibroids in the uterus, your doctor may do an *operative hysteroscopy*. In this procedure, the doctor inserts small instruments through the scope to remove the abnormal tissue. Your doctor may perform this procedure in his office, or in the hospital if more extensive work needs to be done. You may have a nerve block, such as an epidural, or general anesthesia for an operative hysteroscopy done in the hospital.

Laparoscopy

A *laparoscopy* involves placing lighted telescopes and other instruments through the abdomen, as shown in Figure 10-4. The incisions made are very small, about ½ inch or less, and the procedure usually involves one to three incisions. Endometriosis and scar tissue can be removed during a laparoscopy. Fallopian tubes that are infected and dilated also can be removed this way.

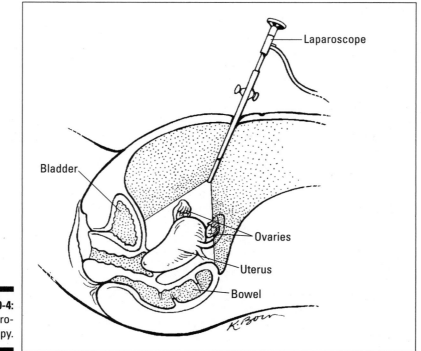

Figure 10-4: A laparoscopy.

A laparoscopy is usually done as an outpatient procedure in a hospital or surgical center. The most common problems after the surgery are pain (usually minimal) from the incisions and pain in the right shoulder from the carbon dioxide used to inflate the abdomen. The recovery period is usually short, less than a week. (This is the same kind of surgery that is done for tubal ligations, and is often referred to as "Band-Aid surgery".)

Post-coital tests

Post-coital testing, also known as the Huhner test, is done around the time of ovulation. It is a diagnostic test done to evaluate the ability of your partner's sperm to survive in your cervical mucus. Timing of this test is very important to correctly evaluate the results. Your doctor will want you to have sex around the time of your LH surge (determined by blood levels or ovulation predictor kits) and come into the office the next morning, anywhere from 4 to 12 hours later; different doctors have different opinions on the exact timing.

The doctor or a nurse takes a sample of mucus from your cervix for the test, so don't take a bath, douche, or use lubricants, such as KY Jelly, for sex. The doctor puts the mucus on a slide and looks at it under a high-powered microscope. You hope that the doctor sees six to ten sperm moving forward per high-powered field. You *don't* want to see a few inert sluggards or a bunch of sperm seemingly stuck together; stuck-together sperm may mean that antisperm antibodies are present. (See the section "Testing for immune disorders," later in this chapter, for more information about antisperm antibodies.)

In addition to checking out "the boys," your doctor also examines the mucus itself, which should be clear in color, make a leaf-like fern pattern under the microscope, and be very stretchy, a quality known as *spinnbarkeit*. Good ovulation-time mucus can be stretched about 4 inches, but nobody will blame you if you don't want to check this out yourself! All these qualities are required for sperm to swim rapidly through the vagina without being mired down or destroyed.

Sometimes the mucus seen doesn't live up to all these great qualities; here are a few possible reasons why it may not:

> ✔ You may not be ovulating. If your predictor kit says that you're having a surge but your mucus is thick, your kit may be wrong. Your LH level could be high in conjunction with a high FSH level; this is common in premature ovarian failure or perimenopause.

✔ You may have a cervical infection. With cervicitis, normal cells are destroyed, and the squamous cells that grow in their place don't make good cervical mucus.

✔ If you're taking Clomid (a fertility drug), it may be affecting your mucus. (See the section "Passing the clomiphene citrate challenge test (CCCT)," later in this chapter, for more on Clomid.)

✔ If you've had any procedures done on your cervix for abnormal Pap smears, your mucus-producing cells may have been destroyed. Such procedures include cone biopsy, in which a wedge-shaped piece of cervix is cut out and sent to be tested for cancerous cells; loop electro-surgical excision procedure (LEEP), in which a piece of cervix is removed by using a fine wire; laser; and freezing.

Many fertility experts have recently given up the post-coital test. This is because women with poor post-coital tests can still get pregnant, and the treatment for most simple infertility involves the use of intra-uterine insemination (IUI), in which the sperm are injected directly into the uterus, thus by-passing the cervix entirely.

Sonohysterogram

A *sonohysterogram* is very similar to a hysterosalpingogram, except that a saline solution, rather than a dye, is injected, and ultrasound, rather than an X-ray, is used to show uterine abnormalities such as polyps or fibroids. The test can be done in the doctor's office and requires no medication in most cases.

A sonohysterogram is very effective for evaluating your uterus but not as effective as an HSG for looking at the fallopian tubes. It's commonly used to verify findings discovered by the HSG, and as a follow-up to previous surgeries. It's generally much less uncomfortable than an HSG.

Taking Your Blood

It's never fun to have blood drawn, but there's a wealth of information in those little tubes. Blood tests are one of the most non-invasive ways to see how you're doing, reproductively speaking, by testing your hormone levels at different times of your menstrual cycle to see if you're "measuring up" to fertility standards.

Baseline blood tests

"Let's get some baseline bloods," your doctor may say when you first start looking for an answer to the "why am I not pregnant" question. This test is one of the simplest tests you can have done. You simply wait until your period starts, go to the lab on day two or day three of your period, and have blood drawn. Within a day or two, you usually receive the results, which give you quite a bit of information about your fertility. Here's what the tests reveal:

- **Estradiol:** Estradiol on day 2 or 3 of your period is normally greater than 10 but less than 80. An estradiol level that is very low, less than 10, may indicate that your ovaries are suppressed and may not respond well to stimulation to make a normal egg (however, it may be normal). An estradiol level that is over 80pg/ml on day three may indicate ovarian cysts. It's also a bad sign for pregnancy happening in that particular cycle.

- **Progesterone:** On day two or three of your period, your progesterone levels should be low, less than 2. Progesterone levels go up in the second half of your cycle, after you ovulate, and should be over 10 ng/mL after you release an egg. Progesterone comes from the *corpus luteum,* the left-over shell of the follicle after you ovulate, and is necessary to help the embryo implant.

- **Luteinizing hormone (LH):** The LH level is usually about 5 on day two or three; women with polycystic ovaries (we discuss this in the section "Polycystic ovary syndrome (PCOS)," later in this chapter) may have an LH level that is significantly higher than their follicle-stimulating hormone level on day two. LH levels rise later in the cycle, usually going over 40 when you're almost ready to ovulate.

- **Follicle-stimulating hormone (FSH):** Your FSH level should be less than 10 or 11, depending on your lab, on day two or day three. A higher than normal FSH level may indicate that you have diminished ovarian reserve, or may mean you're going into perimenopause, the period a few years before menopause; you may also not be making eggs every month. We discuss FSH in more detail in the section "FSH and Inhibin B," later in this chapter.

Your partner's hormone levels, especially LH, FSH, and testosterone, also need to be normal for good sperm production. Most doctors don't test the levels unless your partner's semen analysis is abnormal because a good semen analysis means his hormone levels are normal.

FSH and Inhibin B

Follicle-stimulating hormone is necessary for the production of an egg each month, but, like other things in life, sometimes too much of a good thing is a problem. FSH rises above normal levels when production of estrogen by the ovaries wanes, similar to what happens in many other parts of the human body; this is a feedback loop reaction. FSH is cranked out in larger quantities, trying to get the ovary to understand and put out estrogen, reflected as a higher blood level of FSH. Because the estrogen stays low, no egg is matured. Your doctor may say that you're in *perimenopause,* which is the time from two to ten years before menopause.

Many doctors feel that a single high FSH reading, meaning anything over 10 or 11mIU/ml — the exact number varies with your lab — means that you have diminished ovarian reserve. If you're under 40 years of age and the FSH is over 20, you may be diagnosed with premature ovarian failure (POF). If you're over 40, your doctor may consider this rise in FSH as a normal reaction to aging ovaries. In any case, FSH over 20 can indicate difficulty getting pregnant with your own eggs.

You may wonder why normal ranges for FSH vary from lab to lab. The reason is that many labs establish their own norms based on their specific patient population. The instruments used in the lab can also cause variations from one lab to another.

In certain cases of POF, some doctors try to bring down high FSH levels by fooling the ovary into thinking that the estrogen level is rising. This is done by giving a type of synthetic estrogen. The ovary reduces the amount of FSH produced because it "sees" the estrogen rising, which may give your ovary a chance to start producing an egg, either on its own or with the help of medication. This has worked for some women, and may be worth trying, especially if the patient is young (under 40).

An Inhibin B blood test is done on day three of your period and may give an idea of how your ovaries are functioning. A low level of Inhibin B may indicate that your ovarian function is decreased. This test may be considered to be complementary to the FSH test. It does not appear to be superior or have any more predictive value, and for this reason, the day 3 FSH test remains the "gold standard".

Passing the clomiphene citrate challenge test (CCCT)

The CCCT, or clomiphene citrate challenge test, is a measurement of estradiol and FSH (see "Baseline blood tests" for a description of each) taken on day two or three of your period and then measured again after you take a medication called clomiphene citrate for five days. This drug, marketed under the brand names Clomid or Serophene, is a fertility medication that stimulates egg production. You then recheck your estradiol and FSH levels. Your estradiol level should rise by the fifth day, but if your FSH level is elevated on either day two or after five days, you'll be told that you had a failed CCCT. Your doctor may feel that a failed CCCT means that you have a decreased ovarian reserve, which decreases your chance of getting pregnant.

Hyperprolactinemia, or high prolactin

Although less than 1 percent of women have high prolactin levels, high *prolactin* (the hormone responsible for maintaining breast milk production) levels are found in 10 to 40 percent of premenopausal women who have stopped menstruating due to anovulation.

Women who are pregnant or breast-feeding should have high levels of prolactin. If yours is elevated at any other time, it may suppress ovulation. A tumor is found on the pituitary gland in about 30 percent of women with high prolactin levels; these are almost always benign. Many drugs can cause high prolactin levels, including antidepressants and antihypertensives.

A pill called Parlodel can be given to lower your prolactin levels so that you'll start ovulating again.

Thyroid tests

The best state to be in with your thyroid is *euthyroid,* which means that your thyroid is in balance. Thyroid problems are very common, with one out of eight women diagnosed with a thyroid problem at some point in their lives; men can also have thyroid disorders, but women are five to eight times more likely to be affected. Your thyroid can be either overactive (hyper) or underactive (hypo). Both hyper- and hypothyroid conditions can cause infertility problems in men and women.

A thyroid that is hypoactive usually causes fatigue, dry skin, and weight gain. A hyperactive thyroid causes a rapid heart rate, anxiousness, sweating, and weight loss.

In men, thyroid problems can cause a low sperm count and decreased sperm motility. Women may experience an increased rate of miscarriage, lack of ovulation, or irregular periods. Hypothyroidism can cause an increase in *prolactin,* the hormone responsible for maintaining breast milk production in pregnancy. High prolactin can cause a decrease in fertility.

Thyroid imbalances can be treated by daily medication, radiation, or, in severe cases, surgery. Your thyroid medication may need to be adjusted if you become pregnant.

Testing for immune disorders

Immune testing in infertility is considered controversial. This is because rigorous studies have not definitively proven a role in infertility. However, some doctors feel that it can be valuable.

In most cases, only a blood sample is required. Interpretation of the results isn't always simple, however, and different doctors have different opinions of the importance of immune testing in infertility. Some tests are widely done and the results almost universally accepted. Other tests are done only by doctors specializing in immune disorders, and not all doctors believe the results are important. Here are some of the most common immune tests, with information on what the tests mean and how you're treated if the tests are abnormal.

Antisperm antibody (ASA)

Many fertility centers do antisperm antibody (ASA) tests on all their patients. Both you and your partner may be positive for ASA. Women are tested through a blood test, and men are tested through a semen specimen.

Antisperm antibodies in either partner are thought to cause problems with fertilization. Males with ASA may need to do IVF with ICSI (intracytoplasmic sperm injection, or the injection of one sperm into an egg) if they have more than 20 percent antibodies because the antibodies cause the sperm to clump together instead of moving forward. (We discuss ICSI in more detail in Chapter 11.) About 70 percent of men who have had a vasectomy reversal have antisperm antibodies; they're also common in men who have had injury or insult to the testicle. Ten percent or so of infertile men have ASA. Some IVF programs routinely perform ICSI if the man has a history of vasectomy reversal or high levels of ASA.

Antisperm antibodies are less common in women; less than 5 percent of infertile women have antisperm antibodies. They're found in the cervical mucus as well as the blood. The antibodies attach to the head of the sperm and make it hard for the sperm to penetrate an egg. The treatment is IVF with ICSI.

Antiphospholipid antibodies (APA)

You'll most likely be tested for antiphospholipid antibodies (APA) if you've had multiple miscarriages or repeated failure with IVF. The test for APA actually tests for a number of different antibodies; a moderate or high reaction to two or more antibodies is considered a positive reaction. Treatment is either baby aspirin, heparin (an anticoagulant, or blood thinner), or a combination of the two. Antiphospholipid antibodies can interfere with the embryo implanting or can cause miscarriage; they disrupt the normal clotting of blood and the adhesion of the embryo to the uterus.

Antinuclear antibodies (ANA)

A high positive antinuclear antibodies (ANA) test can mean that you may have a disease called systemic lupus erythematosus (SLE). At lower positive levels, especially if the pattern is speckled, ANA can increase your risk of miscarriage. A positive ANA level may be treated with low-dose steroids, but this therapy is not proven to decrease miscarriage rates.

Antithyroglobulin (ATA)

Antithyroglobulin antibodies (ATA) can cause problems with your thyroid function. Because the thyroid is so important in maintaining your hormone levels, antibodies that interfere with the thyroid's functioning have been hypothesized to cause problems with egg production. As with other antibodies, a high ATA level may be treated with steroids.

Antiovarian antibodies (AOA)

If you're in premature ovarian failure or early menopause, you may be tested for antiovarian antibodies (AOA).

Leukocyte antibody detection (LAD)

Foreign bodies are usually rejected because they're attacked by antibodies; this would be true of a fetus if it didn't have the protection of *blocking antibodies,* which you make in response to the genetic material from your partner that is present in the embryo. Therefore, it has been suggested that if you and your partner have DNA that is too similar, those antibodies won't be activated, and the fetus is more likely to be rejected. A positive leukocyte antibody detection (LAD) test is good; it means the antibodies are present.

If the test is negative, patients were advised to undergo leukocyte immunization (LI) therapy, which injects white blood cells from the male partner into you by using a small intradermal needle, similar to a tuberculin test. At present, LI therapy has been stopped by the U.S. Food and Drug Administration.

Natural killer (NK) cells

NK cells are part of white blood cells that attack and destroy anything they see as a foreign substance in the body. They're an important part of keeping cancer cells from spreading. A normal NK cell range is about 2 percent; if the count is higher, the cells are thought to be too aggressive, and it has been suggested that they may attack a growing embryo. Treatment for high NK cells is intravenous immunoglobulin therapy (IVIG), which is also used in cancer therapy. IVIG is quite expensive (over $1,000 per treatment), quite controversial among infertility specialists, and often not covered by insurance. (We talk more about IVIG therapy in Chapter 20.)

Enbrel, a drug created for treatment of rheumatoid arthritis, has also been used to treat NK cells. Its value in the treatment of recurrent miscarriage is also unproven.

Considering the Possibility of Endometriosis

More than 5 million American women have endometriosis, a common, complicated condition that affects 30 to 40 percent of all infertility patients. Despite its prevalence, it's often underdiagnosed and undertreated. (See *Endometriosis for Dummies* [Wiley, 2006] for the full scoop on endometriosis, and see Chapter 6 for more on getting pregnant with endometriosis.)

Endometriosis is the presence of endometrial tissue, which lines the inside of your uterus, in places it has no business being. Endometriosis can be found throughout the pelvis — around the fallopian tubes and ovaries — but it has also been found in the lungs, skin, and brain. No one is quite sure how endometriosis travels so far, but theories are that it travels through the circulatory system or the lymphatic system.

Because endometriosis is endometrial tissue, it reacts to hormone changes the same way your uterine lining does. So when you get your period or have midcycle spotting, endometriosis tissue also bleeds. Because this tissue doesn't have a handy exit point the way your uterine lining does, the blood stagnates, causing inflammation, irritation, and eventually scar tissue.

You might suspect that you have endometriosis if you have any of the following symptoms:

✔ Chronic or recurring pelvic pain

✔ History of ectopic pregnancy or miscarriage

✔ Backache or leg pain

✔ Nausea, vomiting, diarrhea, or constipation

✔ Rectal bleeding or bloody stools

✔ Blood in urine

✔ Urinary urgency or frequency

✔ Chest pain or coughing up blood, especially at the time of your period

✔ High blood pressure

Because the symptoms are so broad and sometimes nonspecific, endometriosis may be confused with the following:

✔ Appendicitis

✔ Irritable bowel syndrome

✔ Bowel obstruction

✔ Ovarian cysts

✔ Pelvic inflammatory disease

Endometriosis can be diagnosed by laparoscopic surgery or a laparotomy; endometrial lesions can often be removed at the same time.

Ovulation Issues

You can have all the right reproductive parts in all the right places, but if they're not functioning properly, pregnancy will never occur. Getting pregnant is dependent on the release of a healthy egg capable of being fertilized by a healthy sperm. If your menstrual cycle is messed up, your egg production and release may be, too. (We take a closer look at menstrual disorders in Chapter 2.) Your menstrual cycle is one of the first things your doctor will probably ask you about when trying to get to the bottom of fertility issues.

Amenorrhea — not getting your period at all

Amenorrhea is the absence of menstrual periods. If you've never had a period, undoubtedly you've been evaluated sometime during your teenage years to see whether a structural problem, such as absence of the uterus, malformation of the vagina, or undeveloped ovaries, is the cause.

However, many women have periods at one time and then quit having them. This may happen if you have Asherman's syndrome (discussed earlier in this chapter in the section "Seeing the complications of scar tissue") because little normal tissue is left and the exit path from the uterus may be blocked with scar tissue, or maybe you aren't ovulating any longer. If you've had periods previously and no longer do, have a checkup to see whether anovulation (failing to ovulate) is the problem.

Failing to ovulate

If you're not getting your period at all, or if you're having irregular periods, you may not be ovulating, a condition known as *anovulation*. Many factors, including emotional factors and stress, can cause anovulation.

Looking at your weight . . . or lack thereof

One cause of anovulation is weight gain or loss. Of course, most women don't want to look at their weight. But even a slight deviation — about 15 percent — either up or down may create menstrual irregularities and subtle infertility issues. After your weight falls into normal limits, your chance of getting pregnant without any other therapy may increase.

In today's culture, where thin is in and "you can't be too thin" is a widely accepted standard, overweight women are far more likely to consider their weight a problem than the underweight. The fact is, however, that being underweight is equally as damaging as being overweight if you're having fertility problems.

Frequent, strenuous exercise can also cause anovulation if it causes the body fat percentage to drop to less than 22 percent, the amount needed to keep menstruation occurring.

Factoring in stress

You may wonder about the role stress plays in anovulation. Stress can alter your body functions, which can affect your menstrual cycle. Lowering stress levels is easier said than done, but if you're under severe stress, you may want to consider therapies such as biofeedback to decrease negative response to stress.

Reducing stress and maintaining normal weight may help correct some cases of anovulation, but not all.

Polycystic ovary syndrome (PCOS)

Between 3 and 5 percent of women have a condition called polycystic ovary syndrome (PCOS). Many of these women have difficulty getting pregnant because many women with PCOS ovulate irregularly or not at all.

Often your doctor will test for PCOS if you're overweight (50 percent of all PCOS patients are obese) and are hairy where you shouldn't be, a condition that may be caused by an overabundance of male hormones called *androgens*.

If your doctor suspects that you have PCOS, he may do a pelvic ultrasound. Women with PCOS have lots of small follicles on their ovaries that are visible on ultrasound. Your doctor will probably check your hormone levels as well; PCOS patients often have a baseline blood LH level that is higher than normal. The high LH levels can cause abnormalities in eggs and also increase miscarriage rates. Insulin levels are often high as well, but these can be treated by taking oral diabetic medications such as Glucophage. PCOS patients have a higher chance of developing adult onset diabetes.

Many women with PCOS respond well and begin ovulating if treated with Clomid or with injectable gonadotropins to induce ovulation. In resistant cases of anovulation, your doctor may suggest laparoscopic laser ovarian drilling, a procedure in which your doctor makes small punctures in your ovary during laparoscopic surgery. Between 70 and 90 percent of women start ovulating after this procedure, although the effect may be temporary. Risks of the surgery are infection and scar tissue formation. (See Chapter 6 for more about PCOS and its effect on fertility.)

Chapter 11

All About the Boys

*Y*ou always knew men were different — but you might not have known *how* different! When it comes to reproduction, everything about men is different is — from the way they let it "all hang out" to the way they produce gametes (both eggs and sperm are called gametes.)

In this chapter, we hang out with the boys, examining their reproductive organs, their sperm-producing mechanisms, and the ways things can go awry in the sperm production department.

Analyzing a Semen Specimen

You may find your partner acting a little funny when it's time to "check out the boys," but because male-factor infertility accounts for about 40 percent of infertility, semen analysis is a necessary step.

Undergoing semen analysis

Semen analysis can be done at your doctor's office, if he has the proper tools, or in a laboratory. There's no special preparation for a semen analysis, although your partner should have abstinence (no ejaculation) for two to five days.

Usually semen samples are produced on site; some clinics or offices may provide "visual aids" to ejaculation such as magazines or movies. Can you "help" with production? Only if you promise to use no lubricants or saliva, which can mess up the sample!

If it's absolutely impossible for your partner to produce on site, you can bring in a sample produced within the last 15 minutes to half an hour in a sterile container.

Most any laboratory can do a "screening" semen analysis. However, the determination of morphology (proportion of "normal" forms), especially by the criteria of Kruger (see the section "Evaluating sperm"), takes a high level of expertise, and is generally only available at a bona fide fertility program.

If you're bringing in a semen sample, keep it at next-to-body temperature — holding it under your armpit is ideal. Make sure that the lid's on tight!

Evaluating sperm

Sperm are extremely small, but under the microscope, you can see how complicated they really are. A normal sperm (see Figure 11-1) has three sections: a head, a midpiece, and a tail. All three parts need to be normal for a sperm to be considered normal according to the strict Kruger morphology, a system for evaluating sperm that was developed in Africa by Dr. Thinus Kruger.

- ✔ **Head:** Contains all the genetic material, so a sperm with an abnormal head — either a round head, pinhead, large head, or double head — isn't capable of fertilizing an egg.

- ✔ **Midpiece:** Contains fructose, the energy the sperm needs to move rapidly.

- ✔ **Tail:** Needed for propulsion. Sperm with no tail, two tails, or coiled tails are all considered abnormal.

The World Health Organization (WHO) has set standard parameters for a normal semen specimen, so this is what your sperm should have to be graded A+. Your doctor probably won't go into these fine points of your sperm with you, but you can always ask about morphology or forward progression if you want to dazzle him with your knowledge!

- ✔ **Volume:** Should be 1.5 to 5 ml, or approximately a teaspoon.

- ✔ **Concentration:** Should be greater than 20 million sperm/ml, or a total of greater than 40 million per ejaculate.

- ✔ **Motility:** More than 40 percent of the sperm should be motile, or moving.

- **Morphology:** More than a certain percentage of the sperm should be normally shaped, as determined by the lab technician. If the lab is using the WHO criteria, the normal cutoff is 30 percent. If the lab is using Kruger criteria, which are more strict, the normal cutoff is 14%, with a value of 4 percent to 13 percent considered "borderline." Less than 4 percent is considered poor prognosis.

- **Forward progression:** On a scale of 1 to 4, at least 2+ means a good number of sperm moving forward.

- **White blood cells:** Should be no more than 0 to 5 per high-power field. More could indicate infection.

- **Hyperviscosity:** Should gel promptly but liquefy within 30 minutes after ejaculation.

- **Ph:** Should be alkaline, to protect sperm from the acidic environment of the vagina.

There are some other tests that the doctor may order, although these are not normally performed during the initial evaluation:

- **HOS, or hypo-osmotic swelling, test:** Greater than 50 percent of the sperm tails should swell when exposed to a hypo-osmotic solution; this swelling is a sign of normal functioning.

- **Antisperm antibodies:** A normal semen sample contains no antisperm antibodies. Antibodies cause problems if they're attached to the sperm tail, because they interfere with movement, or to the head, where they may make it difficult for the sperm to penetrate the egg.

- **Zona-free hamster-egg penetrating test:** Human sperm cannot penetrate the egg of another species. This is because there are specific binding sites on the zona pellucida, the outer layer or "shell" of the human egg. However, a normal human sperm can penetrate a hamster egg after the *zona,* or outside layer of the egg, is removed. The ability to penetrate the hamster egg has predictive value for the sperm because sperm that can penetrate the hamster egg can generally also penetrate intact human eggs. The Kruger morphology assessment is so good that many fertility programs use it in place of the hamster test.

- **Acrosome reaction test:** The head of the sperm is covered with two layers of membranes, called the *acrosome.* It contains enzymes that allow the sperm to penetrate the egg. In order for the enzymes to be released, the sperm needs to undergo an "acrosome reaction.". The proportion of sperm that have undergone the acrosome reaction can be assessed in the laboratory and this result is thought to be predictive of fertility in the male.

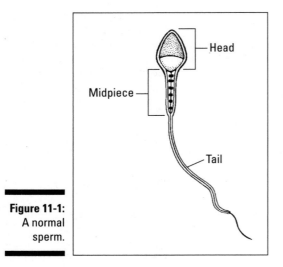

Figure 11-1:
A normal
sperm.

It takes three months for sperm to properly develop, so if your partner was sick, taking medication, or had anything else unusual going on three months ago, his specimen may be abnormal. Check a second specimen in a few weeks to see whether anything has changed.

Interpreting Your Partner's Test Results

With some of the test results back, you may be even more confused than you were before. If your partner's semen analysis comes back with some results askew, he may be too embarrassed to ask what the results mean. Sometimes it's easier to look up the problems in a book, so here you are!

Semen samples can vary from month to month, or even day to day. That's because it takes about 72 days for sperm to develop. Unlike eggs, which are present from your embryonic days, sperm are replenished all the time.

Sperm are produced in the testicle, then collect in an area called the epididymis, and from there they must be transported via the vas deferens to the ejaculatory duct. The prostate adds the seminal plasma, the thick liquid which then carries the sperm via ejaculation into the outer world. There are lots of things that have to happen to make sperm come out, and therefore, there are lots of factors that can cause variability from ejaculate to ejaculate.

Because men are constantly producing new sperm, one "bad" semen analysis should be followed up with another in a month or so to see if the problem was a temporary one. An illness, injury, or medication or drug use a few months before may make one sample not so superior, but checking again a month later may show an improvement.

Making too few sperm

Sometimes a semen analysis shows a very low number of sperm, less than 20 million, a condition called *oligospermia*.

While 20 million sperm may sound excessive — why isn't one or two million enough? — large numbers of sperm are needed in the ejaculate because many sperm are abnormal even in a good sperm sample, and it's a long way to the ovulated egg, so many don't make it all the way.

There are many causes of oligospermia, ranging from varicoceles (see "Correcting Varicoceles") to lifestyle issues (check out "Lifestyle Changes to Improve Sperm Production"). Other causes might be:

- Hormone imbalances, which can be checked by a simple blood test
- Chromosomal abnormalities such as a congenital deletion of part of the Y chromosome
- History of lymphoma or testicular cancer or chemotherapy (see chapter 6 for more about fertility and cancer treatment)
- Diabetes
- Sickle cell disease
- Kidney disease
- Liver disease

You can get pregnant without fertility treatments if your partner has oligospermia, but your chances of pregnancy are higher if you do one of the following:

- **Intrauterine insemination (IUI):** The sperm will be concentrated and "washed" so that the best sperm are used for insemination. (See Chapter 13 for more on IUI.)
- **In vitro fertilization (IVF):** This treatment allows fertilization to take place in the lab, where a high concentration of sperm can be put in with the egg. If the sperm are especially abnormal, the lab may need to utilize intracytoplasmic sperm injection (ICSI), the insertion of a sperm directly into an egg. The procedure is done by an embryologist under a high-powered microscope. (See Chapter 17 for more information on ICSI.)

When there's no sperm in sight

If no sperm are seen, it's called *azoospermia*. Between 5 and 10 percent of the male population have either azoospermia or oligospermia.

If your partner has azoospermia, you won't be able to get pregnant conventionally. Different factors can cause azoospermia; either the production of the sperm or the delivery of the sperm can be at fault. Sperm production problems can be caused by the following:

- **Sertoli cell only syndrome:** In this condition, the germ cells that produce sperm in the testes are absent. There is no way for a person with this syndrome to father a child.

- **Anabolic steroids:** Their use may cause a possibly reversible shutdown of the sperm production.

- **Abnormal hormone levels:** Low levels of LH, FSH, or testosterone can cause low sperm production. This problem can be treated with hormone injections, pills, or transdermal patches.

If the problem is obstruction, in general, the sperm production is normal, and the sperm simply can't get to the ejaculatory duct. In these cases, your partner will need a surgical procedure to extract the sperm from the testicle (discussed in the sidebar "If you need a sperm aspiration," later in this chapter). This procedure must be done in conjunction with IVF because the sperm need to be injected directly into the egg. Obstructive problems include the following:

- Absence of the *vas deferens,* the tube that delivers sperm to the ejaculatory duct and the prostate

- Previous vasectomy

- Previous infection that causes scarring and obstruction of the epididymis

- Obstruction from prior surgery

Mechanical problems with getting the sperm where they need to be include the following:

- Retrograde ejaculation, in which the majority of the sperm go into the bladder

- Spinal cord injury that prevents ejaculation

- Previous injury from trauma

- Previous injury from surgery, such as hernia surgery

- A disease such as diabetes

If you need a sperm aspiration

Sperm can be aspirated from either the epididymis, which sits on top of the testes, or from the testes themselves. There are four different types of procedures, each with advantages and disadvantages:

✔ **MESA (microsurgical epididymal sperm aspiration):** This procedure can be done only for obstructive azoospermia, because men with nonobstructive azoospermia rarely have sperm in the epididymis. A small incision is made in the scrotum, and then a dilated tubule in the epididymis is cut open and examined through a lighted microscope. Fluid is collected from the tubule and examined for sperm. This procedure can be done in the doctor's office. You may be given a spermatic cord block and sedation during the procedure. You can generally return to work the following day.

✔ **PESA (percutaneous epididymal sperm aspiration):** This procedure is done in the office. A blind needle stick into the epididymis is used to extract sperm. Local anesthesia and sedation may be given.

✔ **TESE (testicular sperm extraction):** A small incision is made, and a piece of testicular tissue is removed. Testicular sperm doesn't freeze or thaw as well as epididymal sperm but may be the only sperm found in men with nonobstructive azoospermia.

✔ **TESA (testicular sperm aspiration):** This procedure is done in the office, using a blind needle aspiration of the testicle.

All four techniques can cause bleeding and *hematoma* (a collection of blood that can be painful). A biopsy usually requires only a one-day recovery and can be done under local anesthesia or mild sedation.

Congenital absence of the *vas deferens,* the duct that leads to the urethra, is associated with cystic fibrosis in men. Genetic testing will most likely be suggested if this problem is found. One way to diagnose absence of the vas deferens is to test for a sugar called fructose that's usually found in semen; it won't be found if the duct is missing.

Swimming in circles, or not at all

Sometimes plenty of sperm are seen in the ejaculate, but the sperm themselves are abnormal. Sperm are very complicated little creatures. Despite their small size, they contain three distinct sections, and a problem with any section can cause infertility.

The head of the sperm contains the DNA, or genetic material. If the head is abnormally shaped, the sperm is probably incapable of fertilizing an egg because its genetic material is abnormal.

The midpiece of the sperm contains the energy necessary to propel it to the egg. Sperm need a tremendous amount of energy to get to an egg. If they lack this energy, they're not going to make it the whole distance.

The tail of the sperm makes the sperm move rapidly; if the sperm sample has a lot of coiled, rather than whip-like tails, or no tails at all, those sperm may go in the wrong direction or may go nowhere at all — they may just twitch a bit. Again, these sperm aren't going to be able to get where they need to be.

Correcting Varicoceles

A *varicocele* is an abnormal dilation of the spermatic vein. Varicoceles are more common than you may think; about 15 percent of men have them. More varicoceles are found on the left testicle than the right — around 90 percent, in fact. The effect of varicoceles on male fertility is somewhat controversial. However, some doctors feel that they are the leading cause of male infertility.

Varicoceles can lead to decreased fertility in the following ways:

✔ Increased temperature in the testes

✔ Stagnation of blood around the testicles

✔ Hormonal alterations

✔ Decreased sperm production and motility

Varicoceles can be corrected in one of two ways:

✔ **Surgery:** Done as an outpatient; a small incision is made just above the groin, and the offending vein is located and tied off. Recovery time is a week to ten days, but heavy lifting should be avoided for a month or so.

Surgical risks include infection, nerve injury, and hydrocele formation (a collection of fluid around the testicle).

✔ **Radiographic embolization:** Also an outpatient procedure; advantages are immediate recovery with no restrictions on lifting. A small catheter is threaded through the femoral vein in the groin; dye is injected to show exactly where the problem vein is, and then the vein is blocked, or occluded, so that no blood flow can reach it.

In the past, varicocele repair was a very common procedure. Most recently, varicocele repair has become controversial because studies designed to demonstrate improvement in fertility after the surgery have not been able to show the degree of improvement that was anticipated. Only very large and obvious varicoceles tend to be repaired these days. It can take up to 4 months for an improvement in sperm count to be seen after a varicocele repair.

Lifestyle Changes to Improve Sperm Production

Even if your partner's sample doesn't look optimal, take heart; there may be things he can do to improve. Many lifestyle issues can impact sperm production in a big way; consider the following and change what you can:

- ✔ **Smoking:** Cigarette smoking can decrease sperm count, increase the number of abnormal sperm in a semen sample, and some studies suggest that smokers are more likely to be impotent (unable to sustain an erection) than non smokers.

- ✔ **Marijuana:** Marijuana use in men can lower the amount of seminal fluid produced, and can result in decreased sperm production.

- ✔ **Alcohol:** Alcohol, in large quantities, increases the number of abnormally shaped sperm, can change male hormones, and leads to impotence.

- ✔ **Anabolic steroids:** Anabolic steroids suppress testosterone, resulting in small testes, possible impotence, and severe decrease in sperm count, or even a total absence of sperm.

- ✔ **Bicycling:** Cycling seems like a great way to burn calories and stay in shape — and it is. However, studies have shown that cyclists are more likely to have fertility issues related to the pressure of the bicycle seat on the testicles.

- ✔ **Chemical exposure:** Working with chemicals such as pesticides, chemical compounds, or inhalants can result in a decreased sperm count and/or an increased number of abnormal sperm in the ejaculate.

- ✔ **Cocaine:** Cocaine decreases sperm counts, results in abnormal-looking sperm, and may be carried on the sperm into the fertilized egg; this may lead to abnormal development in their children.

- ✔ **Laptops:** Who'd have thought it ten years ago: Your laptop can actually decrease male fertility! This only happens if you hold it on your lap; the heat produced by the laptop can overheat the testicles. Some laptops have gotten hot enough to start on fire! So put something between you and the laptop, or better yet — put the laptop on a desk or table.

- ✔ **Medications:** Many prescription drugs used to treat high blood pressure and depression have negative effects on fertility; if you are dealing with a low sperm count or impotence, be sure to discuss any prescription medications you're taking with your doctor.

- ✔ **Weight:** As with women, overweight men have decreased fertility, according to some studies. If you're overweight, reducing may help increase your sperm count — and give you more energy to chase after your future bundle of joy!

Analyzing the effects of age

For years, it's been considered unfair that men, unlike women, had no age limit placed on their fertility. While new dads in their seventies still make the news from time to time, studies have shown that age may play a part in male fertility as well as female fertility.

Some studies suggest that older men produce fewer mature sperm. Immature sperm are slower moving and lack the strength to "go the distance" to the egg.

Decreased testosterone production in older men may lead to erection difficulties and a weaker ejaculation.

A recent study showed a possible link between older men and the incidence of autism in their offspring; similar studies have shown an increase in offspring with schizophrenia born to older dads. A Canadian study showed abnormalities in DNA in sperm of men over age 45 — in fact, men over 45 had double the number of abnormal sperm found in men aged 30.

Of course, you can't change your age, so if you're attempting pregnancy over age 40, the best thing you can do is maintain a healthy lifestyle to make sure you're producing the best sperm possible.

Two syndromes that affect male fertility

Kleinfelter's syndrome and Kallman's syndrome are two syndromes that affect male fertility.

Kleinfelter's syndrome is far more common than most people realize. One out of 500 to 1,000 males are affected. Symptoms of Kleinfelter's are delayed puberty, decreased facial and body hair, small firm testes, and long legs. Blood tests show an increase in LH and FSH levels and a decrease in serum testosterone levels. Chromosome tests will show an XXY karyotype. Treatment is testosterone. Fertility was thought to be impossible, but recently several live births have been reported after testicular sperm extraction and IVF with ICSI.

Kallman's syndrome is less common but may be familial. Symptoms are loss of smell, delayed puberty, osteoporosis, red-green color blindness, and possibly cleft palate and urogenital abnormalities. Blood tests show high LH and FSH levels and low testosterone levels. Treatment is with hormones such as HCG or FSH and testosterone. Since Kallman's syndrome affects the brain and pituitary gland, and not the testicles, fertility is possible after hormone replacement in these patients.

Considering Erectile Dysfunction Issues: A Sensitive Topic

Abnormal sperm may be a problem you both can deal with. Problems with ejaculation or the ability to sustain an erection, however, may be so difficult to address that you may have a hard time bringing it out into the open. Yet it's a common problem: Ten percent of men between the ages of 18 and 59 have experienced erectile problems in the last year, and 10 percent of men between the ages of 40 and 70 have complete erectile failure.

Plenty of medical-related conditions can cause problems with erection and ejaculation. The following list gives examples of what can cause such problems:

✔ **Medications**

  - Antidepressants

  - Anti-ulcer medications

  - Certain blood pressure medications

- Cholesterol-lowering medications

✔ **Diseases**

  - Diabetes

  - Heart attack (myocardial infarction)

  - Hypertension or other vascular disease

  - Hypothyroidism or hyperthyroidism

  - Leukemia

  - Liver cirrhosis

  - Renal failure

  - Sickle cell anemia

✔ **Surgeries**

  - Abdominal perineal resection

  - Proctocolectomy

  - Radical prostatectomy

  - Transurethral resection of prostate

  - Radiation, trauma, heavy alcohol use, and neurological damage from surgery, stroke, epilepsy, or multiple sclerosis can also cause erectile dysfunction.

Erectile dysfunction may also result from psychosexual problems better addressed by therapy. Whatever the reason, the first step in dealing with the problem is being able to discuss it, especially with an outsider such as a doctor or nurse.

Handling the emotional effect of male problems on both of you

A few decades ago, failure to produce a baby was always considered to be the woman's fault. In many cultures, a man could obtain a no-questions-asked divorce from any woman who didn't give him a child. With the advent of microscopes high powered enough to look closely at sperm, it became obvious that male factors are as important for reproduction as female factors.

Intellectually it shouldn't matter which one of you has a problem, but intellect and emotion are two different matters. Women tend to approach medical problems with a "let's just fix it" attitude, while many men approach medical issues with a "let's just bury our head in the sand" approach. For whatever reason, more men than women have an ego issue when it comes to their reproductive parts. Their sense of personal failure may be more pronounced than yours, and they may also be less willing to face the problem and do what it takes to fix it.

If it turns out that he's the problem, you may have to tread very gently around the issue, especially if you're the one more interested in having a child. He may consider the whole subject closed if he's the problem — no sperm, no child, okay, end of discussion. Not all men feel so closely tied to their semen analysis, but if your partner does, be prepared for some tense moments.

Undoing a Vasectomy: Is It Worth the Pain?

About 500,000 vasectomies are performed each year. As with tubal ligation, many men regret their decision and decide to have the surgery reversed. Vasectomy reversal surgery is often successful in that sperm will be found in the ejaculate in the majority of cases, but the number of sperm may be too small to make pregnancy likely, or antibodies attached to the sperm may make it nearly impossible for the sperm to swim properly or fertilize an egg.

Antibodies are found in 50 percent of men after vasectomy reversal; men with antibodies may need IVF for their partner to become pregnant.

As with tubal ligation, vasectomy reversal success depends on what type of surgery was done. The reversal success rate is higher if:

- ✔ The surgery is done on a straight section of the vas deferens.
- ✔ The pieces to be joined together are of equal size.
- ✔ The reversal is done within ten years of the original surgery.

Your chance of pregnancy after sterilization reversal depends on several factors. Consider carefully whether reversal will be more cost effective and offer a better chance of success than IVF, in which tied tubes can be bypassed or sperm can be removed directly from the testicles via sperm aspiration. Of course, personal preference plays a great role in this decision. The principal appeal of vasectomy reversal is that pregnancy can occur naturally. The main disadvantage is that it may not work, and if it doesn't, IVF will be needed anyway.

A recently reported study showed that there was less pain and less time lost from work with sperm aspirations as opposed to vasectomy reversals.

Chapter 12

When the Beginning Is the End: Early Pregnancy Loss

***

In This Chapter

▶ Understanding the meaning of "a little bit" pregnant

▶ Dealing with a miscarriage or ectopic pregnancy

▶ Recovering after a loss

***

As upsetting as it is not to get pregnant, getting pregnant and having the pregnancy end in loss is even more devastating. Why do so many pregnancies end early, and what does it mean for future pregnancies? And how can you avoid personal feelings of failure when a loss occurs? In this chapter, we discuss how and why pregnancies are lost in the first 12 weeks, and we offer advice on how to pick yourself up and try again if this happens to you.

Being "a Little Bit" Pregnant — It's Possible

Most of you have heard that there's no such thing as "a little bit" pregnant. This statement is true in one sense, but at times, you do feel that you're "almost" pregnant . . . and you may be right.

Understanding chemical pregnancies

Even after embryos successfully implant, a large percentage (depending on the age of the mother) stop developing before they develop a heartbeat. Most of these early miscarriages, up to 30 percent, take place before the time when you would notice any signs of pregnancy. If this happens, you may have no pregnancy symptoms at all, not even a missed period. Or you may have very early pregnancy signs, such as breast tenderness, which suddenly disappear. These signs may be followed by a slightly late, heavier-than-normal period, which is actually the passing of a very early pregnancy. You may pass more clots than normal (for you), or you may feel "crampier" than usual. You probably wouldn't even realize that you had been pregnant unless you did a sensitive early pregnancy test, such as a blood test.

If you're under treatment by a fertility doctor, you may be asked to do a blood pregnancy test, called a beta-HCG (this stands for the beta sub unit of the HCG molecule, the hormone of pregnancy produced by the implanting placenta, or "beta" for short), about two weeks after ovulation or embryo transfer. Your beta number may be positive (most labs have a sensitivity of 5, meaning that anything over 5 is considered positive; some labs have a sensitivity of 2, or even 1.5) but very low when first tested, and it may be negative a few days later, at the second test. Your doctor may say that you had a *chemical pregnancy* if this happens.

Testing for possible fixes

At least 50 percent of the time, chemical pregnancies are caused by the implantation of a chromosomally abnormal embryo, but other factors can also cause very early miscarriage. Your doctor may do tests, such as checking your progesterone level, to see whether there are other reasons why the embryo isn't "sticking." In a normal pregnancy, the *corpus luteum,* or leftover "shell" of the ovulated egg, produces a hormone called *progesterone.* Progesterone is necessary for the implantation and growth of the early embryo. If your progesterone is lower than normal, the embryo may not be able to grow properly.

A simple blood test can check your progesterone levels. Alternately, your doctor can do a biopsy to see if the uterine lining (the endometrium) is responding to the progesterone that is in your system. In a biopsy, your doctor takes a tiny scraping of your uterine lining and sends it to a lab to see if the response to progesterone is adequate. If the tissue sample shows less than a normal response to progesterone, your doctor can recommend supplementing progesterone in the form of shots, pills, or vaginal suppositories. The biopsy needs to be done just before the period. Since you may be pregnant at this time, it is usually done after a negative pregnancy test; it needs to be done within a day or so of the test because it will not be accurate if your period has started.

So even though people may say that you can't be a "little bit" pregnant, the truth is that a pregnancy can start to implant and then stop before you even miss a period. You may not realize this is happening to you without a very early blood pregnancy test. If your doctor suspects that you're having chemical pregnancies, he or she will order further testing to see whether an easy fix, such as adding progesterone supplements, can solve the problem.

Suffering a Miscarriage

A *miscarriage* is a pregnancy loss that occurs after you know you're pregnant but before the fetus is *viable,* or able to live on its own.

Miscarriages are very common: About one in four women has a miscarriage during her reproductive years. But knowing that miscarriages are common events and not likely to recur doesn't make them any easier to deal with.

The vast majority of miscarriages occur in the first 12 weeks of pregnancy. Based on this fact, many couples decide not to shout the news to friends and relatives before this time has passed.

Understanding different terms

Doctors call all miscarriages *abortion;* that term doesn't have the same meaning as what you're used to. There are different types of miscarriages, and they're tied to the type of symptoms you have:

- ✔ **Threatened abortion:** The first sign of possible miscarriage is usually spotting. But because spotting is common in pregnancy (occurring in one in five women), doctors don't always take it as a dire sign. If spotting and cramping stop quickly, the chances are excellent that the pregnancy will carry to term. Most doctors restrict sex and heavy exercise if some spotting has occurred. Your doctor may call cramping and spotting a *threatened abortion.* Bleeding can be caused by implantation of the embryo or by the sloughing off of the lining around the area where implantation has occurred. An internal exam will show whether your cervix has started to open. An ultrasound done around six weeks will show whether a fetus is in the uterus and may show a heartbeat. A heartbeat *should* be seen by vaginal ultrasound by seven weeks at the latest.

- ✔ **Inevitable abortion:** If your cervix has started to open, or *dilate,* and you're bleeding, you'll almost certainly miscarry. Your doctor may call these symptoms an *inevitable abortion.* An ultrasound may show no fetal heartbeat. Your doctor will want you to watch for signs of infection, such as a temperature over 100 degrees or a foul-smelling discharge. Hospitalization isn't necessary in most cases of miscarriage. Save any tissue that you pass so that your doctor can send it to a pathologist, who will examine it and make sure there is nothing sinister about the miscarriage. In general, tissue passed at home will not be viable enough to allow an evaluation for chromosomal abnormalities. You'll probably continue bleeding for seven to ten days.

✔ **Missed abortion:** A *missed abortion* occurs when the pregnancy stops progressing but there are no signs of miscarriage, such as bleeding or cramping. Your pregnancy blood levels may be lower than expected, and the ultrasound shows no fetal heart activity. A missed abortion may require a dilation and curettage, a minor surgery, to remove the tissue.

Knowing if you need a D&C

You need a D&C, or *dilation and curettage,* if you don't pass all the pregnancy tissue on your own. This procedure involves opening the cervix and scraping the uterus with a blunt instrument called a curette, or with a plastic tube with an opening connected to suction vacuum, to make sure that no tissue is left, because leftover tissue can cause an infection. This surgery is done under light sedation, usually as an outpatient procedure. Your doctor may tell you not to take tub baths, use hot tubs, douche, or have sex for a week or two. You may be asked to return for a follow-up visit to make sure that you're healing normally. There won't be any stitches to remove after a D&C.

Don't be upset if your doctor calls your miscarriage a *spontaneous abortion,* or SAB. This is the medical term for a miscarriage.

Finding the cause

More than 50 percent of miscarriages are due to chromosomal abnormalities. In these cases, no amount of rest or anything else that you do — or don't do — will prevent them. The good news is that the vast majority of these are considered "random" and "non-recurrent," which means that the next time you get pregnant, there is no reason to think the same thing will happen.

In trying to understand chromosomal abnormalities, you can compare a growing fetus to a house being built. If a builder orders a lot of lumber but no roofing materials, a house's walls can be built, but only up to the point where the roofing materials are needed. If the genes needed for the baby to develop are processed wrong at the time of conception, the baby will develop to the point where it needs those genes to keep growing. Without those genes, the fetus can't continue to develop. Its "walls" will be built, but without the "roof," it can't continue to grow. Two types of chromosomal errors are listed below.

Blighted ovum

A blighted ovum is the most common outcome (other than a chemical pregnancy) of a conception that has a chromosomal error. *Blighted ovum* occurs when the placenta and amniotic sac develop and put out pregnancy hormones but the fetus itself doesn't develop. So you may test pregnant, but there is no fetus. You and your doctor may discover this fact when you start spotting and the doctor tests for fetal activity and finds no fetus. Since most fertility doctors perform routine ultrasound testing of all pregnancies, a blighted ovum (or "empty sac") may also be picked up at the time of a routine evaluation. The most frustrating part of a blighted ovum is that the HCG is produced by the placenta, and therefore may be quite high, with associated pregnancy symptoms — morning sickness, breast tenderness, tiredness — and yet there is no baby.

Molar pregnancy

Another, somewhat rare type of chromosomal anomaly is called a molar pregnancy. Molar pregnancies, also called a *hydatidiform mole,* occur in one in a thousand conceptions in the United States; *Molar pregnancies* result when the egg is abnormal; it has no chromosomal content to pass on, so there is no fetus, only a placenta. The placenta usually grows very quickly; you may show signs of pregnancy very early and have unusually high beta levels.

Molar pregnancies are treated with a D&C to evacuate the abnormal cells. In some cases, the cells can transform into *choriocarcinoma,* a rare disease that behaves like a cancer in that it can spread to other parts of the body. In these cases, you may be given methotrexate, a chemotherapy drug, to stop the abnormally fast cell division. After a molar pregnancy, you will be advised to avoid another pregnancy for 6 to 12 months to be sure that no abnormal cells remain in the body and that a choriocarcinoma does not develop.

Other common causes of miscarriage, such as abnormalities of the uterus, lack of progesterone support after ovulation, or vaginal infection, can be evaluated before you try to get pregnant again.

You should know, though, that regular cigarette smoking can increase the rate of miscarriage by 30 to 50 percent, so cutting down drastically or stopping smoking is a good idea if you want a successful pregnancy.

Evaluating chromosomes

Even though most miscarriages are caused by chromosomal abnormalities, don't expect your doctor to always be able to prove this. Sharon remembers this as one of the most frustrating things about having a miscarriage–the fact that no one could give her a reason why. The tissue may be sent for analysis, but the cells may not grow (the cells must be viable and divide in the lab in order for the chromosomal testing to be done). Other times, the mother's own cells may overgrow the cells of the placenta, and the chromosomal analysis simply confirms that the mother was normal (46 XX); this is called *maternal contamination.*

Whereas the vast majority of chromosomally abnormal conceptions are caused by random errors and are non-recurrent, there are some mistakes that are caused by rearrangements in chromosomes that are passed on by the parents. Even if you have the right number of chromosomes (46), two of them, or parts of two of them, may have gotten "stuck" together. Now imagine what happens when you try to make an egg (or a sperm), and put half of your chromosomes into the gamete (remember you only get to contribute half of your chromosomes, and your partner provides the other half). If two of your chromosomes are "stuck" together, instead of contributing 23 chromosomes, you may only be able to contribute 22, or 24. Any pregnancy that occurs will always have the wrong number of chromosomes.

Your doctor will recommend chromosomal testing, also called karyotyping, if you have had two or more miscarriages, or if the chromosomal test on one of them revealed a translocation. Chromosomal abnormalities fall into one of several categories:

- The wrong number of chromosomes — either too many, or too few

- Translocations, or rearrangements, of chromosomes

- Data added to or subtracted from certain chromosomes

Playing the blame game

Are you feeling guilty about your miscarriage because you once sneaked a cigarette, had a glass of champagne at a wedding, had sex, or went skydiving during your pregnancy? Maybe you've been depressed or had an abortion when you were 17. Whatever, now you blame yourself and your careless ways for the miscarriage. Don't. Although some of these actions may not have been the best decisions, the truth is that almost certainly *none* of them caused this miscarriage.

Factoring in age

As in most fertility issues, age is a definite factor in miscarriage rates. Consider these numbers:

- If you're under 35, the miscarriage rate is about 6 percent.

- If you're pushing 40, the miscarriage rate increases to 14 percent.

- If you're over 40, your chance of miscarriage is 23 percent.

- If you're around 43, the rate goes up to nearly 50 percent.

- After age 45, 87 percent of all women are infertile, so pregnancy is rare, making miscarriage rates more difficult to gather. Also, periods are more irregular, so what appears to be a late period could be a miscarriage.

These statistics reflect the increased number of chromosomally abnormal eggs still left as you get older; your "best eggs" have already been ovulated. We discuss age-related fertility issues more in Chapter 1.

Ectopic Pregnancy: When the Embryo Is Developing in the Wrong Place

An ectopic pregnancy is a different type of miscarriage. In an *ectopic pregnancy,* the embryo may be developing normally, but it's growing in the wrong place, usually in the fallopian tube. Like a miscarriage, an ectopic pregnancy ends your hopes for a baby *this time,* but it can cause other problems as well.

Ectopic pregnancies aren't rare — 1 out of 100 pregnancies is ectopic — and the percentage has been rising over the last 30 years. With an ectopic pregnancy, the fetus may be normal but attaches to tissue outside the uterus, usually in the fallopian tube, and begins to grow there. The fallopian tube is much smaller than the uterus, and the baby can't grow beyond a certain point, usually around seven weeks, before rupturing the tube, causing severe complications. Ectopic pregnancy is the leading cause of maternal death in the first trimester of pregnancy.

What to do if you suspect an ectopic pregnancy

Any time you have severe one-sided pain, severe shoulder pain, or a feeling of lightheadedness and weakness a few weeks after missing a period, you *must* go to the emergency room to make sure that you don't have an ectopic pregnancy. A positive pregnancy test and an ultrasound showing no fetus in the uterus can confirm an ectopic pregnancy. If you have no physical symptoms, an ectopic pregnancy may be suspected if the BSU is lower than it should be; rarely, the pregnancy test can also be negative. An ultrasound will show nothing in the uterus — no sac, placenta, or fetus.

What your doctor will do

Treating an ectopic pregnancy involves either dissolving the developing pregnancy with a drug called methotrexate, the same drug used for molar pregnancies (see the section "Molar pregnancy," earlier in this chapter), or removing the pregnancy through surgery. Surgical removal of an ectopic pregnancy can also cause more infertility problems; the fallopian tube may need to be removed, and adhesions or scar tissue may develop after the surgery. An ectopic pregnancy can be a life-threatening event. If the fetus gets too big, the fallopian tube will burst, and you could be in danger of bleeding to death.

Methotrexate causes the pregnancy to dissolve by stopping the rapid cell division necessary for a fetus to grow. Four percent of women taking methotrexate have diarrhea, mouth soreness, or stomach irritation because these cells are also fast-growing and affected by the disturbance in cell division. Serious side effects, such as liver toxicity or lung problems, are rare.

Stop taking folic acid while on methotrexate because it may interfere with the action of the methotrexate.

Methotrexate successfully dissolves an ectopic pregnancy 90 percent of the time, but it must be used before the fetus grows larger than 3.5 cm (a little over an inch). After that, surgical removal is necessary.

If surgery is required, your doctor may try to save the fallopian tube if possible. If the fallopian tube has to be removed, you can still get pregnant. An egg can even be released from the right ovary and find its way to the left tube if the right tube is gone.

Can the pregnancy be moved somehow from the fallopian tube to the uterus? Because the placenta and the tissues involved with growth are "dug in" to the tube, removing the fetus from the tube and reattaching it to the uterus are impossible at this time.

Understanding why ectopic pregnancies happen

Although anyone can have an ectopic pregnancy, ectopic pregnancies are more likely in women who have any of the following risk factors:

- If you have a swollen, dilated fallopian tube, called a *hydrosalpinx,* you're six to ten times more likely to have an ectopic pregnancy. Hydrosalpinx is frequently caused by pelvic inflammatory disease (PID), often associated with a chlamydia infection. (See Chapter 2 for more on chlamydia.) Even if you have IVF, in which the embryo is placed directly in the uterus, it may migrate back up into the hydrosalpinx and implant there! This is one of the reasons a hydrosalpinx should be removed prior to IVF.

- If you smoke, you're one and a half to four times more likely to have an ectopic pregnancy.

- Have you had a previous tubal surgery? You have a 15 percent chance for an ectopic pregnancy. If you've had a prior tubal sterilization reversed, the risk is about 5 to 10 percent (it's less than after surgery for diseased tubes because, in most cases, tubal ligation is performed on healthy tubes, and they should be healthy again after the reconnection.)

- Previous use of an IUD slightly increases the chance of an ectopic pregnancy. (If you currently have an IUD and you get pregnant anyway — not likely if you're reading this book, by the way — the risk that the pregnancy is in the tube is about 20 percent.)

✔ Current use of progestin-only birth control pills also increases the chance of an ectopic pregnancy.

✔ If you've had a previous ectopic pregnancy, your chance for another is 20 percent. Your chance of being infertile is about 30 percent.

✔ If you douche regularly, at least three times a week, you're more likely to have an ectopic pregnancy.

Other origins of ectopic pregnancies

Most infertility treatments are associated with a higher rate of ectopic pregnancies. In fact, just being a patient in an infertility doctor's office increases your risk of ectopic pregnancy! Twin, triplet, and other multiple pregnancies are also associated with ectopic pregnancies; in some cases, one fetus may implant in the uterus and another in a tube, a condition called a *heterotopic pregnancy.*

Recurring Miscarriage: Why It Happens

Two percent of all couples suffer *recurrent miscarriage,* which is the loss of three or more early pregnancies. After three losses, the chance of a fourth loss increases to 45 to 50 percent. What causes this repeated heartbreak?

✔ Uterine problems, such as fibroids that intrude into the uterine cavity, scar tissue in the uterine cavity (Asherman's syndrome), or malformations of the uterine cavity shape, can result in a miscarriage. If your mom took DES, a drug to prevent miscarriage, in the 1950s and 1960s, you may have an unusually shaped uterine cavity. Between 15 and 20 percent of recurrent miscarriages are caused by uterine problems. (We discuss this topic in depth in Chapter 7.)

✔ An incompetent cervix is responsible for 5 percent of all recurrent miscarriages. An *incompetent cervix* is a cervix too weak to stay closed during pregnancy. The cervix dilates painlessly, resulting in the loss of the pregnancy; this usually occurs after 12 weeks, when the growing fetus puts more weight on the cervix. An incompetent cervix can be diagnosed on ultrasound; the cervical length will measure less than 20 mm. An incompetent cervix can be caused by DES exposure before you were born, trauma to the cervix (such as a cone biopsy done to diagnose possible cervical cancer), or congenital deformities. Pregnancy loss can be prevented in most cases by placing a stitch, called a *cerclage,* through your cervix to keep it from opening too soon. This is usually done after 12 weeks.

- ✔ Chromosomal abnormalities in either you or your partner cause 5 percent of recurrent miscarriages. Chromosomal karyotyping, performed as a blood test, on you and your partner can be used to diagnose chromosomal abnormalities.

- ✔ Immune problems, including diseases such as lupus, may be a factor in a miscarriage. Antibodies called antiphospholipid antibodies, which cause clotting problems, and many other possible immune deficiencies are currently a hot topic in fertility workups. (See Chapter 7 for more information about immune issues.)

Pregnancy loss is an issue of biology, not morality. Fertility problems are not a punishment for anything; they're the result of biology gone awry.

Suffering the insensitive remarks of family and friends

What's worse after a miscarriage than friends who become pregnant? Or friends who continue to be pregnant when you're not? How about relatives who try to jolly you out of depression with stories of how miscarriage was probably a blessing and that you should be thankful for the children you have? Or what about women who regale you with stories of their own miscarriages?

Everyone has her own way of dealing with people you can't avoid. Some women politely ask that it not be discussed. Other women not so politely ask the offender to please shut up. Yet other women agree and pretend that they're feeling better. Try to remember that people are feeling awkward and don't know what to say, but they're trying to make you feel better because they care about you. Spouses may be having an equally difficult time because few men discuss miscarriage with their friends; if they do, they may find little sympathy for an early loss. They may also feel out of the loop and uninformed about exactly what happened, and may not want to question you for fear of upsetting you more. If you can bring yourself to talk about it, a little conversation goes a long way toward making your partner feel more like a partner and less like a hindrance during this difficult time.

Picking Yourself Up after a Loss

As if you haven't heard it enough, your body needs to heal after a miscarriage. However, also remember that miscarriage is a common event, and is a part of reproduction. Women have been having miscarriages for millennia.

Your doctor may recommend waiting up to three months before trying to conceive again. However, a recent study evaluated the risk of another miscarriage in women who conceived in the first month after a miscarriage — without a single intervening period — and found no increase in a second miscarriage as compared to women who waited longer. Therefore, there is no reason to wait longer than one month before trying again. This is especially important if you're over 40. Remember, time is not your friend!

If you're still bleeding after a miscarriage (or a D&C), your cervix may still be open, and your body is telling you that it is not yet ready for conception. So you probably want to avoid intercourse until the bleeding stops. After that, you should be fine. If you bleed for longer than two weeks after a miscarriage (or a D&C), call your doctor and get an ultrasound. There may be some tissue left behind.

Time truly does heal, or at least dulls the pain. Each passing day will help to make your next pregnancy a joyous experience completely its own, not a shadow of the fear and doubt of your early pregnancy loss.

Even the most optimistic of you will experience those times when your hope button is stuck on "off." This phase is a temporary, albeit painful, condition. Rebooting your emotions can go a long way toward resetting your physical condition as well.

What to do while you're waiting

Just like your body needs to repair itself, your spirit needs some help as well. As you count the days until you can begin trying again, consider using this time to help your future child in another way. Here's your to-do list:

- ✔ **If you have already been blessed with a child or children, take a moment to appreciate them.** A hug from your precious one can right many of the world's wrongs.

- ✔ **Allow yourself the time to grieve.** Trying to pretend that you're back to normal when you're not may make you feel temporarily better. In the long run, however, covering up grief rather than expressing it and working through it will cause it to resurface again, possibly during your next pregnancy, in the form of resentment or guilt. Take the time to heal.

- ✔ **Do something wonderful for yourself.** Whether it's a special purchase, a dinner out with your partner, or an ice cream sundae, indulge a whim.

- ✔ **Do consider professional help if your sadness is debilitating or lasts longer than three months.** A counselor can help guide you through the minefield of emotions that you're facing.

You and your partner are allies, not enemies, no matter how differently you process the stress and grief of your loss. Helping your partner deal with his own emotions will help you come to terms with your own feelings as well. This experience can make you a stronger team if you work together.

What not to do

Taking care of yourself during this time and allowing others to care for you should be your first priority, if not your only one. Part of this task, which may seem daunting enough, is to keep in touch with your own feelings and stay in touch with those who care about you. To help accomplish this, here's our list of things to avoid:

- ✔ **Don't force yourself to do anything that you don't feel up to.** You may need to decline an invitation to a friend's baby shower, christening, or family gathering, and that's okay. This time is about getting better, emotionally and physically. Don't do anything to compromise your recovery.

- ✔ **Don't go into hiding.** You'll want to skip some events, but don't completely isolate yourself. Your community of friends and family can help you heal. Although pain is unavoidable, suffering, particularly alone, is optional.

- ✔ **Don't redecorate the nursery or wander through baby stores.** These types of behaviors are similar to picking at a scab. The temptation to do these things is great, and you can talk yourself into believing that these actions will be cathartic. In actuality, they'll most likely cause you more pain and prolong your healing process.

An early pregnancy loss does have somewhat of a silver lining. It confirms that you can conceive, which can often be more than half the battle.

Part IV

Moving Up to High-Tech Conception

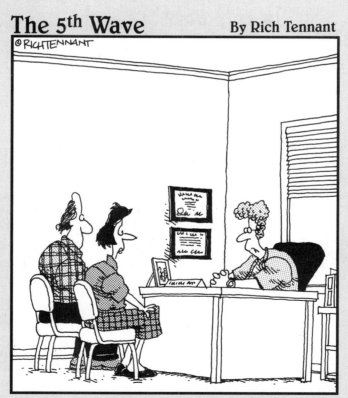

The 5th Wave   By Rich Tennant

"I realize the diagnosis is serious and raises many questions, but let's try to address them in order. We'll look at various treatment options, make a list of the best clinics to consider, and then determine what color ribbon you should be wearing."

In this part . . .

This part explains what high-tech infertility treatments are, from injections to vitro fertilization. We guide you through the complicated maze of finding the right clinic and take you through the stimulation process and the egg retrieval itself. We visit the embryology lab after your egg retrieval and give advice on how to get through the "two week wait" for your pregnancy test without losing your mind. We also discuss the dollars and sense of infertility, what different processes may cost and how to maximize your funds, your insurance and your resources.

Chapter 13

A Little Help from Dr. Specialist: Intrauterine Insemination and Fertility Injections

*S*tarting an IUI (intrauterine insemination) cycle or a stimulated medication cycle is a big step up from just trying to figure out when you're ovulating and planning to have sex accordingly. IUI cycles involve monitoring blood and ultrasound results, and often involve injecting potent hormone stimulators called gonadotropins.

In this chapter, we explain how IUI and stimulated cycles work and discuss some of the testing involved and the medications you may be taking. We also help you find those expensive gonadotropins as cheaply as possible, and we give you tips on how to inject them as safely as possible.

Deciding How Much Treatment You Need

There are several roads to travel when seeing a fertility doctor, and on which one Dr. Specialist (see Chapter 7 for more on how to find the right Dr. Specialist) places you depends on the reason for your infertility. If the problem is diagnosed as mild male factor (a slightly lower than normal sperm count or motility), Dr. Specialist may suggest doing an IUI (see "Artificial Insemination? No, It's Real!" for details on IUI) to give the sperm a "leg up" on getting where they need to be by washing them and placing them directly into the uterus.

If you're not producing an egg or not releasing an egg, you may be prescribed stimulating medications to increase egg production. If you're getting your period less than two weeks after you ovulate, your doctor may prescribe progesterone for a suspected luteal phase defect, which we explain in the section "Treating Luteal Phase Defects."

Even if your partner's sperm is fine, you're ovulating, and your tubes have been tested and found to be open, you may still be faced with so-called "unexplained infertility." Many studies have shown that couples with unexplained infertility have substantially higher chances of pregnancy if the woman takes fertility medications and the sperm are placed in the uterus with an IUI.

If you've gone several months without a positive pregnancy test, you may end up doing all three: IUI, gonadotropins (stimulating medications), and progesterone supplementation.

"Take two Clomid and call me in three months"

The prescription Dr. Basic hands you (if you can decipher it) at the end of your first visit may say "Clomiphene citrate 50 mgm qd X 5 days, #10. Refills 3." Or it may simply say "CC 50mg qd d 3-7." What does this mean?

Clomiphene citrate, more commonly called Clomid or Serophene (two brand names), is given to help you make an egg or to help you make a *better* egg; it may also help sustain a pregnancy by creating an egg whose corpus luteum (see Chapter 2 for more about the function of the corpus luteum) produces higher progesterone levels. Normally, you take Clomid for five days. Some doctors start you on it on day three of your cycle, and others start you on day four or five. The exact timing isn't important; the point is to start it before your ovaries start to develop one dominant follicle.

Usually your doctor will give you one pill a day the first month or two and then move up to two or three tablets a day if you still don't seem to be ovulating regularly. Clomid comes in 50 milligram tablets, so if your doctor starts you at a higher dose, 100 to 150 milligrams per day, you'll need to take more than one. After you stop taking the pills, you can check for ovulation by using your old friends, the basal thermometer and the ovulation predictor kits.

Clomid works by fooling the body into thinking it's not making enough estrogen. When your hypothalamus thinks that you're low on estrogen, it releases GnRH (gonadotropin-releasing hormone), which stimulates the release of FSH (follicle-stimulating hormone) into your blood. The FSH stimulates the ovary to produce estrogen, so that a follicle will begin to grow.

Eighty percent or so of women taking Clomid ovulate in response to this stimulation. Clomid works best for those whose ovaries are capable of functioning normally but need a little tune-up. If you're already ovulating a mature follicle regularly, Clomid can help by increasing the stimulation to the ovary, or even by causing you to ovulate more than one egg. In the latter cases, the Clomid is generally combined with an IUI.

Your doctor may want you to have an ultrasound before starting Clomid each month to make sure you don't have any ovarian cysts. Most pregnancies from Clomid occur in the first three to six months of therapy if the drug is taken for anovulation.

Clomid has a few drawbacks, including the chance for multiple births. Between 5 and 10 percent of all Clomid pregnancies are twins, 1 in 400 is a triplet pregnancy, and 1 pregnancy in 800 results in quadruplets. Obviously, you may be delighted to have a twin pregnancy, but triplets or quads may not be so thrilling. Higher-order multiples (triplets and above) have a very high rate of premature delivery and significantly higher than normal maternal and infant complications. Multiples result from Clomid working too well and stimulating more than one follicle to grow.

Some doctors monitor you with ultrasounds while you're on Clomid to be sure that you're not making too many eggs. If you're making a large number of eggs, you may develop ovarian hyperstimulation syndrome, which can cause a very high estradiol level, making hospitalization necessary. If you're on Clomid and feel very ill, with a sudden weight gain, severe bloating in your abdomen, or abdominal pain, call your doctor immediately. This is a rare side effect of Clomid.

Clomid also has some less serious side effects, some annoying, some potentially detrimental to pregnancy. For example:

- Because your body has been fooled into thinking that it doesn't have enough estrogen, you may have some of the same symptoms women have when they enter menopause and their estrogen drops: hot flashes, headaches, nausea, or blurred vision. Some doctors may give you estrogen to decrease your symptoms.

- Clomid can also interfere with your production of cervical mucus because it locks into all the estrogen receptors, including those in your cervix, so they don't make mucus in response to rising estrogen levels like they normally do. Because estrogen also builds your uterine lining, some women on Clomid don't make a thick lining. If you have either of these side effects, you may need to take estrogen after you start making a follicle. If your cervical mucus is decreased, an IUI may be in order to bypass the mucus altogether and deposit the sperm directly into the uterus (see Chapter 5 for more information on the importance of cervical mucus).

"Artificial" Insemination? No, It's Real!

Artificial insemination may sound like it's a fake procedure, but it's the real thing. _Artificial insemination_ (another term for "insemination", which in today's day and age means "intrauterine insemination" or IUI) means simply that sperm is placed into the uterus to give it a "leg up" on getting where it needs to go, which is to your egg.

You may or may not be taking stimulating medications to create more eggs during an IUI cycle. Some doctors start with Clomid, a pill given to increase your egg output, and move up after a few months to stimulation with gonadotropins. In the past, some doctors would simply monitor your normal cycle and inseminate, hoping to fertilize the one or possibly two follicles you produce each month. This may be okay if you're using donor sperm; however, there's no evidence that an IUI without stimulation increases the chances of pregnancy in unexplained infertility.

Measuring your chance for success

Artificial insemination will not increase your chances over timed intercourse if you have a normal semen analysis and normal ovulation (see Chapter 11 for more about semen analysis). Nor will IUI be effective if the problem is severe male factor (a very low sperm count or antisperm antibodies) or blocked tubes.

Although statistics reported for IUI seem to vary widely, most studies have shown about a 10 per month success rate for women under age 35, using clomiphene plus IUI, with decreasing success as your age goes up. Injectable medications produce more follicles per month and thus, the per cycle success rate with their use along with IUI is a little higher, about 15 percent for women under 35. Many experts believe that your chance of getting pregnant after six failed IUI cycles is slim unless you do in vitro fertilization.

Collecting sperm

When your partner is directed to produce a semen sample in a cup, you may have a mental picture of a little paper drinking cup. Of course, no clinics use paper cups to collect sperm — at least, we hope they don't. Clinics give the guys a plastic sterile container for this purpose.

Semen collection and concentration are a big part of IUI. Several methods are used both to collect and to concentrate the sperm:

✔ **Clean container collection:** A sterile container is used to collect the sample obtained through masturbation.

✔ **Condom collection:** A special condom containing no lubricants or spermicides is used if the semen sample has to be collected during intercourse. This method is useful for those whose religious beliefs prohibit masturbation. This method is not as good as masturbation, because less of the specimen is collected, plus contact between the semen and the penis inevitably introduces bacteria into the specimen.

✔ **Withdrawal:** Other men who cannot masturbate may be able to ejaculate as a result of intercourse and withdraw at the last minute to collect the specimen into a sterile cup. This takes a certain presence of mind! This method is also not as good as masturbation for the same reasons as the condom collection method, but may actually result in a slightly better collection and a slightly cleaner specimen than the condom method.

Don't be insulted if the andrologist (the person who deals with sperm) asks whether there was any spillage. This isn't a comment on your general clumsiness or the look of your sample! The first part of the semen has the highest concentration of sperm, so if any was lost, your semen sample may not be as good as it should be.

Sperm need to be "washed" before they're ready for IUI. Washing must be done because the unwashed semen specimen contains not only the sperm, but also the seminal plasma. This liquid, which originates in the prostate gland, is designed to protect the sperm from the acidic environment of the vagina. It is alkaline, forms a sticky clump to keep the sperm in the vagina, and contains large amounts of prostaglandins, chemicals that cause smooth muscle contractions. None of these qualities are favorable for a trip directly into the uterine cavity. If a large amount of semen — more than 0.2 ml — is injected unwashed into the uterus, the prostaglandins can cause severe cramping at the least!

If you're picturing the washing process being done in a little machine with a spin cycle, you're partially right! The semen specimen is first diluted with culture media (a sperm nutrient solution) and the sperm are spun down into a little pellet in a centrifuge before being placed in the uterus. One method spins the sperm in a centrifuge, and another puts the sperm on the bottom of a test tube and allows the best sperm to swim up, and third method combines the two: centrifugation followed by swim-up. Another common method used puts the sperm on top of several layers of washing media; the tube is spun down, and the pellet on the bottom will contain the largest amount of motile, healthy sperm. The sperm pellet is then placed via catheter into the uterus. All methods have in common the concept of isolating the sperm from the seminal plasma.

The main risks of doing IUI are risk of infection and risk of multiple births if you're taking medication to stimulate growth of more than one follicle.

Checking out your egg

IUI and timed intercourse (timed for your ovulation) will work only if the sperm arrives in the right place at the right time — when you have a mature egg. Making sure that you're making a follicle and checking it for maturity before an IUI increase your chances of pregnancy.

Monitoring your hormone level

One way to be sure you're making a good egg is to monitor your hormone levels. As you start to make a mature egg, your estradiol starts to rise. A good egg should produce an estradiol of 150 to 300 pg/ml. About 30 hours before your egg releases, your LH will also start to rise; a good LH surge is usually over 40.

Thar she blows: Ultrasounds before and after ovulation

Many fertility doctors use pelvic ultrasound to monitor the growth of ovarian follicles. Ultrasound works by bouncing high-frequency sound waves off internal organs. Unlike X-rays, ultrasounds don't expose you to radiation. There are two types of pelvic ultrasound:

- **Transvaginal ultrasound:** This procedure uses a long, wand-like probe that can be embarrassing if you're very modest. In addition, the moving probe can cause uncomfortable pressure. This method, which can be done with an empty bladder, gives better images than abdominal ultrasounds in most cases.

  For a transvaginal ultrasound, you undress from the waist down, cover yourself with a sheet, and lie flat on your back with your legs in typical exam table stirrups. The ultrasound technician or your doctor inserts the vaginal probe after covering the tip with transducing jelly and placing a condom over it. The tip of the wand is smaller than a vaginal speculum. Some centers ask you to insert the probe yourself. The technician moves the wand from side to side to record good pictures of your ovaries and uterus.

- **Abdominal ultrasound:** This procedure requires a full bladder. The images aren't usually as clear as the transvaginal ultrasound.

  For an abdominal ultrasound, you pull your pants down to the pubic hair line. Jelly is placed directly on your stomach, and the technician then moves the transducer (a small hand-held device about the size of your hand) over it. Be aware that, because you have a full bladder, this pressure can be uncomfortable.

  A full bladder is needed for abdominal ultrasound for this reason: The uterus and ovaries normally lie behind the intestines, but a full bladder moves the uterus back and pushes the intestine up, so the uterus and ovaries can be seen more clearly. The bladder also provides a fluid contrast that makes the uterus easier to identify.

There are no known side effects from ultrasound. When your ultrasound is finished, you can go home with no special instructions.

If your doctor does ultrasounds during the first two weeks of your cycle, you'll see your follicle growing as your estradiol rises and your LH surges; usually the follicle is about 22 to 25 millimeters at the time of ovulation. Many centers do an ultrasound the day of IUI and the day after, to make sure that the egg has released from the follicle; when this happens, the follicle shrinks on ultrasound. Without a release ultrasound, you may be making a good follicle but not having the egg release. Pregnancy can't occur unless the egg releases. Some clinics will ask you to come back for a second IUI if the follicle is still there, hoping that it will ovulate before you come back the next day.

Getting the timing right

Timing is all important when doing IUI because washed sperm don't seem to live as long as sperm ejaculated into the vagina. At best, washed sperm are thought to live 24 hours, while ejaculated sperm can live up to 3 days normally, and as long as 5 days in optimal mucus. What this means is that IUI timing has to be well coordinated, with egg release and sperm placement timed so that the short lived sperm can get to the egg at the right time.

Sharon remembers talking to an out-of-state friend who was not a patient about her IUIs and suggesting to her (she still blushes at her audacity about this!) that she talk to her doctor about the timing of her IUIs, since she hadn't gotten pregnant in three cycles. She did; he (what a great doc!) listened to her, changed the timing slightly, and she got pregnant the next cycle — with triplets!

Moving Up to Controlled Ovarian Hyperstimulation

Clomid is usually the first drug given to start your follicles growing because it can be given orally and has fewer side effects than injections. If Clomid isn't working for you after a few months, your doctor may suggest moving up to the big time: injecting gonadotropins, a technique called *controlled ovarian hyperstimulation,* or COH for short. We talk about gonadotropins in the section "Defining gonadotropins," later in this chapter.

Understanding the need for injections

With COH, the goal is to make more than one or two follicles. The reasoning is that if you make a few more follicles, you have a better chance of getting pregnant each month.

Obviously, taking injections is a big step. Not only do you have a possibility of making too many follicles when taking injectable stimulating medications, but you also have to deal with the logistics of COH, including going in for frequent blood tests and ultrasounds and finding someone to give you your injections. Some clinics may offer to give the injections, usually for a small fee, but others want your partner or someone else to come in and learn how to give the shots. Fortunately, with newer formulations of the gonadotropins, many can be given subcutaneously (called "sub-cu" for short, it means that the shot is given with a small needle just under the skin, much like an insulin shot that may be taken by a diabetic. It's physically easy to self-inject these medications; of course that doesn't account for the psychological difficulties!

Getting injections from your partner

Believe it or not, most partners do very well giving injections — after the first few times, that is. Giving shots is a learning experience, and unfortunately, *you* are the learning tool in this experience.

Your clinic will probably show you and your partner how to give injections, and it may send you home with a video and an informational tearsheet that you'll refer to frequently in the first few days.

Is it really safe to put a needle in the hand of a totally untrained person and tell them to have at it? Statistically speaking, yes. Millions of diabetics inject themselves every day or have someone else do it. The biggest risks are from infection and hitting a nerve. You can prevent infection with a careful sterile technique, and hitting a nerve can happen to anyone, even a professional, because your anatomy may not look like the textbook picture.

If at all possible, insist on doing your first injection in front of someone at your clinic, so a person skilled in this procedure can critique and give pointers. Also, after you and your partner have done it once, your partner is less likely to pass out the first time you do an injection at home.

Giving yourself shots

Sometimes, for whatever reason, you may have to give yourself the shots. Maybe you don't have a partner, maybe your partner is locked in the bathroom refusing to give you a shot, or maybe you travel a lot. You can inject yourself, although it's a bit trickier.

If you know that you'll be doing your own injections, ask your doctor if he can give you subcutaneous gonadotropins. These are injected with a very tiny needle — like a diabetic needle — and can be used in the top of your leg, in your stomach, or in the back of your arm, although this latter site is a hard place to inject yourself. Subcutaneous gonadotropins are *recombinant* or *purified*, so they can be injected subcutaneously without causing a rash. The medication your doctor orders depends primarily on personal preference, since there are no studies proving the superiority of one medication over another.

If you end up taking intramuscular injections, such as Repronex, made from human urinary proteins, standing in front of a mirror when you give them may be helpful. Or ask your clinic if you can inject them into the top of your leg.

Your doctor may recommend that you take all medication intramuscularly if your body mass index (BMI) is over 30, so that the medications will be absorbed better.

Defining gonadotropins

Gonadotropins are stimulating medications (see Chapter 22 for the most commonly used ones), meaning that they make follicles grow. Each follicle contains an egg, so making five follicles each month rather than one or two gives you a better shot at getting pregnant.

Gonadotropins contain either all follicle-stimulating hormone (FSH) or a combination of FSH and luteinizing hormone (LH). Some doctors prefer that you have a little LH because they feel it aids stimulation, while others prefer a pure FSH product. Urinary products are cheaper and some need to be injected intramuscularly, although most of the newer medications are injected subcutaneously.

Some doctors have definite preferences about which type and brand of drug you should take. Sometimes the preference is medical, and sometimes it depends on which drug company representative has been in the office most recently. The reality is that studies that have tried to compare the various medications have consistently failed to demonstrate the superiority of one medication over another.

Exploring the side effects

Because these drugs are hormones (which stimulate your ovaries to make more hormones), you can expect to be more "hormonal" when taking them. The most common side effects are headache, bloating, weight gain, and mood swings. Obviously, the hormone changes are going to be a big part of making a stressful situation worse for some people.

Deciding which medication to use

All gonadotropins are purified in the laboratory from a raw protein product. This product can be either the urine of menopausal women, or the product of a cell culture which has been bio-engineered to make gonadotropins. The cells which are used for this are Chinese hamster ovary cells which have had the DNA for the gonadotropins injected into them. When the cells grow, they make FSH, LH, or HCG, depending on which DNA is in the cells. The choice between medications depends on several things:

- ✔ With which medication does your doctor feel most comfortable working? If your doctor has a preference, ask him why. He may have done or read studies that have influenced his opinion that one is better than the other.

- ✔ Do you have drug coverage? Which medication will it cover? If your prescription plan covers only one type of injectable, that's probably what you'll get. If you have no drug coverage, you may want to go with what's least expensive.

- ✔ How needlephobic are you? If you're extremely needlephobic, you'll need to go with subcutaneous medications (see the section "Giving yourself shots," earlier in this chapter) or risk being a wreck for two weeks, dreading each shot.

- ✔ Do you have someone to give you your injections? If you'll be doing most of your shots yourself, you'll probably want to do subcutaneous injections.

- ✔ Have you taken one or the other in the past? How did you respond? If you've taken stimulating medications before, you have some kind of track record. Did you do well on that medication? If not, you'll probably want to try something different. If you did well, you may want to do the same, because changing to something else may change your results.

Mimicking nature with a minipump

When all else fails, some fertility specialists may use a rarely-used method of ovulation induction: stimulating the pituitary with an infusion pump. The pump, which can administer either intravenous or subcutaneous doses of gonadotropin-releasing hormone (GnRH), attempts to mimic nature by releasing a small dose of GnRH every 90 minutes. This stimulates your body to produce LH and FSH.

The benefits of the pump over LH and FSH injections are the following:

- ✔ It doesn't require daily injections.

- ✔ Ovarian hyperstimulation syndrome, described in the section "Ensuring proper monitoring throughout your cycle," later in this chapter, is not as common.

- ✔ You have less chance of a multiple pregnancy.

Disadvantages of the pump are the following:

- ✔ It's expensive.

- ✔ It must be inserted and refilled by a physician.

- ✔ It increases the chance of infection.

Injecting HCG to mature your eggs

The last injection you'll take when doing COH is called HCG, or *human chorionic gonadotropin,* a luteinizing hormone substitute given to mature your eggs and help them release from their follicles. It's usually given a day or two before your IUI.

The HCG injection is not always necessary. Most of the time, when you take gonadotropins, this affects your ability to release LH at the right time and in quantities sufficient to induce follicle release. For this reason, HCG is given as a substitute LH surge. However, in some cases, LH release does take place. The risk is that your IUI may be timed on the basis of the HCG injection, and if you have already ovulated on your own, the timing will be wrong. Therefore, some fertility clinics ask the patients to monitor their LH surge with a urinary ovulation kit, and others instruct the patients to have intercourse every other day during the gonadtropin stimulation "just in case."

HCG helps the eggs in the follicles to mature and complete the cell division needed before they can be fertilized. HCG is made by several companies (see Chapter 22) and is usually given intramuscularly; a newer laboratory-created HCG called Ovidrel can be given subcutaneously.

Don't take nonsteroidal anti-inflammatories such as aspirin, Motrin, or ibuprofen during the middle part of your cycle. They may inhibit prostaglandin production, which may keep you from ovulating.

Ensuring proper monitoring throughout your cycle

If you're taking stimulating medications of any kind — injectables or Clomid — your clinic may want to monitor you to make sure that you're not making too many eggs. Some centers will cancel your IUI or insist that you do in vitro fertilization if you're making a lot of eggs because the risk of hyperstimulation and getting pregnant with triplets — or more — is increased.

Ovarian hyperstimulation syndrome (OHSS) is a serious complication that could land you in the hospital. It starts when you take injectable stimulating medications and make a lot of follicles. If your estradiol rises over 1500, OHSS may occur; it's more common with IVF but can also occur with IUI cycles. Some symptoms of OHSS are the following:

- ✔ Difficulty urinating
- ✔ Difficulty breathing
- ✔ Sudden weight gain of ten pounds or more

If you have OHSS, your clinic may want to monitor your blood count, liver function, weight, and urine output. OHSS may not resolve itself for several weeks, and symptoms may worsen if you're pregnant.

OHSS isn't the only complication of taking gonadotropins or Clomid; multiple pregnancies of five or more babies are usually the result of stimulating medications. Albeit rare (there's a reason why they make the evening news!), these high-order multiples are more often the result of IUI or timed intercourse than IVF because IVF can control the number of embryos put back into the uterus, whereas IUI can't. The number of follicles you have is the number of babies you could end up with!

Treating Luteal Phase Defects

Luteal phase, in fertility circles, means the two weeks after you ovulate and before your period starts. You may be diagnosed with *luteal phase defect* (LPD) if your period starts ten or so days after you ovulate, rather than the normal two-week period. If you've been monitoring your BBT (basal body temperature), you may see an early drop in your temperature as well, but this is not considered a reliable indicator of LPD. LPD can be caused by the following problems with the corpus luteum or with the uterine lining.

After you ovulate, the leftover shell of your follicle, now called the *corpus luteum,* starts to produce progesterone. Progesterone stimulates the uterine lining to produce extra blood vessels so that the embryo has a good supply to support its growth if it attaches.

A poorly developed follicle, or one that releases an abnormal egg, won't put out enough progesterone to properly develop the lining. In this case, the treatment is not more progesterone after you ovulate, but stimulating medications to produce a better-quality follicle.

Some women have a uterine lining that doesn't respond normally to progesterone, and in these cases, progesterone supplements may be helpful. The best way to evaluate your lining is to have an endometrial biopsy done; an ultrasound done a week after you ovulate can also show if your lining is changing to a pattern needed for implantation.

If you get your period less than two weeks after you ovulate, it's important to have a biopsy done to check your progesterone. An *endometrial biopsy* involves scraping a little of your uterine lining with a small curette. The scraping is then checked to see whether the lining has responded appropriately to the progesterone and whether it is capable of supporting embryo implantation. A biopsy is done in your doctor's office, usually the day of a negative pregnancy test before your period starts.

Boosting Progesterone

Because progesterone is essential to maintain pregnancy, many doctors give progesterone supplements in pill, suppository, or injection form to all their infertility patients on an "it can't hurt and might help" basis. Most doctors want to see a progesterone blood level of at least 10 and preferably 15 ng/ml after ovulation.

Another way to raise progesterone levels is to give HCG "boosters," usually a 2,500 IU injection of HCG every few days. HCG stimulates the corpus luteum so that it puts out more progesterone. The disadvantage to boosters is that your pregnancy test will be positive, even if you're not pregnant, for up to ten days after the last HCG injection. Furthermore, HCG injections increase the risk of ovarian hyperstimulation syndrome (OHSS).

If you've taken gonadotropins, you may be given both progesterone and estrogen supplements after you ovulate. Your doctor may prescribe them because gonadotropin administration can affect embryo implantation by interfering with normal hormonal production after ovulation.

The main problem is that when gonadotropins are given to stimulate follicle development, the luteal phase is very often shortened as a result of estrogen and progesterone secretion dropping prematurely. In other words, both estrogen and progesterone secretion drops off earlier than the two weeks which are thought to be needed to allow good embryo implantation. For many years, progesterone alone was given and it is probably enough by itself. More recently, because of the strong stimulation used in conjunction with IVF, both estrogen and progesterone have been used. Either way (progesterone alone or both estrogen and progesterone), the idea is to extend the duration of the luteal phase so that embryo implantation has the best chance of occurring before the lining starts to break down in the next menstrual cycle.

Getting Your Medications for Less

As any smart shopper knows, it's always best to avoid paying the retail price. Instead, look for outlets, sales, and other bargains that can help you get the same product for less money. In this section, we discuss some of the "deals" available when purchasing fertility medications.

Shopping at mail-order pharmacies

Many doctors suggest that you order your medications from one of the mail-order pharmacies now specializing in fertility medications. (See Chapter 22 for a list of some of the biggest mail-order pharmacies.) These pharmacies carry all fertility medications, can ship quickly, and often offer the best prices. In addition, they may provide 24-hour access to nurses or pharmacists who can answer questions for you and Web sites that address common concerns. Many mail-order pharmacies offer overnight shipping at no additional cost with a minimum order. Many mail-order pharmacies also provide booklets, tapes, and hotlines to provide you with information any time of the day or night.

Another added benefit is virtual anonymity. You won't risk standing next to a nosy neighbor who's certain to share your fertility battle with the neighborhood, if not the world. Mail-order pharmacies are subject to the same Food and Drug Administration (FDA) regulations as your corner drugstore and are completely safe to use.

Making a quick trip over the border

For those adventurous types who would rather use the drive-through to get low-cost medications, should you consider a trip over the border? Mexico and Canada are both sources for lower-cost medications, and for some people, they're only a car ride away. Do remember, however, that the standard in the United States, set by the FDA, is quite rigid, and you have no guarantee that other countries will employ the same quality controls. The more Westernized a country, the more likely it is to maintain standards similar to those of the United States. But if you want the security of homegrown products, the only option is to stay home!

When we speak of going over the border to buy medications, we're not referring to scoring fertility drugs from the guy on the corner. Your only source should be the local pharmacy. Some individuals and couples join forces and elect a representative to travel across the border and fill prescriptions for the group.

Turning to drug studies

Another option for low-cost or no-cost medications is to get involved in a drug or protocol study, which is generally run by larger institutions or drug companies. Ask your doctor if he is aware of any existing studies for which you may qualify. Internet bulletin boards also have this information, and other fertility patients often pass along information on studies that their doctors or others are conducting. Studies usually provide only free medications. You would still be required to pay for any procedures, such as IUI or IVF.

Deciding How Long to Keep Trying COH and IUI

Because statistics vary so much on successful COH plus IUI, it can be difficult to know when to say "enough." You may also notice that every doctor has a different take on your odds for success. Although most doctors quote you numbers that reflect their *own* success with any given process, they may also alter them a bit to better reflect your age or your response to treatment so far.

Many doctors use the "three strikes and you're out" rule. In other words, they have you try a particular method three times and then move on to something else if that approach doesn't work. Others point out that if a particular protocol hasn't worked by (for example) the fourth try, the odds of success are greatly diminished.

Jackie and her husband were beyond her doctor's statistics, which showed that 87 percent of his patients became pregnant by IUI #4, if at all. In fact, it was the baker's dozen, the lucky stimulated cycle #13 (IUI #7), that finally stuck!

But, regardless of whether you're on IUI #1, 4, or 40, after a while, it *all* becomes a bit too much.

Growing sick of getting stuck

Perhaps you grew sick of waiting when the first home pregnancy test read negative. But even if you're more patient, what if a month, or two or three, of nightly injections of hormones is just about all you can handle?

First off, be assured that your impatience and irritability aren't a reflection of your winning personality, but more likely the side effects of the drugs you're taking. Most women find that acknowledging that their moods or mood swings are largely chemical in nature does lessen the burden. If you haven't confided in a friend about your fertility struggles, perhaps now is as good a time as any. You'll find that friends or relatives in the know will treat you with kid gloves right about the time that you're ready to pull out the boxing gloves.

Another thing to remember is the numbers game that is human reproduction. One of our favorite stories is that of a professional basketball player who smiled and clapped every time he missed a free throw. When asked about this odd behavior, he responded, "With every miss, I'm one shot closer to success." Consider *your* shots the same way.

Being sensitive to your partner's feelings

Just as you may find the fertility rituals to be all-consuming, your partner may be sharing your views, more than you know. The partner being treated may feel that he or she is undergoing the lion's share of discomfort and disappointment. But remember, even if your partner isn't experiencing every needle stick or test result, that person is watching you go through it. "Big deal!" you scoff. Well, it can be. Watching another person experience pain or sadness can be as difficult as going through it yourself. The silent partner also must suffer with feelings of inadequacy and powerlessness in being unable to relieve your discomfort. Partners of terminally ill patients often need their own support networks as well. And, as a recent study reveals, fertility patients, due to the sometimes long nature of their treatment, share some of the same issues faced by the chronically and terminally ill.

Encourage your partner to share his or her feeling with friends, family, or a professional. Although you may feel as though you're losing your sanity, your partner may feel as though he's losing you.

Chapter 14

Welcome to the Big Time: In Vitro Fertilization

In This Chapter
▶ Moving up to in vitro fertilization
▶ Finding the right clinic
▶ Funding IVF

*I*n vitro fertilization (IVF) and the other assisted reproductive technologies (ARTs) represent the top of the high-tech mountain of infertility treatments, so naturally, you may be a bit nervous about moving into an invasive, expensive, no-guarantees treatment. The good news is that high-tech fertility has come a long way and is no longer a shot in the dark. Pregnancy rates can approach or even exceed 50 percent per attempt in good prognosis situations, and even if you are not under 35, IVF still represents your best chance for fertility even if all simple treatments have already failed.

The term *in vitro fertilization* means fertilization (the joining of egg and sperm) that occurs in the laboratory; that's where the term "test tube baby" comes from. Before you get to the fertilization point, you have to make eggs with the help of stimulating medications called gonadotropins and retrieve them from the follicles they grow in during an egg retrieval procedure. Twenty years ago only a handful of clinics performed IVF. Now more than 400 clinics offer this service (just in the U.S. and Canada, never mind the hundreds of clinics around the world), and IVF has become a big (and lucrative) business.

In this chapter, we help you evaluate different IVF clinics, decipher the confusing statistics about IVF success rates, and give you some help in deciding whether IVF is the next step for you.

Reaching the Top of the Mountain: What In Vitro Fertilization Means for You

For those of you who just basically need to know when to show up at the clinic, here's the scoop on IVF:

- IVF is expensive.
- IVF is time consuming.
- IVF is unpredictable.
- IVF does not guarantee success.
- IVF involves injections.
- IVF requires frequent ultrasounds and blood work.
- IVF can be frustrating; you will scream at the IVF nurses at least once during your treatment.
- IVF can make your whole life stressful; you will scream at your partner at least once, and then *he'll* scream at the IVF nurses.

That's all you really need to know — you can pick up the rest along the way. But we thought you'd like some insights.

Perhaps the most intimidating part of IVF is the notion that you're at the end of the technologic line, the top of the fertility treatment mountain in your quest for a biological baby. While part of you may feel enormous excitement anticipating that you've finally found the magic path, the other part may fear what will happen if IVF doesn't work. If it fails, you may find yourself going back to less-technological methods, or you may move forward to other means of creating a family, such as donor egg or adoption. Think of IVF as a beginning and one step closer to your dream, however it may be attained.

Understanding that IVF isn't for everyone

Although IVF gets a large share of publicity when it comes to infertility, the fact is that only about 2 percent of infertile couples actually end up doing IVF. (In 2003, approximately 122,000 IVF cycles were done in the United States.) Because the techniques used and the ethical issues are still considered cutting edge, media coverage of IVF far exceeds that of, say, intrauterine insemination. So it may seem that way more people are doing in vitro than really are.

Publicity for every celebrity IVF baby may also make it seem like IVF is a sure-fire success method, but of course, media coverage is almost always oversimplified. However, the national statistics for live births per initiated IVF cycle are about 35 percent — and that's for women under age 35. The national statistics break down this way (even though individual clinics may do a little better):

- ✔ **Under age 35:** A 37 percent chance of a live birth per IVF cycle
- ✔ **Ages 35 to 37:** Approximately 30 percent chance of taking home a baby per IVF cycle
- ✔ **Ages 38 to 40:** A percent chance of a live birth per cycle
- ✔ **Ages 41 to 42:** An 11 percent chance of a live birth per cycle
- ✔ **Over age 42:** A 4 percent chance of a live birth per initiated cycle
- ✔ **Over age 45:** Virtually no chance of pregnancy unless you use donor eggs

If you want to see all the national statistics for ART, check out the following Web site: www.cdc.gov/ART/ART2003/section1.htm.

The cost of one IVF cycle is about $8,000 to $10,000, which may or may not include your medication and blood draws. It does generally include monitoring, including ultrasound tests, egg retrieval, embryo culture, and embryo transfer. Most centers charge extra for additional laboratory procedures, like intracytoplasmic sperm injection (ICSI). Of course these items may not be covered by insurance.

Looking at the preceding success rates, you can see that it may well take two or more cycles to get pregnant with IVF, and the cost equals or exceeds a new car. Plus, you have no guarantees of success. Sounds like a great way to spend money, eh?

On the brighter side, if your insurance covers IVF, including medications and ultrasounds, the only thing you have to lose is time.

Looking at the risks of IVF

Although IVF has become a familiar and accepted way of dealing with infertility, it's not entirely without risk. Some risks are well established, and others are not as clear-cut. Before you decide to move on to IVF, consider these factors.

High rate of twins or triplets

The best documented risk of doing IVF is the high rate of twins or triplets. Because more than one embryo, usually two to four, is placed into the uterus at one time, the risk of getting pregnant with more than one baby is high. In the normal population, twins occur a little over 1 percent of the time, or about 1 in 90 births in the United States. Contrast this with the fact that about 25 percent of IVF births are twins! You may see this as an advantage — two for the price of one — but the price tag on multiple deliveries is high.

About one-half of twins are born prematurely, (before 35 weeks gestation), or with a low birth weight. Up to half have a lower than expected birth weight, compared to 10 percent of single babies. One-half or more of twins are delivered by cesarean section, as compared with about 30 percent of the normal population. (Of course, for reasons that are not clear, the cesarean section rate after IVF, even for singletons, is substantially increased. It may be that after all that work getting pregnant, more women are likely to simply schedule their delivery and accept the cesarean as part of the deal.) Mothers of twins are twice as likely to have preeclampsia (high blood pressure and fluid retention, factors that can lead to preterm delivery and in extreme cases can cause maternal seizures).

Neonatal deaths are rare these days. Nevertheless, premature infants in general are three to six times more likely than full-term infants to die in the first year of life. Premature babies also have a higher risk of vision problems, cerebral palsy, and learning difficulties. And you thought that getting pregnant was the only thing you had to worry about!

Ovarian hyperstimulation syndrome

Ovarian hyperstimulation syndrome (OHSS) occurs in 1 to 5 percent of all stimulated cycles in which gonadotropins, medications that stimulate growth of follicles, are taken. OHSS can generally be managed with fluids and pain control, but in extreme cases can cause serious maternal illness, including blood clots and pulmonary emboli. Your doctor will monitor you for the development of this serious complication, whether you are doing COH for IUI or for IVF. In severe cases in association with IVF, pregnancy is intentionally avoided by freezing all of the embryos and allowing the ovaries to return to normal size before trying the embryo transfer. If you have OHSS, keep in touch with the doctor's office. Serious complications have been reported after severe OHSS, including stroke.

Birth defects

An increase in the rate of birth defects is a controversial and as yet unproven possibility in IVF. Some studies show an increase in birth defects in IVF pregnancies, while other studies don't support this claim. This may be because babies born after IVF tend to be scrutinized more than the general population. It's also not clear if an increase in birth defects is associated with IVF or simply with infertility. Much more research will undoubtedly be done in this area as IVF children become older. Techniques such as ICSI and assisted hatching (see Chapter 12 for more on assisted hatching) have been done only in the last ten years, so the children conceived are still young.

It's logical to expect that men who need to do ICSI for male factor issues may pass the gene responsible to their sons, who will most likely also need to do ICSI (or whatever the equivalent technique is) 20 or 30 years from now.

Deciding Whether to Stay with Your Current Doctor

The clinic you've been going to for IUI or monitoring may also perform IVF. And if you're comfortable with the staff and the doctors, know the routine, and have all your insurance coverage set up there, you may decide to stay with that clinic.

You should, however, think about it and do some reading before deciding to stay with your current center. More than 400 U.S. clinics do IVF, and they range from little more than the "weekend dabbler" that does maybe 30 to 40 egg retrievals a year to the megacenters that do more than 1,000 or even 2,000 egg retrievals a year.

Bigger isn't always better, but when it comes to high-tech procedures such as IVF, success rates are highly dependent on the quality of the IVF lab. It stands to reason that a small center doing 30 or 40 retrievals a year may not have the same lab setup as a center doing 1,000 a year. (This is why many small centers actually use a lab that is associated with a large IVF center. You need to ask and find out what the individual setup is.)

You can evaluate centers by:

✔ **Comparing their statistics and what they offer via the Society of Assisted Reproductive Technology (SART).** SART is the professional society for doctors and clinics performing IVF. At the very least, you should be sure that the center with which you work belongs to SART. A condition of membership is that every center sends all of their IVF data to a central organization, which compiles and publishes them. Since member clinics also voluntarily agree to have their data audited periodically, SART is, in effect, the statistic watchdog of IVF. We describe in detail what it monitors and how the statistics are compiled in the section "Sorting through SART statistics," later in this chapter.

✔ **Talking to patients who are currently doing IVF there and to your doctor or the nurses.** Sometimes the nurses are more candid about whether you should stay or move on, especially if they've gotten to know you, like you, and want what's best for you. If the nurse slips you a little note about another clinic a few towns away, pay attention!

Moving On: Finding Dr. Magic's Clinic

Sometimes the decision to move on to another clinic is easily made. For example, if your current clinic doesn't take your insurance, you don't like the staff, or its hours aren't convenient for the more intensive monitoring of IVF, you know you need to switch doctors. Or maybe you need or want specialized treatment that your present clinic doesn't do, such as sex selection, preimplantation genetic diagnosis (PGD), or sperm aspiration. Luckily for you, Dr. Magic most likely has a Web site, a good place to start looking for your IVF doctor.

Searching through IVF Web sites

Most medium to large IVF clinics have a Web site. At the very least, the Web site should tell you the following information:

- ✔ How many egg retrievals the clinic does in a year
- ✔ How many embryo transfers the clinic does in a year
- ✔ Pregnancy rates for all age groups, broken down per egg retrieval and per embryo transfer
- ✔ Whether it freezes embryos
- ✔ Whether it does ICSI
- ✔ Whether it transfers three-day embryos or blastocysts (see Chapter 12)
- ✔ How many doctors do IVF
- ✔ The educational level of the doctors and whether the doctors are reproductive endocrinologists
- ✔ Whether the clinic cycles patients through all the time or you have to wait for the next group
- ✔ Whether the clinic has a donor egg or embryo program

You may have other concerns pertaining to your own situation. If you can't find the answer on the Web site, you may be able to call the center and ask to speak to an IVF nurse. Usually they're happy to answer any questions you have about their program, and you won't feel as committed as you might after talking to a doctor. (You don't have to give your real name, either!)

Sorting through SART statistics

The Society of Assisted Reproductive Technology (SART) is an organization affiliated with ASRM (American Society of Reproductive Medicine), the organization for healthcare professionals involved with reproductive medicine. SART's members are the approximately 430 IVF clinics in the United States that submit the following information to SART for publication each year:

✔ The number of cycles they do

✔ The types of infertility their patients have

✔ The outcome of their cycles

✔ Pregnancy rates

✔ Multiple pregnancy rates

✔ Miscarriage rates

✔ Cancellation rates

In short, the clinics provide information on just about anything and everything concerning their patients' IVF cycles.

SART takes the information and compiles a booklet of information about every one of the 437 clinics and distributes it to its members; it also publishes the data on *its* Web site. SART data is also found with other data from the Centers for Disease Control and Prevention (CDC).

Clinics that are members of SART can be audited and their data checked for accuracy. The amount of information required by SART is astounding: Your age, Social Security number, infertility type, and type of cycle are reported to SART for every IVF cycle that you do. In most medium to large clinics, compiling and reporting SART data take a tremendous amount of time.

SART confirms clinic-reported data by visiting about 30 clinics a year and auditing selected patients' charts to make sure that the submitted information is accurate.

Individual clinic statistics presented on their Web sites can be difficult to read because not all clinics report their numbers in the same way. For example, one clinic may report pregnancy rates per retrieval, and another may report per transfer. One advantage of the SART data is that it does allow you to compare apples to apples when sifting through SART data. But remember that statistics do not tell the whole story. For example, SART statistics don't tell you anything about the clinic population except for its breakdown by age. A center dealing with only the crème de la crème of patients, the place everyone else calls the "Mecca," certainly has higher pregnancy rates than the center that treats everyone, including patients rejected at the Mecca.

Looking for a clinic

Although SART statistics make interesting reading and may help you decide which clinic to use, they don't tell the whole story. You also need to check into the following information:

- The clinics that are nearest to you. Long-distance IVF is possible but complicated.
- The clinics that are accepting new patients.
- How much clinics charge if you don't have insurance.
- Whether the clinics take insurance — not all do!
- Whether the clinics treat patients like you, an important consideration if you're over age 40 or have been turned down by another clinic.
- The kind of feeling you get from the clinic. For the answer to this question, you'll probably need to make a consultation appointment with a doctor. The clinic usually charges for this appointment. However, compared with all of the other costs associated with fertility treatment, the cost of the initial consultation is a relative bargain! You will have uninterrupted "quality" time with the doctor for 45 minutes to an hour. Before deciding on the clinic with which you are going to work, you should seriously consider visiting two or three that you picked out. You will find that this is a worthwhile investment of time and money.

You don't need to commit to a program at your initial consultation. It never hurts to go home and think everything over before you go any further. Remember, also, that if you're at one of the big-name clinics, you're also being sized up as a candidate for its program, and you could be turned down for treatment if you don't fit the clinic's criteria. Some centers don't want to give you false hope if they don't believe that they can help you, and others don't want to bring down their statistics.

Whether you need or want to know everything about a clinic before you go there depends on your personality. You may be happy to go wherever it was that your best friend went, or to go where your insurance tells you to go, or to go to the clinic around the corner. There's nothing wrong with trusting your instincts and other people's personal experiences. However, if you're already filling up infertility notebook number three, your family doctor's recommendation that you just go to his golfing buddy probably isn't going to convince you.

Evaluating a clinic's personality

IVF clinics have personalities just like people do, and just like with individuals, you may find your personality is a better fit at some clinics than at others. Usually, but not always, the head honcho or main doctor at the clinic sets the tone for the whole office. Sometimes instead of one main doctor, a clinic has a team of fairly equal doctors, all of whom leave their impression on the way the clinic functions. Here's a rundown on the most common types of offices and what you may encounter when you enter their doors:

- ✔ **The razzle-dazzle office:** They have the name recognition and reputation as the "Meccas of infertility." These places are selective and often expensive, but you'll probably feel like you're in first class if you go there. And because their reputation is based on success, you may well get pregnant here — if they'll take you as a patient.

- ✔ **The serious office:** Dr. Serious and his cohort, Dr. Seriously Published, take infertility very seriously indeed. Their offices are quiet, well organized, and feature conversations peppered with statistics. If you're a serious type yourself, you'll love Dr. Serious.

- ✔ **The gloom-and-doom office:** If you have a naturally pessimistic nature, Drs. Gloom and Doom will foster your natural tendencies. They want to make sure you understand all the problems you'll have getting pregnant, so they dwell on them in great detail. A visit with Dr. Doom and Gloom may cause you to need antidepressants before each visit.

- ✔ **The chaotic office:** They lost your appointment, can't find your chart, and dropped your blood down the sink by mistake? Welcome to Dr. Chaotic's office, where nothing ever seems to go the way it should. However, because Dr. Chaotic is often an original thinker with great ideas, wade through the chaos if you think he can help your unique situation. Just keep duplicate copies of everything.

Why IVF Costs So Much — Especially Without a Free Toaster

No, you won't get a free toaster at your IVF clinic, but you may feel like you should. Why on earth does IVF cost so much? Although supply and demand may have a bearing on costs — in other words, doctors respond to market pressures — the fact is that IVF costs are high because IVF is a high-tech procedure and high tech costs money. An IVF lab costs over a million dollars to set up, and you will see lots of employees — nurses, lab personnel, ultrasound techs — when you go for your consultation.

However, it's hard to feel sorry for your fertility clinic when you're the one who will be pouring thousands of dollars into its coffers. In the next sections, we help you get every penny out of your insurance company to which you're entitled to help pay for your IVF cycle.

Discovering what your insurance plan really covers

Even if you have insurance coverage, you may be amazed to see how little of your IVF bill is covered. Some insurance plans cover only monitoring, meaning the frequent blood draws and ultrasounds. Because these can run well over $2,000 per cycle, this coverage is a help. Other plans cover only the medications, which is a help, but not by any means relief from the total cost.

Nor is it easy in some cases to decipher your insurance plan. Check out your plan before you start treatment. Even if you live in a state with mandated coverage, your particular employer may find several loopholes to slip through. Finding out you're not covered at the pharmacy the night before your cycle is supposed to begin isn't a good way to start treatment.

Many insurance companies require preauthorization even if you do have coverage. Preauthorization can take several days to complete, so don't leave this step until the last minute!

You may be covered only if you go to an "approved" clinic. But what if you don't want to go to this clinic? Maybe it doesn't offer treatments you want, or it doesn't have high success rates. In that case, you'll be forced to make an unpleasant choice: Will you go for care that costs you less but may not succeed, or will you pay more for a higher chance of success? These decisions would have had even King Solomon, the master of wise decisions in the Old Testament, in a quandary.

Insurance 101: The differences between types of insurance

You may be confused over whether your insurance is public or private, group or individual. Public insurance is paid for, at least in part, by the government. Medicaid, for those on public assistance; Medicare, for those over age 62 or disabled in some way; and CHAMPUS, for military families, are public insurances. Private insurances are paid for by you, either directly or indirectly. If your employer pays the costs for you as part of a benefits package, you have group insurance. If you pay the entire cost yourself, you have an individual policy, which is usually quite expensive.

Changing jobs or changing insurance to get infertility coverage

People have been known to change jobs to get better insurance, or to drop insurance at their place of employment and pick up coverage under their spouse's policy, even if it costs more per month.

Is it worth taking a lesser-paying job to cover IVF costs? If the drop in pay isn't too much, it might be. Three or four IVF cycles could certainly cost you more than $40,000 over a year or so.

Consider a part-time job as another means for establishing fertility coverage. Some companies offer insurance to part-time (20 or more hours a week) employees — insurance that may cover fertility treatments.

For a listing of major companies that offer infertility coverage (of some sort), visit http://www.inciid.org/article.php?cat=benefits&id=243.

You still need to confirm this information with the organization (after you get the job, that is!) to determine the specifics of the plan. And remember, most companies have a waiting period, which could last from 30 days to one year, prior to the time when you are eligible for insurance. So don't cancel your old policy until/unless you know that your new policy kicks in. Going from one group insurance plan to another gives you an automatic acceptance regardless of pre-existing conditions. You don't want to get caught with a lapse in coverage, however. Not only is that a precarious situation for your health and your finances, but it could also affect what your new insurance will or will not cover.

Before you throw away your law career or consider moonlighting, you may want to check out any other insurance your company may offer. Some companies offer a choice of plans. You may pay more for a plan that covers infertility, but the savings may be worth the extra cost.

Some companies allow you to change insurance only at certain times of the year; this is usually called *open season*. Check out your choices ahead of time so that you can have your insurance in place before you need to start using it.

Getting coverage from professional associations

So your insurance company won't give an inch, and the option of a new or second job is just not an option at all. Is it over? Maybe not.

States are in charge — for now

No federal mandate for insurance coverage for infertility treatment exists at this time, although a few bills were sent to Congress in 2002. When you consider that the federal government has spent years arguing over general health care coverage for U.S. citizens, one can only imagine how bogged down a specific coverage for infertility treatment would become in Washington.

For now, it's up to individual states to pass and enforce infertility coverage. States can force employers to cover treatment in two different ways:

- They can mandate companies to cover infertility treatment.
- They can mandate that employers *offer* coverage.

If your employer is only mandated to offer coverage, you'll usually have to pay extra for the coverage, in the form of a *rider,* or extra policy, attached to your main insurance coverage.

That flier inviting you to your industry association dinner may come in handy after all. Many organizations have professional associations that offer open enrollment programs for insurance, meaning that if you're a member (you pay the monthly dues), you can't be turned down for insurance. Because these associations generally boast large memberships, you benefit from group coverage, which may include some of the extras not found in smaller companies or individual plans. You can start by checking out associations within your profession.

Long-time resources for the self-employed, who often have trouble getting coverage of any kind, professional and trade organizations are a popular way to cover yourself. Associations can be found in almost any field, particularly those that tend toward the self-employed or those underrepresented in business. Examples include the National Writers Union, Graphic Artists Guild, Public Relations Society of America, American Marketing Association, and Women in Communications. Often, you must be a member for a period of time before you can enroll in an insurance program. Sometimes, the insurance policy may have a one-year preexisting condition rider as well.

The type of insurance available to you will also depend upon where you live, even if you are part of an association or professional group. Typically, the tri-state area of New York, New Jersey, and Pennsylvania tends to offer more plans for freelancers and the self-employed. These plans are not necessarily available for those that live outside of the area.

Touring the States That Mandate Fertility Coverage

As of this writing, 15 states mandate some sort of reimbursement for in vitro fertilization. No consensus exists between states on how coverage should be applied or who has to offer it. This coverage is still a mixed bag for the average patient; even if your state mandates insurance coverage, your employer may be exempt from offering coverage if he meets certain requirements listed below.

States that currently have some infertility coverage mandates are Arkansas, California, Connecticut, Hawaii, Illinois, Louisiana, Maryland, Massachusetts, Montana, New Jersey, New York, Ohio, Rhode Island, Texas, and West Virginia.

Remember, state mandates affect the states where your employer/corporation reside. So, even if you are a sales representative living in a covered state, if your employer is based out of a noncovered state, your insurance will reflect the laws of your employer's domicile, not yours. The opposite applies as well. You may live/work in a state that is not mandated but your company headquarters are in a state that is. Don't just assume. That's what human resource departments are for!

Here are the state requirements:

- ✔ **Arkansas:** Requires coverage for infertility, including IVF up to a lifetime cap of $15,000.

- ✔ **California:** Employers must make available a policy covering infertility treatment, excluding IVF but covering gamete intrafallopian transfer (GIFT), a type of IVF in which the egg and sperm are placed in the fallopian tube before fertilization takes place. This avoids the religious/ethical difficulty of having embryos in the lab, but adds a laparoscopy to the mix, which adds cost and invasiveness to the procedure.

- ✔ **Connecticut:** Must offer a policy covering infertility, including IVF.

- ✔ **Hawaii:** Requires coverage, including one cycle of IVF.

- ✔ **Illinois:** Requires coverage of diagnosis and treatment of up to six IVF cycles. Employers with fewer than 25 employees are exempt.

- ✔ **Maryland:** Requires coverage for IVF after certain conditions are met; HMOs and companies with fewer than 50 employees are excluded.

- ✓ **Massachusetts:** Requires comprehensive coverage.

- ✓ **Montana:** Requires HMOs to cover infertility as part of "preventive care."

- ✓ **New Jersey:** Requires coverage, including IVF.

- ✓ **New York:** Requires coverage of diagnosis and treatment as part of a correctable medical condition.

- ✓ **Ohio:** Requires HMOs to cover infertility under "preventive care."

- ✓ **Rhode Island:** Requires comprehensive coverage but allows a 20 percent co-pay for consumers.

- ✓ **Texas:** Requires certain insurers to offer coverage for IVF only.

- ✓ **West Virginia:** Requires HMOs to cover infertility costs.

Some states exempt HMOs from mandated coverage. Some states make HMOs cover infertility treatment. Some states cover everything except IVF; others cover IVF but not medications.

After you get past what is and isn't covered, in some states your employer can refuse to pay for infertility treatments if:

- ✓ The company has fewer than 50 employees.

- ✓ The company doesn't cover maternity care.

- ✓ You haven't done at least several cycles of intrauterine insemination (IUI) before moving to IVF.

- ✓ You've had a vasectomy or tubal ligation.

- ✓ You're over a certain age.

- ✓ You haven't had two years of documented infertility.

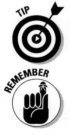

If you are still unsure of your state's policy, you can always contact your local RESOLVE chapter (www.resolve.org) to find the information for your area.

State mandates are always an issue under consideration in the legislature. If you are feeling particularly motivated or vocal in trying to get your state covered for infertility, contact your local RESOLVE chapter. They are generally on the front lines when it comes to advocacy in this area. They can let you know "what's on the table" and how you can help.

Fighting City Hall: Insurance Appeals

Insurance appeals need to attack one of the three basic reasons insurance companies give for not covering infertility treatments:

- ✔ Infertility is not an illness.
- ✔ Infertility treatments are not medically necessary.
- ✔ Infertility treatments are experimental.

You need to address one of these issues to win your claim. In some cases, your doctor may write a letter of "medical necessity" for some of your treatment.

A policy with vague wording may be easier to appeal than coverage that specifically excludes infertility treatment.

Take it up the ladder. Don't just settle for a "No" from the first person who gives it, particularly if you feel that there is a legitimate "Yes" that should apply instead. Generally, decisions or reversals get made at a higher level. Keep asking for a supervisor's name (and their supervisor, and their supervisor, and so on). If you're going to get turned down, put up a good fight and besides, you just might win after all!

When Having Insurance Doesn't Help

You can have the world's most comprehensive infertility insurance that can end up being worth nothing to you if your clinic is not on the preferred provider list. This is why the best kind of insurance is the type that pays a certain amount, regardless of where you go. Why would a clinic choose not to contract with an insurance company? For one thing, the amount the insurance offers isn't enough, in the eyes of the clinic. Clinics that won't take insurance are usually the "Mecca" types; they're the best, they know it, and they don't see why they should accept the typically low payment that your insurance offers. But there are other reasons. Insurance contracts are convoluted, may require the doctors to fill out special forms, and the insurance company may refuse to pay for a given treatment because some procedure was not followed correctly. Because the contract is between the clinic and the insurance company, this is not your problem, but it may be a serious enough problem for the clinic to cancel that particular insurance contract.

Some clinics take your insurance amount but require you to pay the rest of the bill out of pocket. If a clinic is a preferred provider for that insurance, it's generally required to accept the amount offered as payment in full. If a clinic doesn't want to accept the amount offered, which is usually quite a bit below what most clinics charge for high-tech treatments (such as IVF), it may simply refuse to take the insurance at all. But this is not allowed if the clinic is on the preferred provider list! So double-check the list and contact the insurance company if you see the clinic there.

Getting Creative When You're Out of Other Options

If you don't have insurance or if your insurance doesn't pay anything toward IVF treatment, you may need to get creative. There are ways to have your IVF cycle paid for if you meet certain requirements and are in the right place at the right time!

Donating eggs to reduce costs

A few clinics have innovative donor egg programs that let you donate half your eggs to another couple in return for treatment. The recipient of your eggs pays for your medications and your IVF retrieval and transfer. You need to pay for your own pretesting (such as infectious blood work and a hysterosalpingogram), blood and ultrasound testing, and the cost of freezing any excess embryos you have.

Usually you must meet certain requirements to be an egg donor. Generally, you must be under 35 years old and have a normal follicle-stimulating hormone (FSH) level. Usually a donor list is sent out every month or so by the clinic, and you need to be picked by a recipient to be able to do a retrieval cycle. The donors and recipients need to be matched ahead of time so that their cycles can be synchronized, thereby ensuring that both the donor and the recipient can have a fresh embryo transfer.

Your chances of getting picked are highest if you meet the following requirements:

- ✔ **You're young, preferably under 30:** The younger you are, the better the chance that you'll make a lot of eggs.

- ✔ **You're of normal weight and height:** Overweight donors aren't usually a first choice. Recipients may worry that obesity is hereditary and also may be concerned that they may have infertility problems, such as polycystic ovaries, a condition in which many eggs are made but the egg quality may be lower than normal.

Very short donors may also not be picked as quickly because, given a choice, more people choose to have a taller donor (and hopefully taller children).

✔ **You have proven fertility:** If you have children already, you're more likely to be picked as a donor.

✔ **You have a male-factor issue:** If your only fertility issue is male factor, you may be picked because you don't have any fertility issues yourself.

✔ **You have a good family background:** You have lots of brothers and sisters with lots of children, no genetic diseases, and no mental illnesses. These factors make you a prime candidate.

Everyone has some problem in her background — after all, our grandparents had to die of something. So if your grandfather died of cancer at 85, that's not likely to be a deterrent to getting picked. If your mom died at 40 from breast cancer, you may have more problems being selected.

✔ **You're a nonsmoker:** Evidence exists that smoking can damage eggs, plus nonsmokers are perceived as healthier people who take better care of themselves.

Egg recipients are often looking for someone whose blood type matches theirs and who has certain physical characteristics or racial background, so you may be selected faster if you have what a lot of people are looking for: a common blood type, or a rare one if someone on the list is looking for that.

Your savings as a donor could equal between $8,000 and $12,000, but you need to be comfortable with the idea that your genetic child could be growing up with another family, or that the recipient could get pregnant with your egg and you may not. Only you can say whether you can accept the emotional repercussions of donating eggs to another couple.

Some women say that they don't feel a genetic connection because their egg isn't being fertilized with their partner's sperm, so the child created isn't the same as the offspring from their own relationship. Other women become very angry when their recipients get pregnant and they don't. This is another one of those times where "know thyself" is of the utmost importance.

Joining a drug study

Some doctors' offices are well connected to certain drug companies and do frequent drug studies for compensation. The compensation may be made to the office as well as the patient. Patients may receive anything from a free cycle of medication to an entire paid IVF cycle, including blood work, ultrasounds, and egg retrieval costs.

Some studies have very specific requirements for age, weight, and infertility problem. Others are less strict with their requirements and let the clinic select patients whom they feel are suitable.

In most studies, a new drug not yet approved by the FDA is being tested. If you sign up for the study, you need to understand that you may get fewer eggs or less fertilization than you would from proven drugs. Most studies require that you sign a document stating this. You may also have to keep a journal of all side effects and have frequent interviews with the person running the study.

Centers selected to run drug studies are usually the larger centers, so you may want to check and see whether the clinics you're considering ever participate in drug studies.

Scoring freebies from the drug companies

With the growth of the infertility industry and the volume that the participating drug companies realize, some have taken an extra step to help educate and even finance their clients' efforts.

Serono, Ferring and Organon, three of the larger infertility drug companies, have started services manned by health professionals to answer basic questions on infertility (but don't expect them to give you recommendations on your particular protocol, lay odds on your success, or adjust your meds!). Another interesting facet of these services is the financial aid that they have developed by donating cycle medicines to patients who are in need and have limited resources to pay for the drugs that they require. This "scholarship program" is run on a case-by-case basis and you must contact the company directly to find out the requirements and how to apply. Be aware that you may need to show proof of income such as an income tax return, which may be more information than you want to have to supply.

Shopping for "sales"

Clinics and drug companies can also be helpful when financing IVF is an issue. The following deals may appeal to you!

Going for the money-back guarantee

Some clinics try to overcome resistance to the high cost of IVF by offering a money-back guarantee. This offer sounds good, but it does have a few catches.

Some centers call these "shared risk" programs. The specifics vary, but usually you pay an upfront fee, such as $15,000, for three or four IVF cycles. If you get pregnant in any one of the cycles, the clinic keeps all your money. If you don't get pregnant at the end of the last cycle, you get your money back (or at least a large part of it). You must pay extra charges for intracytoplasmic sperm injection (ICSI) or using an egg donor or gestational carrier.

Patients must meet certain requirements for acceptance into the programs; usually you must be under a certain age and have a normal uterine cavity and normal baseline blood test results.

Are these programs a good deal? That depends. Obviously they try to hedge their bets somewhat by selecting patients they feel have a good chance of success. If you get pregnant on the fourth try, you'll have gotten a good price per try. If you get pregnant on the first try, you'll have spent a great deal of money for one cycle, far more than you needed to. But if you get pregnant on the first try, will you care about the cost? Only you know the answer.

If you're able to look at a pregnancy on your first try as an incredible blessing and not count the cost, this program may be for you. After two cycles, the clinic begins to break even on you, so if you get pregnant on the fourth cycle, this is a good deal for you financially.

Taking 'em up on a twofer

Other clinics advertise a "twofer" deal, offering two cycles for the price of one for a limited time when they open a new office. As long as the office is a reputable one, you have nothing to lose by signing up for this offer. If the clinic doesn't have a proven track record or a good success rate, you may not be getting a good deal no matter how many free cycles it gives you.

ASRM (the American Society for Reproductive Medicine) has supported shared risk programs as a way to decrease costs to patients if they don't get pregnant. If you do get pregnant on the first try, you're basically subsidizing other people's third and fourth tries.

Ask your doctor whether his or her practice offers this type of quantity discount (or any discount at all for that matter). For specific information on networks of physicians who offer this type of pricing, visit your local search engine on the Internet. One such organization is www.arcfertility.com, but other such networks are available as well.

Going overseas for IVF

As you may have heard, the term *medical tourism* now describes a new type of travel, one that can certainly benefit those pursuing lower cost infertility treatments.

South Africa, South America, Mexico, and certain parts of Europe have infertility programs that provide higher tech options such as IVF and Donor Egg at lower prices, with some clinics quoting IVF cycles under $10,000, inclusive of travel, and Donor Egg cycles under $15,000, inclusive of travel. Before you rush to make your reservations or shudder at the thought of a back alley operation, keep a few things in mind:

✔ While not FDA regulated, most countries have their own federal board of standards that require that certain conditions be met to insure safety and efficacy. When researching a clinic abroad, you might want to directly contact one of the regulatory agencies in the region. South Africa has SASRSS (South African Society of Reproductive Science and Surgery) and the South African Department of Health; European countries may be regulated by ESHRE (European Society of Human Reproduction and Embryology. If you're not sure what agency to contact, start with the country/government Board of Health. You can also contact the local docs at ASRM (American Society of Reproductive Medicine) to get the latest on which countries or clinics are the best regulated.

✔ For donor egg programs, you want to be assured that the donors are being screened for Infectious Diseases and/or Sexually Transmitted Diseases as well as basic genetic mutations.

Make sure that the price(s) that you are being quoted are inclusive of all necessary medical services. Is anesthesia extra? You might want to know. Some programs include the price of air travel in their package. Make sure to find out what the travel arrangements are and that they meet your needs.

Lastly, take some time to enjoy the scenery! One of the benefits of "infertility tourism" is the tourism part. Ask the clinic to recommend good hotels and/or activities that you might enjoy.

Chapter 15

Let the IVF Cycle Begin!

*I*n vitro fertilization (IVF) is the high-tech method of getting pregnant. During an IVF cycle, you take stimulating hormone medications called gonadotropins so that your ovaries are willing to make more than one or two eggs. Then you go through an egg retrieval, a minor surgery to take the eggs out of the follicles in which they grow. After that, the eggs are fertilized in the lab and then put back into your uterus so they can grow.

The treatment sounds complicated, and it is — but not so complicated that you can't understand the basic idea and walk into your clinic confident that you know what to expect.

So, if you've sent in your payment for in vitro after hassling with the billing office a few times, gasped at the hole left in your wallet, spent days on the phone arguing with your insurance company, bought all your medications, and gasped again at the cost, you're ready to start an IVF cycle. In this chapter, we discuss how to get through an IVF cycle with the least amount of frustration, explore what egg retrieval involves, and explain how your best friend's cycle may be completely different from yours and why you shouldn't worry about it.

Starting an IVF Cycle: A Roller Coaster Ride of Emotions

In vitro fertilization is a complicated process. It involves injecting potent medications with possibly serious side effects for several weeks, taking time out of your schedule to have blood work and ultrasounds done, and undergoing surgery, albeit minor, to retrieve your eggs. And that's just the beginning! Every step of the way through IVF is crucial, and every day brings news that will either thrill you or bring you to your knees in despair. Is it any wonder that you're feeling scared?

Experiencing the emotional ride

Even though you're scared to death, you're also excited. You've probably been through a lot to get here, you've spent buckets of money, and you have high hopes that high tech will not fail you.

Behind the excitement may be depression. This is where you've ended up. You've tried all the simpler methods of conception, and they failed. This is your last shot, and it may seem that there's nowhere to go from here. Before you got to IVF, you always knew you had one last thing to try. Now you're trying IVF, and if it fails, you don't know what you'll do next.

From the emotional side, rely on that support network that you've been building. Many women on chat room sites, in Resolve meetings, and in mind-and-body classes find "cycle buddies," literally other women going through IVF (or any of the lower-tech measures) at the same time. (For more details about Resolve, turn to Chapter 8.) You may find comfort in sharing your experiences, good and bad, with someone else who is going through the same thing at the same time. Remember, though, to share and not compare! You're not in competition with anyone. You're trying to have *your* baby.

And try to get your partner to read this chapter, because he's going to be bewildered by the roller coaster ride. Your partner is experiencing much of the IVF process secondhand (with your "hand" being the first line of defense). You're the one dealing directly with the physical discomfort, the scheduling madness, and the emotional ups and downs, so your partner will likely relate to the experience much differently than you do.

Looking at your protocol

When you first sit across the desk from an in vitro fertilization specialist, you may come to think of him as Dr. Magic. He'll probably give you a stack of totally incomprehensible papers that you'll promptly file in your fertility notebook — you know, the notebook that every patient seems to carry around with her. One of those undecipherable papers is probably your protocol. A *protocol* is nothing more than a blueprint or schedule of how your cycle will be done. It includes the medications you'll be taking, instructions on how to take them, and the procedures you need to follow throughout the cycle.

Dr. Magic may review your protocol with you, or he may mumble something about the IVF nurses going over the protocol with you. If he reviews it that day, you'll probably be too excited, nervous, or scared to remember exactly what he says. Patients have described to co-author Sharon protocols that they swear the doctor gave them that resembled no IVF protocol on the face of this earth.

Reading your protocol

So it's time to take out your protocol. Step Number 1: Read the protocol. You would think this would go without saying, but it doesn't. Read the protocol!

Now, your cousin Mary out in Duluth may be going through IVF too, so you call her up and start comparing your protocols. Even though you're only four months apart in age, and everyone says you're more like sisters than cousins, you have two completely different protocols! How can this be? Has one of your doctors made a mistake?

Relax. Doctors rely on a few standard IVF protocols (we list them in Table 15-1), and most doctors prefer to use one over the other. Here are some possibilities:

✔ If you're under 35 and your baseline hormone levels are normal, your doctor could choose to start you on a down regulation cycle, starting leuprolide acetate (which has the brand name Lupron) a few days after you ovulate. (Some clinics like to start birth control pills on the third day of your menses, and then overlap the pill with the Lupron shots; this takes a little longer but you avoid having to monitor your ovulation.) Lupron shuts down your normal hormone receptors and encourages the growth of many follicles instead of one or two. The drug also keeps you from ovulating before retrieval. You start your hormone-stimulating drugs when your period starts. Some centers call this a "long Lupron" cycle, and others call it a "down regulation" cycle. Lupron is a GnRH (gonadotropin-releasing hormone) agonist; it shuts down your normal growth of one dominant follicle by suppressing your pituitary gland.

Instead of stimulating a dominant follicle, like you would normally do, Lupron allows multiple follicles to develop at the same time.

✔ Your doctor may prefer to use a drug called ganirelix, a GnRH antagonist (with the brand name Antagon), or cetrorelix (with the brand name Cetrotide) in conjunction with follicle-stimulating medications; this drug also suppresses your LH surge so you won't ovulate before your egg retrieval. (The difference between the GnRH agonists and the antagonists is that the agonist must be started sometime before ovulation would normally happen in order to prevent its occurrence, whereas the antagonists work right away and prevent ovulation on the same day that they are given.)

✔ If you're over 35, many centers use a modified Lupron protocol, sometimes called a "stop Lupron" cycle because you take Lupron for just ten days following ovulation and then stop when you start your stimulating medications. This protocol is to decrease the suppressing effects of Lupron, which can be detrimental to those over 35 or women who are known to produce fewer eggs. Some doctors may administer a GnRH antagonist prior to ovulation to make doubly sure the patient doesn't ovulate prematurely. Or you may be given a "microdose Lupron" protocol, in which Lupron is diluted in normal saline so that only a minute amount is given each day; this protocol is used for women who didn't stimulate well in a previous cycle or those who have an FSH (follicle-stimulating hormone) level above normal (10.5 to 15, depending on your lab's values). In this case, the Lupron is used for its stimulatory properties, as opposed to its suppressive properties (as in the long Lupron protocol).

✔ You could also be doing a natural protocol, with very little or no medication. This protocol isn't common, but it's used in women who can't tolerate large doses of stimulating medication due to age or previous illness, such as breast cancer.

In addition, your doctor will prescribe gonadotropins, or follicle-stimulating medications, usually taken twice a day, although some centers give only one daily injection. *Recombinant or highly purified drugs,* are typically more expensive but are able to be injected subcutaneously, which means they're given with a very tiny needle. (Follistim, Menopur, Bravelle, and Gonal-F are examples of such drugs.) Some, like Follistim, Gonal-F, or Bravelle are nearly pure FSH, without any luteinizing hormone (LH) in them. Menopur is the only highly purified medication that contains equal doses of FSH and LH. Older gonadotropins, such as Repronex, are made from purified urine from postmenopausal women; they need to be given intramuscularly, with a longer needle, because they're more likely to cause irritation to the tissues. They're equal parts LH and FSH. They're usually (although not always!) cheaper than the recombinant or highly purified medications.

Your doctor will prescribe the protocol and medications he feels most comfortable using for your particular case. Try not to compare what you're getting to what anyone else is using. Birth control pills may be used in association with any of these protocols to help cycle scheduling or to suppress the occasional ovarian cyst. The duration of birth control pill treatment is quite variable and is not included in the table.

Table 15-1	Common IVF Protocols at a Glance		
Protocol	*Used For*	*Average Days on Medication*	*Vials of Medication Needed*
Long Lupron	Women under 35; good responders	21+ days total, including at least 10 on Lupron alone	About 40, plus one 14-day Lupron kit (for one cycle)
Antagon or Cetrotide	Women who are oversuppressed on Lupron; patients of any age	10 days on stimulating medications; start ganirelix on day 6 of stimulating medications	About 30 to 40 vials of stimulating medications plus 5 to 6 prefilled syringes of Antagon or Cetrotide
Microdose flare	Poor responders; women over 35	10 to 12 days of microdose Lupron and stimulating medications	60 vials of stimulating medications; one bottle of microdose (diluted) Lupron
Short flare	Women oversuppressed on long Lupron	10 days of Lupron; start stimulating medications on day 5 for 5 to 7 days	One 14-day Lupron kit; 24 to 30 vials of stimulating medications
Modified long Lupron (also called stop Lupron)	Women over 35; poor responders	10 days of Lupron; then approximately 10 days of stimulating medications	60 vials of stimulating medications; one 14-day Lupron kit

Reviewing your protocol

After you've read your protocol over a few times, you're ready to call the doctor's office to discuss it and make sure that you understand it. Some offices have an orientation class for IVF patients to review protocols and policies. Some centers make attendance mandatory for their patients. Other centers schedule injection instruction sessions for you and your partner to review your medications and show you how to inject them. Having your partner inject medications is one of the scariest parts of IVF — for you *and* for your partner. Make sure that you get very clear instructions on how to do this.

If your IVF center is large, nurses probably take care of only IVF patients. If your program is smaller, the nursing staff may take care of both non-IVF and IVF patients. Some programs have only one IVF nurse with whom you deal throughout your cycle; others have so many nurses you can't tell who's who without a scorecard!

Try to figure out how your center works and to whom you should be talking before your cycle starts. In many centers, the IVF nurses draw blood and also do your ultrasounds; larger centers have a separate staff that draws blood and ultrasonographers who do the ultrasounds. Make sure that you talk to the right person when you have a problem or need help.

Following the trend toward less medication

Some doctors are advocating using less stimulating drugs and developing (doctors may use the word "recruiting") fewer follicles. The reason for using a low stimulation protocol may include the following:

- Less cost to the patient
- Less risk of hyperstimulation, or OHSS (see "Avoiding the risks of hyperstimulation")
- Possibility of recruiting better eggs (some doctors feel that hyperstimulation can be bad for eggs)
- Less chance of producing more embryos than you can ever use, along with the ethical considerations that accompany an overabundance of embryos

Dealing with a disappearing doctor

After your initial consult appointment, you may wonder where your doctor went. In smaller centers, doctors may do callbacks with your blood results; some also do their own ultrasounds. In larger centers, you may feel as though your doctor has vanished from the face of the earth because all your instructions come from the nurses. This system of patient communication can be upsetting if you came to a center specifically to deal with a particular doctor. Rest assured that your doctor *is* reviewing your callbacks and instructing the nurses on what you should do next, but in bigger centers, doctors simply don't have the time to do more than 50 callbacks a night. Some centers have even gone to a system where you don't talk to *anybody:* Your instructions are left on a message tape you can access.

If your center has more than one doctor doing IVF procedures, you may also feel like you've lost the doctor you came to see. Many centers rotate doctors through IVF on a one- or two-week cycle; you may never see the doctor with whom you had your consultation again! Sometimes you can request that a certain doctor do your procedure, but granting that request may not always be possible. Your doctor may be doing outside surgery or seeing patients for new appointments the week of your retrieval.

The doctor you saw on your initial visit to the clinic may not be the doctor who is managing your IVF procedure. Try to find out what your center's policy is for scheduling doctors and whether you can request the doctor of your choice.

Taking your medications without having a nervous breakdown

Suppose that you had your injection class a week ago, and on this beautiful bright Sunday morning, you're ready to begin taking your medications. Your partner, with shaking hands, opens the first vial to mix your first injection. "No, no!" you scream, as he proceeds to draw up the liquid. "That's not how she said to mix it!" He stops, and both of you stare dumbfounded at the boxes, the needles, and each other. In one week you've forgotten every word the nurse said. You look at the film you were given on giving injections again, read the colorful pieces of paper that tell you how to mix and inject, and still feel confused, scared, and totally out of control. And it's a Sunday. What on earth are you going to do?

Being confused: Par for the course

First, take a deep breath. Of course, giving yourself injections is hard to do. Do you think doctors and nurses were born knowing how to mix and inject medications? Most people are scared the first time they give a shot or mix a medication. Your reaction is normal.

Second, call your center. Some centers do IVF procedures on weekends, and if yours does, you may be able to talk to someone who can talk you through the mixing and injection.

If no one is there, you can call the answering service and ask for the doctor on call, who may be annoyed but can at least give you some guidance. Some centers also have nurses who carry beepers so they can answer questions when the office is closed. If you got your medications from a large mail-order pharmacy, it may have a nurse on call who can also give you instructions.

Call the main number and ask. Remember that medication confusion (dosing, mixing, injecting) are considered bona fide "emergencies" at a fertility center. Do not hesitate to call! Or maybe you never got to know the doctor or nurse who lives next door? Now might be as good a time as any to strike up an acquaintance! Such a person is likely to be more adept than you at handling a needle and walking you through your first shot.

If you can't get anyone, take a little break, compose yourself, and then go back and try again. The procedure probably won't look quite as overwhelming the second time.

Monitoring your progress (more poking and prodding)

After a few days of injections, you'll start to feel like a pro, your partner will have his injection techniques down pat, and your protocol will start to make sense to you. It's time to find out how well this is working. It's time to have blood drawn and do an ultrasound.

Most centers monitor you every few days to see how you're responding to the medication. If your follicles are growing nicely and your estradiol is rising, your medications will probably not be changed. If you're stimulating too well, or not stimulating well enough, your medications may be decreased or increased.

Avoiding the risks of hyperstimulation

Stimulating too well can be another example of too much of a good thing. The goal of IVF is to have a number of follicles grow so that more than one egg can be retrieved. This result will, it is hoped, prevent you from having to do multiple cycles of IVF to get pregnant, because your extra embryos may possibly be frozen and used later if you don't get pregnant on your first try. With some women, especially those who have polycystic ovaries (see Chapter 6 for more about this condition), hyperstimulation can get way out of hand very quickly. If your estradiol rises too fast, or if you make too many follicles — 20 or more — you run a risk of developing OHSS, or ovarian hyperstimulation syndrome. Patients with OHSS can be very ill after egg retrieval, with fluid buildup in the pelvis and around the lungs. Some women become sick enough to require hospitalization. In the past, a few patients have even died from severe OHSS, which causes fluid volume shifts through your whole body and can make your blood very thick and prone to clotting.

Because OHSS is so potentially serious, most centers watch patients on stimulating medications quite closely, monitoring their blood and ultrasound results every few days. If your clinic thinks that you're in danger of severe OHSS, you may have to freeze all your embryos after retrieval and not do an embryo transfer. OHSS becomes worse if you become pregnant, due to the rising hormone levels from the pregnancy. Some centers may not do egg retrieval at all, and simply cancel the cycle, because the hCG trigger given before retrieval also makes OHSS worsen.

On the other hand, you may not be stimulating well, and your clinic may be increasing your medication to see whether you can do better. This situation also requires closer monitoring because your medications may require frequent adjustment. See Table 15-2 for a typical IVF stimulation cycle, but remember that your cycle may vary.

As a rough guide, you'll probably be on stimulating hormones ten days before you're given hCG to mature the follicle for your retrieval. During those ten days, you'll probably have blood work and ultrasounds done four times, or maybe more or less depending on your circumstances. Some centers insist that all your blood work and ultrasounds be done at their facility; others allow patients to be monitored at outside facilities closer to their homes. You need to find a place capable of doing same-day reports and willing to fax results to your clinic.

Table 15-2	A Typical IVF Cycle — Yours May Vary		
Day of Cycle	*Monitoring*	*Medication*	*Time Taken*
2	Blood and ultrasound	FSH/hCG (stimulating medications)	2 vials a.m./ 2 vials p.m.
3		Keep taking medications	No change
4		Keep taking medications	No change
5	Blood and ultrasound	Adjust according to monitoring results	Change if clinic tells you to
6		Keep taking medications	No change
7		Add Antagon/ Cetrotide	Add Antagon/ Cetrotide in a.m.

(continued)

Table 15-2 *(continued)*

Day of Cycle	Monitoring	Medication	Time Taken
8	Blood and ultrasound	Keep taking medications	No change
9		Keep taking medications	
10	Blood and ultrasound	Take morning medications/hCG	Morning medications: no change; hCG at exact time clinic tells you
11	Blood work only	No medications	
12	Egg retrieval		

Waiting for the phone to ring . . . again and again

The phone rings at 4 p.m., and you grab it off the hook. "Hi, this is Nancy Nurse," chirps the voice on the other end. Your whole world stops for a second, as you try to decipher from the tone of her voice whether she has good news or bad news.

Setting up your callback

Blood and ultrasound callbacks consume a huge part of your life after you start IVF. You find yourself leaving whole volumes of information on how to reach you that day (cell phone, home phone, don't leave a message with the babysitter, partner's number, don't call before 6, don't call after 6, don't leave a message, I really need to talk to you) on your callback sheets, because this call, whether good or bad news, is the highlight of your day.

If your clinic has a lot of staff, try to cultivate a good relationship with one or two nurses with whom you feel comfortable. It doesn't hurt to ask to speak with that nurse when you call. Most nurses are happy to call you if you personally ask for them. Also, if you get to know one or two people well, you won't have to explain all the ins and outs of your case every time you call in.

You may find it easiest to have the clinic call you on your cell phone, and some clinics prefer that you give them your cell number as your primary source of contact. That way, you can have it with you at all times and don't have to feel tethered to the office phone, home phone, and so on. And what if you have to go to the bathroom!

Knowing what to do if you don't get along with the nurse

What if the clinic has only one nurse and you just don't get along? Try to make it easier for both of you. Maybe you can ask for the doctor to call you; if your personality really clashes with the nurse's, the doctor may be willing to handle your calls. If you have to get your calls from someone with whom you're not happy, ask the nurse to leave your instructions on your answering machine so that you don't have to talk to her on the phone. Or you may want to fax in your list of questions so that the nurse can write the answers on it and fax it back. That way, you get the answers you need with a minimum of aggravation.

Sometimes you can just *feel* it — you've become an annoyance to the nurses. You picture the nurses throwing the phone to each other when you call, in a version of patient hot potato. You feel terrible about this. Everyone wants to be liked, and every patient also wants her questions answered without feeling like a pest.

If you're getting bad vibes, you may want to try to clear the air with the staff. Explain politely (not at callback time, when everyone is busy) why you feel things are strained, and encourage some open communication about how you can best work together. Everyone benefits if the communication between you and the staff is good, and unfortunately you're the one who will suffer the most if you don't get along with the rest of the team.

Feeling like everyone in the waiting room is doing better than you

There you are in the waiting room, listening to the person ahead of you brag about how well her cycle is going, how she's got 20 beautiful follicles, how good her partner is at giving shots, how she loves the nurses so much she's making them each a ceramic something to say thank you, how great her veins are, and how happy she is to be alive. You look at your poor black and blue arms and think about how you have only seven follicles on ultrasound, how your partner seems to hit a nerve every other day, how much you hate all the nurses, and how much you hate this whole process.

In some centers, the waiting room is like group therapy in a psychiatrist's office: All the patients pull their chairs together while waiting for their ultrasound appointments and talk about IVF and life in general. This kind of place can provide you with new friends who know exactly what you're going through, but it can also turn into a sort of golf course with chairs — she got pregnant on the first try, she has the most follicles, she's doing better than she did last cycle, she's having twins, she's having triplets.

Stay out of the comparison contests, if you can. Everyone responds differently to medications, and in the end, the person with three follicles may get pregnant, and the person with twenty follicles may not. Remember that the only statistics that matter are your own.

If talking to other people about your problems makes you feel worse, don't join in. Bring a book and headphones and put an unapproachable expression on your face. Arrive as close to the time of your appointment as you can, get engrossed in the TV, or hide in the bathroom!

On the other hand, if you can listen to other women's tales and not compare yourself to them, the waiting room can be a great source of camaraderie and a place to make lasting friendships.

Why feeling blue is normal

We can't stress enough that mood swings are normal with high hormone levels. You may also experience a letdown feeling when doing an IVF cycle. You've planned for it and fantasized about how things would go, and now it's almost over. It's like Christmas: Sometimes the anticipation surpasses the reality. When you're almost ready for egg retrieval, you can't change things. It's too late to say, "We should have waited another month" or "I should have taken more meds, less meds, or different meds."

Taking a Shot in the Dark: Time for hCG

It's Nancy Nurse on the phone again, and this time you can tell that she's got *really* big news. "It's time for hCG!" she says, and because she sounds so excited, you feel like you should get out the pompoms and do a cheer. If you've read your protocol, you know what hCG (human chorionic gonadotropin) is; if you haven't, here's a refresher course.

Defining the role of hCG

HCG is a crucial part of your IVF cycle. HCG is given 32 to 36 hours before your egg retrieval; its job is to mature your eggs and prepare them to be fertilized. Giving hCG allows the IVF staff to plan egg retrievals for a reasonable time during the day, instead of waiting for your natural LH surge to occur. That's why the timing of your hCG is very important.

Watching the clock: Timing is everything with hCG

The hCG instructions include a specific time to take your injection, and following the directions is absolutely critical because timing really is everything. Your injection may be scheduled for midnight, or even a few hours later, if your center has a lot of egg retrievals to do on one day.

If your injection is scheduled for, say, 2 a.m., you can mix the medication ahead of time and put it on your bedside table; then set your alarm for the time you need to take the hCG. Giving the injection at an odd hour is easier if you don't need to fumble around mixing medications when you're half asleep.

If you normally have a doctor's office, close friend, or neighbor do your injections, you may have a problem getting them to give hCG in the middle of the night. Be aware ahead of time that you need to find someone willing to do this when the time comes.

Going for the Gold: The Egg Retrieval

Almost before you know it, it's time for your egg retrieval. All kinds of emotions are probably churning around inside you and your partner. This is the culmination of several weeks of injections, emotions, and worries. It's your big day! How do you feel?

If you know ahead of time about an event that may conflict with your egg retrieval, tell your doctor about it *before* you start taking your stimulating hormones. Sometimes an egg retrieval can be held off for a few days if you take Lupron or birth control a few extra days before starting your stimulating medications. After you start stimulating medications, influencing the day of your retrieval is harder.

Looking at retrieval schedules

Some IVF centers do egg retrievals every day of the week. Others do retrievals only Monday through Friday and start their patients' medications all at the same time to avoid the weekends. Still others cycle patients through in batches, doing retrievals only every other month or a few months of the year. You probably won't have much say in what day or what time your retrieval is done.

Signing here . . . and here . . . and here . . .

Some centers have you sign consent forms ahead of time for your egg retrieval, but you may be asked to sign the day of the retrieval. Usually a nurse reviews the consent forms with you. Keep in mind that your anxiety level will be through the roof, and the chances that you'll be able to read and comprehend 18 pages of legalese the morning of your retrieval are slim. If possible, ask for the consent forms ahead of time so that you have time to read and understand what you'll be signing.

Some centers let you make changes in the consent forms as long as they know what the changes are ahead of time and can have a lawyer review your changes. Here are the most common concerns that people have with IVF consent forms:

- ✔ Having pictures taken of themselves, their eggs, sperm, or embryos, for use in any type of publication. Many people have no objection to this, but some do.

- ✔ Allowing medical, nursing, or other students in the room to watch the procedure.

- ✔ Using any sperm, eggs, embryos, or tissue for research. "Tissue" can mean fluid from follicles, endometrial tissue, or anything else removed at the time of retrieval or transfer.

- ✔ Freezing of any embryos not transferred on a fresh transfer. Some people have religious objections to embryo freezing, and they want to inseminate only a few eggs, so that they can use up all their embryos and not have any left to freeze. Discuss this step ahead of time with embryology to make sure that everyone understands exactly what will be done.

If you have objections to anything in the consent forms, address them before the morning of your egg retrieval. If your clinic has a problem with your requests, it could delay or cancel your retrieval.

Meeting the retrieval team

A whole new group of unfamiliar people will be with you for the egg retrieval — how wonderful. During the egg retrieval, a nurse or a medical assistant may be in the room helping the doctor. An ultrasonographer may be present, and the embryologist will be nearby. It is hoped, you'll know the ultrasonographers and the nurse. With any luck, you'll know the doctor, too, although, the doctor with whom you had an initial consultation may not do your egg retrieval. The person in whom you may be most interested as you arrive in the IVF area (which you probably have never seen before) is the person who will give you the medication for your retrieval.

Previewing what happens in an egg retrieval

Different centers do things different ways, but in most centers, you're taken to the IVF suite, a part of the building you've never seen before and had no idea existed. You'll change into a gown, hat, and shoe covers because the IVF suite is a sterile area where an attempt is made to keep outside germs from entering.

An intravenous (IV) infusion is started. The purpose of the IV is mainly to have access for giving you medication, but it's also there in case any complications require you to be given large amounts of fluid quickly. If you know that certain of your veins are better than others for the IV, don't be shy about informing the person starting your IV!

The embryologist usually comes in to see you before the procedure starts to ask you to verify your name, Social Security number, and information about your partner. The purpose of checking this information is to prevent any type of mix-up with eggs, sperm, or embryos.

The doctor generally comes in the room at the last minute, introduces herself, one hopes, if you don't already know her, and instructs the person giving you medications to start giving them. The doctor inserts a speculum and washes the vagina and cervix thoroughly, trying to keep the area as clean as possible.

You won't remember the rest, so we explain what happens next. The doctor inserts the vaginal ultrasound probe into your vagina. On the top of the probe is a needle guide, a plastic attachment which has a hollow narrow tube-like guide along which a long metal needle slides. The doctor locates your follicles on ultrasound with the probe and then punctures the back of the vagina with the needle, entering each follicle and sucking out the fluid. The follicular fluid is given to the embryologist, who examines it under a microscope and says, it is hoped, "Egg one, egg two," and so on. When the follicles are all emptied, you'll wake up and be taken to a nearby bed for a short time to recover. An egg retrieval usually takes about 30 to 40 minutes from start to finish, and you'll be asleep the whole time.

Knocking you out: Anesthesia choices for the retrieval

IVF centers vary considerably in their methods of anesthesia for egg retrievals. Some centers do all their retrievals in a hospital operating suite, so a nurse anesthetist or an anesthesiologist (a doctor who specializes in giving anesthesia) gives your medications. Smaller centers may have only an assistant or the nurse giving medication under the guidance of your doctor. Still others offer you a choice between conscious sedation and MAC, monitored anesthesia care.

With conscious sedation, you receive some version of medication in the valium family, possibly Valium or Versed, and also some type of narcotic, such as Demerol, fentanyl, or morphine. The degree to which you're awake during your procedure varies quite a bit between individuals. If you've taken narcotics frequently in the past, you may develop a tolerance to them, and they may not make you comfortable. Some women are much more sensitive to all drugs and need very little medication to put them to sleep. Your vital signs, including your heart rate, blood pressure, and respirations, are carefully monitored during your procedure.

If you have MAC, an anesthesiologist or a nurse anesthetist must give it to you. Either of those professionals is qualified to give the medication propofol (Diprivan is the brand name), which will put you in a deep sleep for your retrieval.

Certain medications, such as Versed, have amnesiac properties, which is a fancy way of saying that you won't remember what went on during the retrieval. This effect lasts for a short time after the procedure as well. Nearly every IVF patient wakes up after the procedure and asks, "How many eggs did

I get?" at least three times before she's actually awake enough to remember the answer! You may not remember walking from the table to a bed, either, but you did!

Doing His Duty: Your Partner Is Busy, Too

While you're snoozing away in the IVF suite, your partner will be watching the movies most centers helpfully provide to make it easier for him to masturbate to produce a semen specimen. This can be a tricky issue for some men and downright impossible for others. If you think that your partner is going to suffer from performance anxiety on retrieval day, consider the following ways to take the pressure off:

✔ You can have him freeze a specimen ahead of time. Most centers prefer to use fresh sperm, but if your partner knows a frozen backup is available, he may have an easier time in the producing room. And if he can't, the lab can use the frozen specimen; not as good as the fresh, but a whole lot better than nothing!

✔ He can go to a nearby hotel, or home, if you live close enough — within 15 to 20 minutes away — use a sterile cup the andrologist will give him, and produce there.

✔ You can help him produce. You may feel uncomfortable going in with him, but believe us, it's no big deal — people do it all the time. But andrologists enforce two rules: no saliva and no lubricants. Either one can mess up the semen specimen. Make sure the specimen goes directly from the penis into the cup to maintain sterility as much as possible; no collecting it in your hand or elsewhere!

Answering Common Post-IVF Questions

After a retrieval, almost everybody asks these questions:

✔ **Can I see my eggs before I go home?** You can't see your eggs because they can be seen only under a microscope, and no embryologist in the world is going to let a patient still lurching around in an anesthesia daze mess around with his extremely expensive microscope or those precious eggs!

✔ **Why can't my partner come back to the retrieval room?** In some centers, partners are allowed to be present at the egg retrieval. Other centers don't allow anyone else to be in the room for the retrieval, although they're often allowed in for the embryo transfer. Usually the rooms are too small to allow extra people, and no one wants partners feeling woozy in the retrieval room and knocking over the ultrasound equipment if they fall.

✔ **Do I have to have an IV?** Yes.

✔ **Are you *sure* you won't mix up my eggs (or sperm or embryos) with someone else's?** Yes.

Centers are anxious to reassure patients on this topic, since all centers are very aware of the recent cases in the news and are being extremely careful to avoid such an incidence.

Most centers label all dishes, collection cups, and so on with the patient's name, Social Security number, patient number, and sometimes a color code. Egg retrievals and embryo transfers are done one at a time — never two at the same time. Eggs and embryos go from labeled container to labeled container. And catheters used for embryo transfer are never reused, so someone else's embryo won't be stuck in your catheter!

After an embryo transfer, the catheter that was used is examined again to make sure that none of your embryos decided to stay behind. All those little guys should be in the uterus, where they belong!

Chapter 16

The Care and Feeding of an Embryo: Amazing Teamwork in the Lab

*T*he medical advances that enable IVF (in vitro fertilization) clinics to fertilize eggs and grow embryos in a lab are a science but also an art. The embryology team is skilled in working with the most precious of all biologic material: the eggs, sperm, and embryos that have the potential to become your child.

After you've completed the stimulation part of the IVF cycle and gone through an egg retrieval, everything is in the hands of the members of the embryology team. They're the ones who check your eggs, ready the sperm for fertilization, and keep those embryos growing until the day of transfer. They're the bearers of all good news and bad news, and you want to know everything they're doing.

In this chapter, we tell you what goes on in the lab, what the embryologists want to see, and what they *don't* want to see in eggs, sperm, and embryos. We also review your instructions for transfer, explain why you're taking certain medications, and give some insight into how many embryos you may want to transfer.

Recognizing a Good Egg When You See One

Before you go home after retrieval (see Chapter 15), embryology will look at your eggs and may let you know whether they're mature, postmature, or immature. Mature eggs are needed for fertilization to occur, but immature eggs will often mature within 24 hours after retrieval. An egg retrieval may yield eggs that are both mature and immature, especially if you made a lot of follicles. If your eggs are postmature, they may not fertilize. However, the ability to judge eggs right after retrieval is somewhat limited by the fact that eggs are surrounded by a layer of cumulus cells, which protect the egg during ovulation, but limit the ability of the embryologist to see details about the egg. They may not be able to tell you much about the eggs until the next day, when the sperm have dispersed the cumulus layer.

A mature egg is surrounded by a fluffy cumulus layer that allows the embryologist to see through it and identify the outline of the egg. In contrast, immature eggs have a tight, dense cumulus that has not yet expanded, which makes it very difficult to see the inner details of the egg. An immature egg still contains 46 chromosomes because the immature egg has not yet thrown off half of them, a step that's necessary before fertilization can take place.

When hCG is given at the end of the IVF stimulation (or during the LH surge in a natural cycle), the egg, still in the follicle for 36 hours before being collected during an egg retrieval procedure, undergoes maturation. It separates its chromosomes in a process called *meiosis*, and puts 23 of them into a small cell fragment called a polar body. This is what makes an egg "mature," meaning fertilizable. An immature egg has not yet successfully put out its polar body, but may do so during the next day or so in the laboratory, becoming fertilizable at that point.

Embryologists use the term, "Postmature eggs" to describe those that are mature, but may be dark and grainy-looking. They tend not to fertilize, and are sometimes associated with stimulations that go on too long; the embryologists say they are "overcooked." But this may not be the real reason the eggs don't fertilize, and postmature eggs may just be eggs that weren't meant to be embryos.

If your partner's sperm is normal, and your eggs are going to be fertilized in the lab with normal insemination, the next steps will be:

- The sperm are washed and the egg is separated from the follicular fluid. It still has its cumulus, which helps to activate the sperm.

- Your eggs (up to six to eight per dish) and sperm will be placed in a *petri dish,* a flat-bottomed round glass or plastic dish, which will be labeled with your name, lab number, the date, and the number of eggs in the dish.

✔ The dish is placed in an incubator so the eggs and sperm can be kept at body temperature. They're kept in a nutrient solution (culture medium), which provides conditions as similar as possible to those in the body. Different labs use different culture media, and this is one way that labs differ from one another.

✔ Conventionally inseminated eggs are left alone for 16 to 20 hours. The day after the retrieval, embryology takes the dish out of the incubator, strips off the cumulus, (which has by now been greatly loosened by the action of the sperm) and checks the eggs; what they hope to find is two pronuclear (2PN) embryos, or embryos that have two visible circles lined up next to each other (see Figure 16-1). These embryos contain the genetic material from each parent.

If you're planning to freeze some or all of your embryos for use at another time, your clinic may freeze them at the 2PN stage. Some centers grow all your embryos out to blastocyst stage and freeze only those that make it to blastocyst.

Congratulations! You've got embryos!

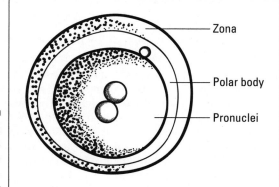

Figure 16-1:
A 2PN (pronuclear) embryo.

Zona

Polar body

Pronuclei

Having atretic eggs

Atretic eggs are dead; they're incapable of being fertilized. What would cause eggs to "die"? Some atretic eggs are postmature; they've been retrieved after their "peak freshness date," so to speak. This can happen when you have many eggs maturing at different rates; allowing time for smaller follicles to "catch up" may mean that a few of the larger eggs may become atretic.

Looking at what can go wrong when egg meets sperm

Good fertilization depends on the quality of the sperm and egg. At most centers, the fertilization rate is about 90 percent of the mature eggs. However, since the embryologists inseminate all the eggs, the overall fertilization rate that you should expect is closer to 60 percent. This reflects the fact that some eggs were not fertilizable. Why do they inseminate all the eggs? For one thing, judging maturity is not a perfect process, and even if an egg is immature at the time of insemination, it may still mature overnight and fertilize then. When embryologists look at the other 40 percent of the eggs, they may see things they'd rather not. For example, they may see the following:

✔ Your embryos may be *polyploid,* meaning that they contain more than two pronuclei. This can occur when more than one sperm has entered the egg (polyspermy), or when the egg doesn't throw off the second polar body (which should occur at the time of fertilization). These embryos are never normal, because they contain too many chromosomes. Since each pronucleus contains 23, a triploid embryo (3 pronuclei) contains 69. Such an embryo will not grow into a baby, and they are not transferred.

✔ The egg may still be immature. In this case, it may still be left in culture, even placed with sperm, with the hope that it will mature and fertilize later.

✔ The egg may be mature, yet show no signs of fertilization. In this case, the egg might be re-inseminated (by putting in some fresh sperm, hoping that the egg was immature when it started, has recently matured, and will now be able to fertilize). Alternately, the embryologists may decide to fertilize the egg by using intracytoplasmic sperm injection (ICSI). Whereas fertilization can be achieved by this method, embryos resulting from "second day ICSI" have a lower chance of implanting, and some clinics feel that it is not worth the effort.

Doing ICSI

If you need to do ICSI for male factor (explained in Chapter 11), the embryologist removes the cumulus and the coronal layers from the egg, washes the sperm in a special solution, and then sits down at the microscope for a most delicate task. ICSI is done under a high-powered microscope and involves holding the egg steady with one pipette, while another is used to inject the sperm into its mid-section.

This task can be time consuming, and if moving, active sperm aren't available, the embryologist tries to pick out sperm for fertilization that are at least "twitching." Sperm obtained during a sperm aspiration (see Chapter 11 for more about sperm aspirations) are particularly notorious for not moving, and the embryologists sometimes put in extra chemicals to get them to twitch so that they can pick out the most viable ones!

ICSI is done with a very fine-gauge needle. The sperm is sucked into the needle, your egg is stabilized, and the needle point is slowly inserted into the egg. ICSI requires very steady hands and a good eye for picking the best-looking sperm.

The process afterward is the same as conventional insemination. The ICSI eggs are left overnight and checked in the morning for fertilization. If the eggs haven't fertilized, ICSI can't be redone.

Some studies have suggested that ICSI embryos may have a higher than normal rate of *aneuploidy,* or abnormal number of chromosomes. This higher rate may occur because men with severe male factor have more chromosomal abnormalities, or because of the way the chromosomes come out the sperm head after ICSI.

Checking Chromosomes with Pre-Implantation Genetic Diagnosis (PGD)

If you carry a genetic disease or sex-linked disease, are over age 35, or have a history of repeated miscarriage, you may want to check your embryo's chromosomes before transferring. Pre-Implantation Genetic Diagnosis, or PGD, makes it possible to check an embryo for some common chromosomal abnormalities and can also determine whether the embryo will be a boy or girl. The procedure doesn't come cheap, however; centers charge between $2,500 and $5,000 (and up!) for PGD, although the cost isn't based on the number of embryos you have — one embryo is the same price as five or six, although that could change at any time.

PGD can be done to make sure the embryo has the right number of chromosomes (or to make sure the embryo carries the right sex chromosomes in gender selection), or it can used to test for a specific gene. For example, sickle cell anemia is a genetic defect in a specific gene, or part of the DNA. During PGD, this gene can be identified, and only the embryos that don't have the disease can be transferred, thus minimizing the risk of passing that gene on to the next generation. PGD can also be done for tissue matching, called HLA matching, to see if an embryo would be a suitable donor of tissue or organs to another person. That is because the HLA genes can be identified in the removed cell.

PGD is done by removing a cell, called a blastomere, from an eight-celled embryo, and then testing that one cell for either the number of chromosomes or for a specific genetic defect (like sickle cell anemia) or a genetic quality (like an HLA tissue match). PGD can be quite labor intensive for the lab, and it is not perfect. It is currently estimated that between 1 percent and 10 percent of the time, the diagnosis is not correct. That is because only a single cell is being analyzed (as compared with amniocentesis, in which hundreds of cells are available). Embryos can also have something called *mosaicism,* which means that the cells do not all have the same number of chromosomes! So the cell that is tested may be abnormal, yet the rest of the embryo may be normal, or vice versa. Not all IVF labs can perform PGD and/or test chromosomes. (See Chapter 2 to learn more about your genes.)

PGD can specifically test for the following, among others:

- Common trisomies (meaning an extra copy of the gene is present) such as Trisomy 13, 18 and 21 (Down syndrome)

- Single gene inherited genetic disease such as cystic fibrosis, sickle cell anemia, and Huntington's disease

- Anomalies of the X and Y chromosomes, such as Klinefelter (male child has 47 chromosomes, including XXY) and Turner (female with only 45 chromosomes; only one X is present) syndrome

- Gender-linked disorders, such as hemophilia

Although PGD sounds like, and certainly can be, a miracle for couples with genetic issues, there are some limitations to PGD, and also some serious ethical concerns. (See Chapter 20 for more about the ethics of PGD.) The limitations are:

- PGD doesn't test for every possible chromosomal abnormality, just the most common ones, which means that 10-15 percent of chromosomal abnormalities may be missed.

- Only one cell is usually tested in the United States, although some centers remove and test two cells (this is controversial; removing one cell hurts the embryo a little bit, taking out a second one may hurt it more). Occasionally, one cell may develop differently than the others, even though at this early stage they should all be identical. Having one cell with chromosomes that differ from the others is called mosaicism; up to 50 percent of embryos may have mosaicism. Mosaicism in a tested call can result in a false diagnosis, either a false positive or false negative.

It's not clear how much damage an embryo sustains from having a cell removed during PGD. Since individual blastomeres frequently die, and the embryo still continues to develop, it's thought that removing a single cell at this early stage of development will have no effect on embryo growth or development.

However, even though abnormal embryos aren't transfer, PGD doesn't increase pregnancy rates. This has been interpreted as meaning that undergoing PGD decreases the per embryo implantation rate by as much as 50 percent. Of course, this is offset by the ability to transfer only normal embryos, and the overall pregnancy rates are maintained. The "absolute damage" rate, meaning that the whole embryo dies during PGD, is small, less than 10 percent.

Results of PGD have to be received quickly, within one or two days, so that a fresh transfer can be done. For this reason, PGD labs frequently work around the clock!

Some studies have shown that embryos with abnormal chromosome testing at day 3 "self correct" by day 5 to have cells with a normal number of chromosomes. Would these embryos have implanted if they had been transferred on day 3? This is just one of the many PGD-related questions that are as yet left unanswered. Much more research is needed into the mysteries of embryo growth at a very early stage.

Answering the Call from Embryology

An embryologist usually calls the morning after your egg retrieval to let you know how many embryos you have and to discuss how many you are thinking you will want to transfer (the final decision will most likely have to be made on the day of transfer, when you will have a better idea of how they're growing). If you're going to freeze some, the embryologist also gives you some help deciding how many to leave out to grow a few days before picking the best few to transfer. Some centers suggest letting six to ten embryos, if you have that many, grow for a few days. They then pick the best two or three to transfer and freeze the rest, sometimes growing the remaining embryos to blastocyst stage before freezing all that survive.

The embryos that are frozen after a few days usually have two to eight cells, and their thaw rate may not be as good as 2PN embryos (embryos frozen the day after egg retrieval).

Two days after retrieval, embryology may call again, this time to tell you how your embryos are growing. One hopes they've now reached the two- to four-cell stage. Figure 16-2 shows a four-cell embryo.

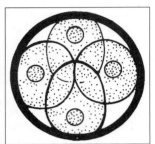

Figure 16-2:
A four-cell
embryo.

You may get a third call from embryology the third day after retrieval if you're doing a three-day transfer. Some centers still do transfers two days after retrieval, and some do most transfers five days after retrieval — at five days, the embryo should have reached the blastocyst stage. (We discuss blastocyst transfer in the section "Blasting Off! Considering a Blastocyst Transfer," later in this chapter.) If your embryos are now four to eight cells, they're ready for transfer. In addition to being graded by the number of cells, embryos are also graded by the equality and roundness of the cells and by the amount of fragmentation, or broken pieces, that are in the embryo. Figure 16-3 shows an embryo with a high degree of fragmentation.

Although a funny-looking embryo doesn't create a funny-looking kid, most embryologists do feel that an embryo with less fragmentation and more even-looking cells has a better chance of implanting. If you do get pregnant from fragmented embryos, the fragmentation does *not* mean that your baby will be abnormal in any way. Some centers remove the fragmented pieces before the embryo is transferred if the embryo has a significant amount of fragmentation. (See Figure 16-3 for a picture of an embryo with fragmentation.) One study suggested that the size and location of the fragments was also important; removing large fragments improved pregnancy rates more than removing small or scattered fragments. However, fragment removal is one of those controversial areas of embryology; if the lab with which you're working doesn't do fragment removal, this doesn't mean they're not up to date. This is why embryology is not just science but also an art. Things that work in one lab may not work in another and may be felt to be unnecessary.

Grading an embryo

At some centers the best-looking embryos on day 3 are graded as an 8A, with 8 being the number of the cells and A through F being the degree of fragmentation. Different centers grade embryos differently, so make sure you understand your particular clinic's grading system.

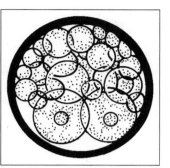

Figure 16-3:
An embryo
with a lot of
fragmen-
tation.

Does a great-looking embryo improve your chance of getting pregnant? Most embryologists would say a cautious yes, depending on your age, uterine cavity, general health, and many other factors. (An "A" embryo in a 40-year-old woman still has a much lower chance of implanting than, say, a "C" embryo in a 30-year old.)

Occasionally, if you're doing a three-day transfer, one or more of your embryos may already be *morulas,* meaning that the cells have pulled together and can no longer be counted. Morulas (from the Latin for "mulberry") usually have a very high rate of implantation, similar to blastocysts; in fact, they're the embryo stage right before blastocyst (see the section "Blasting Off! Considering a Blastocyst Transfer," later in this chapter).

Should you transfer that embryo?

Not all embryos are eight-cell, grade A embryos. In fact, most aren't. But most embryos that are at least four cells and graded B or C have a decent chance of implanting, and every embryologist has seen terrible-looking embryos that went on to become beautiful children. Embryologists suggest discarding the following types of embryos, however, because they're generally chromosomally abnormal:

- ✔ Multinucleated embryos, which contain three or more "bundles" of genetic material: At least 75 percent are abnormal.
- ✔ Embryos with uneven pronuclei: About 85 percent are abnormal.
- ✔ Embryos that develop too rapidly: Many of these have an abnormal number of chromosomes.

Looking at Your Uterine Lining

Embryos will implant only if the uterus is ready for implantation. Many centers look via ultrasound at the uterine thickness and also the appearance of the lining, called the pattern, to decide whether your embryos have a good chance of implanting after transfer. Your lining may be described as triple lined, also called tri-laminar. This pattern description is shortened to TL in most centers and describes the lining most clinics like to see before embryo transfer. Fertility centers differ on what's considered a good thickness, but most prefer to see a thickness of at least 7 millimeters.

The next best lining is an isoechogenic (IE) pattern, and the lining that has the lowest implantation rate is a homogenous hyperechoic (HH) pattern. Different clinics place varying amounts of importance on lining patterns, and your clinic may not even check the pattern.

Most centers, however, do check the lining thickness before transfer; anything over 7 millimeters thick is considered adequate, although pregnancies do occur with thinner linings. Your center's emphasis on the importance of the lining thickness or pattern will vary.

Hatching Embryos — Come on Out, You Guys

Around 1994, embryologists came out with a new technique called *assisted hatching* to help human embryos implant in the uterus. The majority of IVF centers do hatching on at least some of their embryos.

Assisted hatching (AH) is done the morning of your embryo transfer. The embryologist takes a tiny needle with acid on the end of it and barely touches the shell of the embryo, creating a small hole. This helps the embryo "break through" the *zona,* or hard shell, and attach to the uterus, an action that must happen a day or so after the embryo reaches the uterus in nature. Embryos created in the lab are theorized to have harder shells than are seen in natural conception, so the little hole, one hopes, gives them a head start on breaking out and hunkering down where they belong.

Hatching was originally done only on embryos whose zona, or outer shell, was thicker than normal, or on embryos from women over age 37, whose embryos might have a harder time breaking out of the shell. Now, some centers do assisted hatching on almost all their embryos; others still do AH only on certain patients, and some use it on frozen-thawed embryos.

Making embryos stick: Why Super Glue doesn't work

Several IVF centers have come forward with new ideas for "sticking" embryos to the uterine lining. They either coat them with a sticking substance or dig a little hole in the endometrium into which they put them. The IVF community hasn't gone crazy over these ideas because failure to implant usually isn't due to the embryos not sticking to the lining. It's a problem with the embryo or the lining itself. If the embryos, for whatever reason, aren't capable of growing into normal human beings, or the lining itself isn't capable of supporting their growth, forcing the embryos to attach to the lining won't make them grow.

Deciding How Many Embryos to Transfer

Deciding how many embryos to transfer can be difficult. Some centers and some parts of the world don't give you any say in the matter. For example, in England, you transfer two embryos if you're under age 40 — no exceptions. Some centers allow transfer of two embryos for women up to age 30, three embryos between ages 30 and 35, four embryos over age 35, and six or more embryos if you're over 40.

The ideal situation is discussing at your first doctor's appointment how many embryos to transfer, but the trouble is, you won't know at that point how well you'll stimulate, or how your embryos will look. Spending an hour debating about transferring four embryos is silly when you may get only three. If you end up with five embryos with a lot of fragmentation, most doctors suggest transferring more embryos than if they all look good. Some centers don't freeze extra embryos, usually because their labs don't do freezing well. You may have to use 'em or lose 'em, and you may not be willing to discard embryos. At the very least, you can find out your clinic's policies about transfer at your first visit, and keep thinking ahead as you go through IVF about what you'll do at transfer time.

Blasting Off! Considering a Blastocyst Transfer

A few years ago, IVF centers became alarmed at the large number of higher-order multiples (triplets or more) their patients were delivering, and they started looking for ways to transfer fewer embryos and still maintain the all-important high pregnancy rates.

Understanding blastocyst transfer

In most centers, the percentage of live-birth twins is about 25 percent of total births, and triplets somewhere between 5 and 10 percent. Quadruplets and higher are relatively rare, but are considered a problem at almost all clinics because the complication for both mother and babies is very high, and many babies die of prematurity or are miscarried.

Out of that concern came the concept of *blastocyst transfer,* the transfer of a five-day-old embryo. Because only 30 to 50 percent of embryos grow to blastocyst stage (see Figure 16-4), centers felt that only the best embryos were going to be transferred. As it turned out, blastocyst transfer of two embryos results in pregnancy rates in women under 35 that are the same as those achieved by the transfer of three embryos on day 3. However, the risk of triplets was greatly decreased.

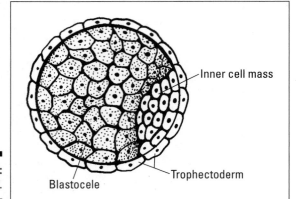

Figure 16-4:
A blastocyst.

Inner cell mass

Trophectoderm

Blastocele

Considering complications

Blastocyst transfer isn't for everyone. Because blastocysts are more complicated to grow than three-day embryos, requiring multiple media changes to keep up with their increased nutritional needs, many centers find it too difficult to grow enough blastocysts to get to transfer. So if your center transfers only blastocysts, you may end up with nothing to transfer.

The second problem comes from the blastocysts themselves. Because they're already "hatching" out of their shells at the time of transfer, blastocysts seem unusually likely to split into identical twins. Although on the surface, having identical twins doesn't seem much different than having fraternal twins, the fact is that identical twin pregnancies are much more problematic than fraternal ones. Because identical twins share the same placenta and sac, *twin-twin transfusion syndrome,* in which one twin gets too many nutrients and the other not enough, is more common, as are cord accidents, in which one baby gets tangled in the other's umbilical cord. The incidence of identical twins is about four to five times higher in blastocyst transfer than in normal conception. Of course, if you transfer two blastocysts and one splits, you're right back to the problem of higher-order multiples again. For these reasons, some centers have stopped doing blastocyst transfer on all patients and instead use it selectively, such as for patients who have had several IVF failures.

Taking Post-retrieval Pills and Potions

You may think that you're all done with medication after your egg retrieval, but you'll receive a sheet full of instructions about everything you need to take starting the day of your retrieval. Yes, the pills and potions go on after retrieval, but most are designed to help your embryo grow. Here's what you'll probably be given:

✔ **Antibiotics:** An egg retrieval is surgery that goes through a "dirty" area: your vagina. Yes, your vagina is considered a dirty area no matter how personally dainty and clean you are, which simply means that in medical terms, the area is not sterile. (By the way, so is your mouth; medically "dirty" simply means that it is not sterile.) So your doctor will probably give you antibiotics for several days, starting the day of your retrieval. Make sure that you mention any allergies or sensitivities.

If you're prone to yeast infections, you can take an over-the-counter pill called acidophilus, which maintains the balance of good and bad bacteria in your vagina. When the good bacteria are killed off with the bad ones, you get an overgrowth of yeast, which causes itching and a white cheesy discharge.

✔ **Steroids:** These may seem like an odd addition to your pill arsenal, but steroids are given to protect your embryo from attack by white blood cells after transfer. Steroids decrease the number of white blood cells in your blood. The dose given is very low and usually for just a few days. Their use is controversial, and most centers don't use them.

✔ **Progesterone:** When it comes to progesterone supplements, you may be given pills, gels, suppositories, or — can you stand it? — injections.

Some centers give progesterone injections to everyone because injections are the best absorbed. But progesterone injections do have a downside:

- **They hurt.** The needle used for progesterone needs to be at least a 22-gauge (relatively thick) variety because the progesterone is very thick, or viscous, and won't flow through a smaller needle. The progesterone is mixed in sesame or peanut oil, and a fair number of women have allergic reactions to the oils.

- **They're hard to find.** Commercially made progesterone in oil is very hard to find. Some small compounding pharmacies make their own, as do some of the large mail-order pharmacies that specialize in fertility medications.

- **Insurance doesn't always cover the cost.** Some insurance companies don't feel that progesterone injections are medically necessary. Costs are reasonable — about $45 a bottle — but can add up if you're using a bottle every five days for several months.

On the other hand, some centers use vaginal suppositories. The downside aspects of these are

- **They're messy.** The suppositories leak, making it necessary to wear a pad.

- **They can cause yeast infections.** Because they keep you continually wet, you're more likely to develop a yeast infection or rash, which can be more than a little annoying.

- **They're hard to find.** Specialty pharmacies usually make them themselves, which means that the amount of medication delivered can vary.

Other progesterone options are the following:

- **Crinone:** This progesterone gel is manufactured by Serono, a drug company that makes many fertility medications. Crinone causes less leakage and irritation than vaginal suppositories. It comes in an applicator that is inserted vaginally. Crinone is more expensive than vaginal suppositories.

- **Prometrium capsules, or compounded capsules:** These are pills, which means that if you take them orally, they pass through your liver after being digested in the stomach. The main disadvantage is that the way they're metabolized causes drowsiness, which can be severe. Some women also complain about dizziness or nausea. The amount of progesterone you get this way is quite small. For this reason, most centers that use these advise patients to take the pills vaginally. The progesterone actually absorbs better than after swallowing them, and they're somewhat less messy than suppositories.

Transferring Your Embryo

When you arrive for your embryo transfer, you'll be taken back to the IVF suite. Many centers allow your partner to come with you, and both of you may need to change into sterile gowns and coveralls. Some centers give you Valium before your transfer, primarily to reduce cramping after the procedure, although relaxing you is a side benefit.

Studies have shown that reducing cramping that you can't even feel can boost the pregnancy rate by 50 percent.

You'll be instructed to lie on an exam table that can be tilted. The worst part of the transfer in most clinics is that you're lying there with a full bladder. A full bladder, uncomfortable as it is, makes it easier to see your uterus under abdominal ultrasound guidance, and many centers now do embryo transfers under ultrasound guidance rather than blindly placing them through the cervix.

Your bladder, lying right over the uterus, pushes your uterus back when it's full; this also straightens the path into the uterus, making the transfer easier. A full bladder is especially helpful if you have an anteverted uterus, meaning one that is normally tilted forward. This is the most common position for the uterus. Remember that the uterus is attached by its base, and its top (the fundus) is therefore free to flop forward or backward. Sometimes, a retroverted uterus is called "tipped," but this is simply a relatively uncommon alternative position. The direction of your uterus makes no difference to whether or not you get pregnant, but it is important to the doctor performing your transfer because he or she must direct the catheter in the right direction.

An embryologist or your doctor may come in to speak with you before the transfer. That person will tell you how your embryos look today, may show or give you pictures, will verify your identity, and will confirm the number of embryos you want to transfer. You'll most likely receive something to sign that says that you agree to transfer X number of embryos, that you understand the risks of multiple birth, that you realize there's no guarantee of success, and that you are who you say you are.

After this point:

- ✔ An ultrasonographer (if your clinic uses ultrasound guidance) will place the probe on your abdomen so that the uterus can be visualized.

- ✔ The doctor or associate (nurses do embryo transfers in some centers) will wash your cervix and remove any mucus from the opening.

- ✔ Leaving a speculum in place, the doctor will let the embryologist know she's ready. Here come your embryos!

- ✔ Your doctor will slide the catheter through your cervix, which may cause a little cramping. If your clinic uses ultrasound guidance for the transfer, the ultrasonographers will let the doctor know how far away from the top of the uterus the catheter is before the embryos are slowly injected into the uterus.

- ✔ The catheter is slowly removed and handed back to the embryologist, who examines it under a microscope to make sure that no embryos are still in the catheter.

A transfer that's traumatic in any way, causing bleeding or severe cramping, may decrease your chance of pregnancy. If you've done a mock transfer (in a mock transfer, a soft catheter is inserted into the uterus, and the depth of the uterus and the angle required to get into it are recorded) before starting IVF, the doctor has a "map" of your cervical canal and uterine opening so trauma is less likely. Ultrasound guidance also makes it easier to see the curves in your anatomy, so your center may not do a mock transfer if it's using ultrasound guidance for your embryo transfer.

After your embryos are in the uterus, you may need to stay on the table with your feet tilted up for a half hour or so. Clinics vary widely in their bed rest requirements, and they may keep you anywhere from no time at all to up to a few hours. After you go home, you'll be instructed to maintain a variable degree of rest for a specified time. Most clinics suggest two days. Others recommend up to a week, and some clinics don't feel that any bed rest is justified.

Embryos are placed directly into your uterus; emptying your bladder or bowels isn't going to dislodge them! Neither will coughing or sneezing. It's easy to get constipated during this time because you're resting. This will make you uncomfortable, never mind more worried about straining! It's best to take a gentle stool softener, like milk of magnesia (which doesn't absorb from the bowel), or extra bran in the diet.

Keeping Your Feet and Your Spirits Up After the Transfer

After you're safely home, you may be on restricted activity for a period of time, depending on your clinic's policies. Try not to compare what you're doing to what anyone else is doing, because different centers have different policies. If you don't follow your center's policies, you're bound to feel guilty if you don't get pregnant, so follow your instruction sheet.

If your center restricts activity after the transfer, you'll be lying around on the bed or couch, getting up only to use the bathroom and eat meals. After your strict rest period is over, many centers still ask you not to lift anything heavy (over 15 pounds is typical), not to do any strenuous exercise, and not to have sex.

Sex is restricted because it can cause uterine contractions, especially if you have an orgasm, so the no-sex rule applies to *any* activity that could cause an orgasm, not just intercourse. Yes, this restriction does include vibrators!

Heavy lifting is another common prohibition that can cause concern, especially if your job requires it or if you have a small child. Most centers will gladly write you a note restricting your work activity, but your 1-year-old probably won't understand a note saying you can't lift him into his high chair. If you have to lift a child, bend with your knees, trying to keep your back straight when you lift rather than bending at the waist and straining your abdominal muscles. This form is good body mechanics, and you should pick up heavy objects, such as children, this way all the time if you want to keep your back in working order.

Mild exercise, such as a leisurely walk, is fine, but forget about aerobics for a while. Use common sense about yoga, tai chi, or whatever else you do to decrease stress and increase endorphins. If you feel guilty doing it, you probably shouldn't be doing it!

Chapter 17

Waiting, Waiting: Surviving the Two-Week Wait after an IVF Cycle

- -

In This Chapter

▶ Surviving the wait for your pregnancy test

▶ Making a backup plan

▶ Steering clear of home pregnancy tests

▶ Handling the news

- -

Finishing up an in vitro fertilization (IVF) cycle brings a whole host of emotions. You're happy that the procedure itself was successful and that the shots are finished or at least greatly diminished. You're ecstatic about having your life back, without the frequent blood draws, ultrasounds, and phone calls. On the other hand, you may feel adrift when the intensity is over and you've gone from constant monitoring to being almost ignored by your clinic.

Now it's time to wait for your pregnancy test. Because the test results won't be accurate for almost two weeks after your embryo transfer, this time period is often referred to by patients as "the two-week wait."

In this chapter, we review some of the do's and don'ts of the two-week wait, and take a little peek into the future when you'll have an answer to the big question — am I pregnant or not? — and what you'll be doing in either case.

Technically, You're Pregnant — Waiting for the Proof

From a purely technical viewpoint, after the embryos are placed into your uterus, you're pregnant — in the loosest sense of the word, at least. You have embryos floating around where they belong, and all they have to do is attach and grow.

This is probably the first time in your infertility history where you can say without a doubt that you've formed an embryo and that it is where it needs to be to grow. You may have known that you made a follicle, and been fairly sure that you got sperm where it needed to go at the right time, but you never knew for sure that the egg and sperm got together. Now you do.

Now comes the waiting period. The two-week wait is a time of "what ifs" and "if onlys" like no other time you've probably experienced. Because this is new territory for you, we give some ideas on how to make it through the two-week wait without driving yourself crazy.

Keeping busy

Although you may be tempted to just relax and wait, unencumbered by other responsibilities, the truth is that sitting around waiting is hard work, a lot harder than keeping yourself busy with everyday tasks. Waiting for water to boil and staring at it as well is a quick recipe for instant irritation, and so is staying idle during these two weeks.

Try to plan as many activities as you can manage (after your post-transfer rest period). If you work, consider it a blessing and immerse yourself in your responsibilities. Many women suggest reading a good book to get you through this time. Try to keep the book as far away from the topic of fertility as possible. Exercise is also a good way to keep busy, but keep it mild, like walking around the block. Many couples find that the two-week wait is a great time to take a vacation. What better way to distract yourself than with a little R&R?

If the tension does begin to run high, assemble your backup plan. What will you do next, pregnant or not? This type of planning often alleviates the fear and uncertainty that accompany the two-week wait.

Making your to-do or not-to-do list

Taking care of yourself during the roller coaster ride of trying to create a baby is crucial. For some women, this may mean a trip to the hairdresser, manicurist, gym, or all of the above. But you should consider a few limitations as you wait out these last few weeks before your pregnancy test.

Coloring your hair

For those whose follicle challenges begin at the top of their heads, hair coloring is more than just a luxury; it's a way of life. To color or not to color has been a long-time topic of discussion among the newly pregnant. According to the American College of Obstetricians and Gynecologists, hair coloring *is* safe during pregnancy. Based on this opinion, coloring your hair during the two-week wait is also presumed to be safe (unless of course your colorist turns your hair orange!). However, keep in mind that the two-week wait is only two weeks. If you're at all concerned, staying off the bottle (of color, that is) for the time being may be the best advice for you.

Having manicures and pedicures

The greatest danger that we know of in manicures and pedicures is for those who give them. You may have noticed that many manicurists now wear masks to protect themselves from the fumes and toxins generated by the products. A simple polish-and-go won't hurt you during the two-week wait. Those with acrylic nails are advised to refrain from having this service during the two-week wait, and those who don't have acrylic nails but want them are better off waiting until after the two-week wait, and after the first trimester of pregnancy for that matter. If you already have acrylic nails, don't panic, but you may consider having them removed before your cycle.

Getting your exercise

Exercise can be a great way to take your mind off your waiting and your worries during the two-week wait. Here are two basic rules to remember with exercise during this time:

- ✔ Don't start up a brand-new routine during the two-week wait. In other words, if you're not a runner, don't become one now. Keep your exercise routine consistent with that in which you engaged before.

- ✔ Keep your heart rate equal to or lower than 140 beats per minute. This rate is also recommended during pregnancy, so this is a good time to get used to keeping track of it. Most fitness stores sell inexpensive heart rate monitors, and certain exercise machines (such as particular brands of treadmills) have a built-in monitor that can read your heart rate when you grasp the metal sensors on the handle bar.

Keep in mind that moderation must become your middle name, in judgment and in exercise. Should you choose the two-week wait as the ideal time to scale Mount Everest? We think not. Nor do we recommend skydiving for novices (or even experts) during this time. Both activities, aside from being highly dangerous, also pose the added risk of high altitude, which may be hazardous for those unaccustomed to it. However, if you live in Denver, the mile-high city, you don't have to move. The two-week wait calls for maintaining the status quo. Leave the new stuff for later.

Having sex during the two-week wait

For those going through the two-week wait after in vitro fertilization, sex is considered a no-no (at least by most doctors). You've had surgery (albeit minor), and the risk of infection may be greater, so hands (and other body parts) off during this time. Another concern is that female orgasm may cause a series of uterine contractions, which are not ideal in creating a hospitable environment for baby embryo. Read a good book instead.

Sensing Every Little Twinge: The Truth about Pregnancy Symptoms

Of course you're anxious. Of course you're anxiously examining every twinge and cramp you have for some indication of whether you're pregnant. If you're taking progesterone, as you most likely are after an IVF cycle, the symptoms of pregnancy can easily be confused with symptoms of progesterone supplementation, because an increase in progesterone is associated with many common pregnancy symptoms. What might you experience, and which signs are good, bad, and meaningless? Here are some symptoms you may experience and what they mean:

- **Sore breasts:** Tender breasts are almost a universal sign of pregnancy, with or without feelings of heaviness or tingling in the nipples. Unfortunately, sore breasts are caused by increased progesterone and estrogen, so sore breasts may be caused by the ovarian stimulation you underwent or your suppositories rather than by a growing embryo.

- **Spotting:** This symptom is very common in very early pregnancy, whether or not you've undergone fertility treatment. Spotting may be caused by an embryo burrowing into the uterus and causing leakage of blood from small blood vessels. If you're taking progesterone suppositories, irritation from the suppositories can also cause some spotting.

- ✔ **Cramping:** This discomfort is typical in the two-week wait and may be caused by the enlarged ovaries if you've done a medicated cycle (taken ovarian stimulating medications, as discussed in Chapter 13). Some centers believe that cramping is a sign of low progesterone, and they may increase your supplements if you have continued cramping.

- ✔ **Fatigue:** This symptom is often related to higher than normal levels of hCG (human chorionic gonadotropin, the injection given 36 or so hours before an egg retrieval) and progesterone, both of which can be from the growing embryo or from your hCG trigger shot. Progesterone pills are particularly noted for causing extreme fatigue. Progesterone also raises your temperature, which may make you more sluggish than usual. Plus you're probably emotionally exhausted from the IVF cycle! This is a perfectly good time to get extra rest.

- ✔ **Nausea:** This symptom is fairly common with progesterone, especially in pill form, and also with high levels of hCG. Higher than normal levels of estrogen can also cause nausea.

So how can you tell whether you're pregnant in the two-week wait? Unfortunately, you really can't. Sharon can name at least a dozen patients who swore they weren't pregnant and were, along with many patients who were sure they were pregnant but weren't. Continue taking your meds even if you're *sure* you're not pregnant, because there's a good chance you're wrong!

Don't be so sure you're not pregnant!

Patients who quit taking their medications such as progesterone on their own when they assume that they're not pregnant make Sharon want to pull her hair out. She usually finds this out when she calls a patient (we'll call her Mary) who inexplicably never came in for her pregnancy test a week or so ago. When Sharon asks the patient why she never came in, she says, "Oh, I got my period, so I stopped my meds." At this point, Sharon's hair starts to stand on end, and she asks if Mary got a full-flow period. Some patients may say yes, but Mary, like most patients, says no — it was lighter than normal. Some women have a very light period even though they're pregnant, so this raises Sharon's voice a few octaves, and she tells Mary to have blood work done. Today. Right now, in fact. Mary voices extreme surprise and a little irritation at this, and says she knows she's not pregnant. And besides, she has something else to do today. You would think that people who just spent thousands of dollars trying to get pregnant wouldn't do something like this, but you'd be wrong. And so is Mary, quite frequently. Don't stop taking your medications until you have your pregnancy test done and someone tells you specifically to stop!

Saying No to Home Pregnancy Tests

Most women find the temptation of a home pregnancy test (HPT) impossible to resist. Those little packaged sticks promise immediate results and an answer to the question "Am I pregnant or not?" Before you go out and buy up your druggist's supply of home pregnancy tests, consider the following:

- ✔ Many home pregnancy tests require a minimum amount of hCG in your system in order to register a positive. Early pregnancy may not result in a high enough number to register, even if you are pregnant.

- ✔ You were most likely given an hCG shot to trigger ovulation before your IVF retrieval. That shot of 10,000 units of hCG doesn't leave your system overnight. Furthermore, it's the same hormone (the pregnancy hormone) measured in home pregnancy tests. For some women, the traces of the hCG shot can take 10 to 15 days to disappear. Your HPT doesn't know that though! This can result in a false positive and a big letdown when the moment of truth arrives.

- ✔ Home pregnancy tests generally require the first morning's urine, which contains the highest concentration of hCG, for greatest accuracy. Many women, pregnant or not, awake in the middle of the night to urinate, making the first morning's urine not the first after all. Unless you want to subject yourself to 3 a.m. wake-up calls for home pregnancy tests, this is yet another reason to "skip the stick."

- ✔ Home pregnancy tests are, first and foremost, over-the-counter devices. They do not replace a *beta HCG* — a blood test that measures the level of hCG. Don't expect the same accuracy or reliability from drugstore pregnancy tests.

Many women get on the HPT roller coaster, allowing their emotions to rise and fall with each subsequent pee stick. It isn't worth it. Wait for the real thing, as hard as the waiting may be. You have no reason to subject yourself to a test that could very well yield incorrect results.

Waiting for the Phone to Ring

It's beta day — the day your blood tests reveal whether you're pregnant or not.

Waiting for the phone to ring is almost always an unpleasant experience — whether waiting for a date to call or a nurse to deliver news of whether your baby is on its way. But modern technology has given us answering machines and voicemail so that you don't have to sit by the phone! Take advantage of this technology.

Deciding where you want the call

If you choose not to be home when the phone rings, alert the nurse or doctor who will be calling you with your results. Do you want that information left on your answering machine? Is there a chance that your little sister, mother, or cleaning person might hear the results instead, and perhaps forget to tell you? Work out these details ahead of time and communicate them to those who'll be delivering your results. Planning to receive this call at work may not be the best idea, unless you have a private area and/or supportive people around you. If you don't want to be called at work, make this fact very clear to the nurses and/or doctor as well. Some choose to have their partners receive the news. If you feel that hearing the news from someone close to you would be easier, consider this option and put it into action. You can't control the news you'll hear, but you can control the way you hear it.

Understanding chemical pregnancy and false positives

False positives are rare in pregnancy tests. You're most likely to get a false positive result on either a home pregnancy test or a beta subunit if it's been less than two weeks since you took hCG. Some doctors give hCG "boosters" during the two-week wait because it helps the corpus luteum, the remnant of your follicle that produced an egg, put out more progesterone.

Although anything over 5 IU is a positive test, the chances of a pregnancy with such a low starting level succeeding are less than if the beta was higher. However, sometimes a pregnancy may implant a few days later than normal, giving an initial low positive. These pregnancies may pick up steam quickly, and the beta will start rising appropriately.

A beta that is positive for only a few days may be called a chemical pregnancy by your doctor; a *chemical pregnancy* is one in which the embryo starts to implant but fails to grow normally, so that a low level of hCG may be picked up for a short time. The beta in these cases may be negative a few days later if you repeat the test. (See Chapter 5 for more about chemical pregnancies.)

Most clinics urge cautious optimism if the first beta level is lower than they would like to see it. Don't broadcast the news to anyone except those closest to you if your initial beta isn't very high.

Responding to Positive News

After you get the call from your center that your test was positive, your initial elation may quickly change to worry: Will everything go well? Are your numbers too high or too low? Should you tell anyone yet? After almost constant contact with your clinic for weeks or months, it can be scary to think that you'll soon be leaving the people you've come to know and trust.

Don't panic. Most clinics continue to see you for a few weeks after your first positive test to make sure that your pregnancy is going well. Some centers even have nurses on staff who deal only with the center's pregnant patients.

Continuing the tests

Some centers continue to check your beta and your progesterone levels for several weeks to make sure that your pregnancy is a good one. Because you may not be able to see an obstetrician for a few weeks, this monitoring ensures that if you have an ectopic pregnancy, you'll be diagnosed promptly, to avoid life-threatening complications.

Your clinic usually wants to see your beta double every two to three days for the first few weeks. The following numbers are typical milestones based on a day-three embryo transfer (three days after the egg retrieval). If you transferred blastocysts on day five, subtract two days. Obviously there are many exceptions to the "rules" here. This list gives only the averages.

- ✔ **9 days post-transfer:** Average BSU 48; range 17–119

- ✔ **10 days post-transfer:** Average BSU 59; range 17–147

- ✔ **11 days post-transfer:** Average BSU 95; range 17–223

- ✔ **12 days post-transfer:** Average BSU 132; range 17–429

- ✔ **13 days post-transfer:** Average BSU 292; range 70–758

- ✔ **16 days post-transfer:** Average BSU 1061; range 324–4130; yolk sac may be visible

- ✔ **By the sixth week of pregnancy:** Average BSU 17,000; heartbeat seen by end of sixth week

- ✔ **End of sixth week:** Average BSU 30,000; embryo seen

If your beta isn't rising appropriately, no one can do much but wait to see what happens. Some clinics monitor your progesterone levels and add more progesterone if your numbers are a little low, but adding progesterone won't save a bad pregnancy if the issue isn't a lack of progesterone.

A beta that starts out high and rises very quickly may mean a twin or triplet pregnancy. In one very unusual case in the clinic where Sharon works, a very high first and rapidly rising beta was caused by a pregnancy growing in an ovary. This is an extremely rare type of ectopic pregnancy.

When will you get to see your baby on ultrasound? Some clinics schedule an ultrasound around six weeks, or two weeks after you've missed a period. Don't expect to see much at this point. The enthusiastic ultrasonagrapher may be able to point out the fetal pole and the yolk sac to you, but these features resemble a blob much more than a baby.

For historic reasons, obstetricians count the "gestational age" from the theoretical first day of the last menstrual period, assuming normal cycles and natural conception. During IVF, the day of egg retrieval is considered the day of ovulation, or 14 days after the last menstrual period. So 6 weeks of gestational age means 4 weeks after ovulation, or exactly 28 days after egg retrieval during IVF. If today is the 31st day after egg retrieval, then your gestational age is 6 weeks plus 3 days.

At this point, you should know whether you have more than one baby, but keep in mind that many times one twin or triplet will disappear by the next ultrasound. Very early losses of one or more embryos are very common, so wait until 12 weeks or so before you tell all the neighbors you're having twins or triplets.

By six to seven weeks you should be able to see a heartbeat, which you may actually recognize on ultrasound as a little flicker, and the embryo will be visible. At this point, your baby will resemble a fish more than a human being. No one will be willing to guess if you're having a boy or girl for another seven or eight weeks. Remember that ultrasound guesses aren't always accurate, so don't decorate the nursery in pink or blue just yet!

One of the most accurate ways of making sure that your baby is growing the way it should is to measure the crown-to-rump length. The embryo can first be measured around six weeks, when it's about 4 millimeters long and the heartbeat can first be visualized. Fetal growth in the first 12 weeks is fairly exact, and your baby's gestational age can be determined from the crown-to-rump length. (This is more important when women are not sure when they conceived, but during IVF it helps to reassure you that the pregnancy is growing according to schedule.) Here are what the measurements should be at different stages. See above for how obstetricians determine gestational age.

- ✔ **Six weeks:** 4 millimeters
- ✔ **Seven weeks:** 10 millimeters
- ✔ **Eight weeks:** 16 millimeters
- ✔ **Nine weeks:** 23 millimeters
- ✔ **Ten weeks:** 31 millimeters
- ✔ **Eleven weeks:** 41 millimeters
- ✔ **Twelve weeks:** 54 millimeters

Saying goodbye to your fertility doctor

Some fertility clinics monitor you through the first few weeks after you become pregnant; others wave goodbye with your first positive beta test. Most clinics don't want to keep you too long as a pregnant patient because they don't want to deal with pregnancy issues. Also, malpractice insurance for gynecologists and reproductive endocrinologists does not cover taking care of patients beyond the first trimester. But you may have a hard time getting an appointment with an obstetrician until you're ten weeks pregnant or so, leaving you in sort of a no man's land of medical care.

Establish yourself as a patient of an obstetrician even before you get pregnant. That way, if you have any problems in the first few weeks, such as spotting, cramping, or severe pain (as in a possible ectopic pregnancy), your obstetrician can take care of you, even if your clinic doesn't deal with these issues.

Defining high-risk pregnancy

Don't think of yourself as a high-risk pregnancy just because you did IVF to get pregnant. Most of the time, IVF doesn't increase the risk of complications in pregnancy. The complications come from whatever caused your infertility, such as your age, uterine shape, or other health issues.

Most doctors consider you high risk for the following reasons:

- ✔ You're over age 35.
- ✔ You have a uterine malformation that may make it hard for you to carry the pregnancy.
- ✔ You have multiples (twins or higher).

> ✔ You have a health history of cancer or a disease such as diabetes, lupus, or heart disease.
>
> ✔ You have a history of incompetent cervix.
>
> ✔ You have had several previous cesarean sections.
>
> ✔ You're significantly overweight.

If you're a high-risk patient, you'll probably be seeing your obstetrician more often than once a month in the first trimester. You may be doing additional testing, such as chorionic villus sampling (CVS), to check for chromosomal abnormalities in the first three months.

Considering the Next Step If IVF Doesn't Work

Every day, a patient asks Sharon how she could *not* be pregnant. "But my embryos looked perfect. My lining looked great, and I did everything I was supposed to. How could it not work?" women say.

Unfortunately, most of the time the answer is, "We don't know." Statistically speaking, if you have a 50 percent chance of getting pregnant, you have an equal 50 percent chance of not getting pregnant, but this isn't the answer a disappointed patient wants to hear. You want an answer, something you can fix in the future. But the truth is that medicine doesn't have all the answers.

Figuring out what happened

What happened? One of several things happened if your pregnancy test was negative:

> ✔ The embryos may not have implanted at all. The most common reason for embryos not implanting is that their development stopped prior to reaching the implantation stage. The older you are, the more likely this is to happen, but the cessation of embryo development is thought to be the most common cause of lack of pregnancy at any age, and in fact, even during natural conception.
>
> ✔ The embryos started to implant and then stopped. Usually this happens because the embryos are abnormal chromosomally. The only way to tell whether embryos have the right chromosomes is to do preimplantation genetic diagnosis (PGD), a procedure in which one cell is removed from

the embryo before implantation and its DNA is analyzed for abnormalities. This procedure is expensive, and not all centers do PGD (see Chapter 16 for more about PGD). Plus PGD has never been shown to improve overall pregnancy rates.

✔ The embryos could be damaged during the process of growth in the lab and in the actual transfer itself. Man-made processes are never going to be as effective as nature intended, and occasionally, a bad batch of medium, which is used to nurture the embryos before transfer, causes the embryo not to grow the way it should.

There might have been a problem with the uterus. There isn't any way to test the endometrium during the actual cycle, because an endometrial biopsy would damage the lining and might actually prevent the implantation, but it is possible to measure the thickness of the lining to make sure it is at least 7 mm. It is also important to check the cavity to make sure there aren't any fibroids or polyps that might interfere with implantation. Other than these two tests, there isn't any other testing that has proven to be useful. Nevertheless, there is always a chance that the embryos found a bad spot in the uterus and failed to implant. This is thought to be a relatively rare situation, however.

Things may have gone poorly during the actual embryo transfer process. As previously mentioned, a traumatic transfer (where there might have been cramping and/or bleeding during the procedure) are associated with decreased pregnancy rates. But even when everything seems to go well, it is possible that the uterus will have cramping and move the embryos to a spot where they're less likely to implant. How to get around this problem? The only way is to try again.

Questions for God and your doctor (who are not one and the same)

An unsuccessful attempt at IVF can be devastating financially, physically, and emotionally. It opens up the floodgates for a host of worries and fears that can be overwhelming. For this reason, your best thinking probably doesn't come on the day of or the day after an unsuccessful attempt. You need to put some time and space between the cycle and your next steps. Remember that your hormone levels are probably off kilter as well. They'll eventually return to normal and probably your mood will, too, as the days pass.

As you prepare your list of questions for your doctor, try to be as specific as possible. "What went wrong?" may be a good question with which to start, but you're better off breaking this broad question down into more specific questions, such as the following:

✔ Did I respond as expected?

✔ How was my egg quality?

✔ What particular stage in the process did you feel posed the most problems?

✔ What did you learn about me and my situation through this process?

✔ What would you recommend as a next step? Why?

Remember that your doctor is not God and doesn't have all the answers that you may want. Fertility is a numbers game, under the best of circumstances. If doctors knew exactly why it all worked or didn't work, they would save you and themselves a lot of time and make a lot more money. Unfortunately, medicine doesn't have all the answers, for anything, including fertility.

Your doctor may be a great source of comfort, but consider taking the "Why me?" question to a therapist, a religious person, or God. Use your doctor for the knowledge that she does have and seek other avenues for the answers that your doctor doesn't have.

Going through the grief process

Perhaps the best way to deal with the morass of emotions brought on by an unsuccessful cycle is by looking at the grief process. Elisabeth Kubler-Ross, the author of *On Death and Dying,* identified the five stages of grief following the death of a loved one: denial, anger, bargaining, depression, and acceptance. The death of a dream, even if it's only a temporary condition, is much the same. You can treat this disappointment as a loss, and some women even liken it to miscarriage. Consider the following stages and how they may apply:

✔ **Denial:** "Maybe the test results are wrong, and I really am pregnant," you may say. Denial is perhaps one of the most time-honored human traditions in dealing with painful situations. Although denial provides you with a brief respite from your pain, it isn't something that can successfully carry you out of your grief. Realizing that you're not pregnant (after your doctor has confirmed it), no matter how much you want to be, is the first step.

✔ **Anger:** "My doctor doesn't care" or "Somebody messed up" may be a typical response. Anger is also a perfectly natural and understandable response to grief. You may find that, as your emotions (and hormones) subside with time, your anger may not seem as urgent. Remember that physical force or verbal intimidation are never appropriate, no matter how angry you are. If you feel this way, you need some time to cool off and perhaps some professional help to do so.

- ✔ **Bargaining:** "If only I could be pregnant, I would never again (pick one) yell at my mother, slack off at work, speed, or engage in any other bad habits." Bargaining is similar to foxhole prayers, those pleas for help that come at desperate times. It's also a normal reaction to grief, albeit not a very useful one. Allow yourself time to move through this stage (as with all of the stages that you experience). This too shall pass.

- ✔ **Depression:** "I'm not pregnant. I'll never have a baby. My life is worthless." Also known as "stinking thinking," depression can cast a cloud over your thoughts and feelings. This is another (normal) stage of grief that often doesn't let you take into account the positive realities in your life. If your depression lasts longer than two weeks, consider seeking professional help, whether from your doctor or a therapist. She or he may prescribe antidepressants to get you through this difficult time.

- ✔ **Acceptance:** Remember that acceptance doesn't equate to agreement. You may accept your circumstances as they are today and yet continue to feel that the situation is unfair — and it is. Remember that you can change your circumstances now that you've passed through your period of mourning.

You may go through these stages of grief more than once. You may skip a stage or repeat it twice before you come to accept what has happened. Regardless, don't rush yourself. You'll get there when you get there, and not a moment sooner.

Taking time out for you and your partner

While you're grieving, your partner may be grieving as well. He may be stuck in a particular stage of the process, such as denial or anger. Look for signs that he may need some additional help to work through his feelings.

After you're both past the initial shock and grief, consider taking some time out to relax and regroup, in that order. Although you may be tempted to resume your normal routine, your body, mind, and spirit will benefit from a little R&R. Your relationship will, too. Grief can be a very personal thing and one that isolates you from the most important people in your life, including your partner. Take the time to reconnect with one another and appreciate those things that you love in each other. A one-month hiatus will not make a difference in the big picture. However, not taking the time to recoup and renew yourself and your partnership could have lasting effects.

Use your follow-up doctor's visit as a springboard to discuss your future plans with your partner. Remember that you're both playing on the same team. If your goals appear to be different at this point, give one another the space and time to consider both sides. If you need help arriving at a mutually agreeable decision, you may want to consider visiting a therapist or a religious adviser.

Keeping Embryos Frozen — What's Their Expiration Date?

If you have embryos frozen from a fresh cycle, you may be concerned that if you don't use 'em, you'll lose 'em. This thought may have you rushing into another cycle before you're emotionally ready, or doing another cycle soon after you deliver Baby Number 1.

While there's nothing wrong with doing a frozen embryo transfer as soon as you're ready, you don't have to worry that your embryos will get freezer burn if left in the tank too long. Embryos have been successfully thawed and created perfectly normal children even after being frozen for ten years.

Some clinics are imposing time limits on keeping embryos frozen because of limited storage capacity. Your clinic will tell you how long they'll store embryos at the time of freezing (and will have you sign a consent form to make sure you understand the implications).

Giving Up on Fertility Treatments? Considering When to Let Go

"When to say when" may come sooner for some infertility patients because of basic reasons: a lack of money, time, or opportunity. But even for those who've figured out ways to juggle limited resources a little bit longer, knowing when to say when still isn't easy. A good friend of hers counseled Jackie one day when she felt she couldn't take the fertility treatments anymore.

"When do I give up?" Jackie cried to her over the phone.

"When you just can't walk another step," her friend replied firmly.

Jackie had moments and even days when she felt that she couldn't take one more blood test or one more ultrasound or answer one more phone call. During those times, the wonderful support of her online network, friends, and family helped her through. It often took what felt like a Herculean effort to do the next right thing when it came to fertility. Along the way, however, Jackie also "gave up" in little pieces. By her last cycle (the one that worked after three-and-a-half years), she had put away her extensive filing system in which she cataloged every test result. Instead of comparing her daily results to past results, she stuffed the files into the bottom of a cabinet and just looked at the day in front of her. Was she giving up or letting go? Perhaps a little bit of both. And although the cycle was successful, she realized that it was not *because* she let go. Letting go at the time was her only option in order to continue taking the necessary steps.

For many people, giving up and letting go are one and the same. For Jackie, both actions allowed her to take the responsibility and the results off herself, where they don't belong anyway. This attitude allowed her to continue without a death grip on every last detail, many of which are truly insignificant in the long run.

Let go if you can, sooner rather than later. Doing so helps you maintain your spirit throughout the process, whether it is short or long. And, if this stops working, and you just can't walk another step, consider your other options.

Part V
The Road Less Traveled . . . So Far!

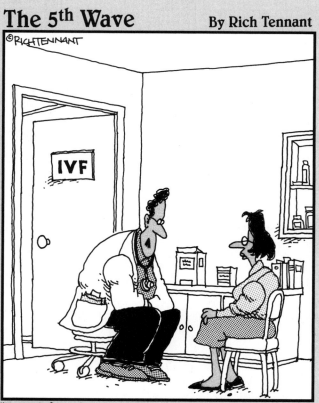

The 5th Wave   By Rich Tennant

"In brief, we'll stimulate your ovaries with daily medications or hormones, perform an oocyte retrieval at the hospital, incubate the eggs in a petri dish at the laboratory, and then sit back and let nature take its course."

In this part . . .

In this part, we look at nontraditional families and methods of conception, including donor egg and surrogacy. We also help you decide when "enough is enough" and discuss the possible alternatives to biological parenthood. Finally, we peer into the future for a look at what's on the horizon for infertility treatment.

Chapter 18

Challenges of Third-Party Reproduction

*T*he traditional family of mom, dad, and 2.7 children has changed considerably over the past few decades. Families today may contain biological children, adopted children, children with single parents of either sex, gay parents, children born with the help of third parties from donor eggs, sperm, or embryos, as well as children carried through pregnancy by their grandmother, their aunt, or a total stranger.

The legal and emotional issues involved with using eggs, sperm, or uteri from someone else can be tricky. In this chapter, we tell you how to decide whether third-party — or even fourth- or fifth-party! — reproduction is right for you, and how to proceed after you make your decision.

Deciding to Use Donor Eggs, Sperm, or Embryos

Deciding to use donor eggs, embryos, or sperm is a difficult decision that opens up a host of emotional issues and legal issues. Usually, you make this decision because you have to — because one or both of you has a fertility issue that can't be fixed. Or you make the decision because you're a same-sex couple or a single parent; obviously, you need some type of donor in these cases.

If you're moving to donor eggs or sperm because you have an unfixable problem, you need to come to terms with your loss before moving on. As an infertility nurse, Sharon saw couples move too quickly to donor eggs and sperm and then struggle with their feelings about being pregnant with a child not biologically their own. Donor eggs or sperm will always be available; don't jump in before you're sure that you're emotionally ready.

If you decide to use donor eggs or sperm, the child created will be related to *one* of you. Is this fact going to be a problem if you and your partner separate down the road? Is it something that one of you might fling in the other's face if the child has a serious health problem, or ends up in trouble with the law? Will the fact that one of you can see family features in your child's face while the other can't become a source of friction? You need to consider these questions, as well as any others that cross your mind, before you make the leap.

Protecting Yourselves — the Least You Should Do If You're Using a Donor

Before entering into any type of donor situation that we describe in this chapter, whether it involves eggs, embryos, or sperm, you need to do several things:

- ✔ **Thoroughly check out the donor's health history but realize that a clean slate is no guarantee against a host of other potential problems.** For starters, we can only test for those diseases that we're aware of today. New communicable diseases and new strains of old ones, not able to be tested for today, may be uncovered in the future.

- ✔ **Be aware of the limitations of genetic tests.** While most centers test for the most common genetic diseases such as cystic fibrosis or sickle cell anemia, they may only test for the most frequently recognized mutations. While this covers the majority of cases, there may still remain as many as 10 percent to 20 percent of rare mutations that are not tested for. Certain populations, such as Native Americans, tend to carry more remote, albeit just as harmful, mutations of diseases such as cystic fibrosis. These would only be found via extensive screening, which would need to be done at your request and on your bankroll as well.

- ✔ **If you're a known carrier of a genetic disease, be sure your donor is tested for these specific diseases.** Less common genetic illnesses, such as Tay-Sachs disease or Maple Syrup Urine Disease are generally not tested for in the standard centers.

✔ **Be aware of the testing differences between donor sperm and donor eggs.** While donor sperm is frozen and quarantined for six months after initial testing, donor eggs are a different egg altogether! Because eggs aren't quarantined after the initial infectious disease testing, there's a small chance that infectious disease could be transmitted to their recipient. While you may be able to rule out the likelihood of certain diseases by your donor's lifestyle, partnership, or health history, remember that you're going on her word and that of the clinic compiling her information.

✔ **Do some soul searching.** Only you know how you really feel about using another person's eggs, embryos, or sperm. Think it *all* the way through — past the cute baby stage into the teenage years and beyond.

✔ **Decide who to tell.** You may change your mind later about telling (or not telling) your child and others that you used donor eggs or sperm. If you must tell someone about your decision, make sure that the person or people you tell are supportive and can keep a secret until you're ready for the news to go public.

✔ **Put things in writing.** If you're using donor eggs, embryos, or sperm, make sure that your clinic's legal documents are thorough. If they're not, get a lawyer to write up a document. Think ahead and consider things such as divorce. You may think that you and your partner will never separate, and it is hoped you won't, but it's always a possibility. You owe it to yourselves and your potential child to be prepared.

If you're using a gestational carrier or surrogate (see "Borrowing a Uterus for the Next Nine Months," later in this chapter), make sure that everything is in writing. *Everything.* Legally controlling another person's actions is very difficult, so bring up just about any possibility you can think of. Having something in writing may save you from some heartbreak down the road.

Reviewing the current FDA regulations for gamete donation

In 2005, the FDA (Food and Drug Administration) implemented stringent new rules regarding donation of oocytes and embryos. The new regulations mean that egg donors must be tested for a number of communicable diseases no more than 30 days before their eggs are retrieved. Couples who may wish to donate their embryos in the future also need to complete testing within 30 days before egg retrieval.

Borrowing from the Bank — the Sperm Bank, That Is

Donor sperm has been used for artificial insemination for more than 100 years. About 50,000 children are born each year as a result of donor sperm insemination, also known as TDI (therapeutic donor insemination) or AID (artificial insemination — donor). Sperm banks are licensed by the state in which they're located, and they have stringent requirements for donors. Sperm banks should be certified by the American Association of Tissue Banks.

Why fewer couples are using donor sperm

Use of donor sperm has decreased since 1992, when it became possible to inseminate an egg with a single carefully selected "ideal" sperm (as ideal as existed in the male's sample, anyway) in a process known as *intracytoplasmic sperm injection,* or ICSI. (See Chapter 11 for more about ICSI.) Men whose sperm counts were very low, or those with poor sperm motility, or move-ment, could now become biological parents — as long as they could afford to do in vitro insemination.

Many couples, however, can't afford, or don't want to do IVF, so they use donor sperm. Also, those men who have no sperm at all, such as those with Sertoli cell only syndrome, (see Chapter 11 for more on this syndrome) still depend on donor sperm to become parents.

Picking "dad" from a catalog

Picking donor sperm can be similar to buying a house; it sounds like fun until you have to really do it! Then the "what if I choose wrong" fears start to set in and the process becomes more nerve wracking than fun.

Choosing the right biological father for your future child is far more impor-tant than buying a house, but many of the same caveats apply. Don't be too heavily swayed by externals, don't let fear of the unknown keep you from making a decision at all, and don't agonize over your decision once you've made it! These next sections can help you understand the donor sperm process and help you choose the best man for the job.

Reviewing donor requirements

In case you were thinking that sperm donation might be a way of making a little extra money, here's a list of requirements for donors from some of the most popular donor sperm centers with the most stringent requirements:

- **Height:** Most people request a donor between 5 feet 10 inches and 6 feet 2 inches.

- **Weight:** The donor's weight should be proportionate to his height.

- **Age:** The donor should be between the ages of 19 and 39.

- **Education:** The donor should be a graduate of a four-year college, or at least have completed two years of college.

- **Sperm specs:** The donor must have 70 percent motile, or moving, sperm, 60 percent with normal appearance (morphology), and a sperm count of 70 million/milliliter. A donor must have better than average sperm because some will be lost in the freeze-and-thaw process.

Donor sperm can be frozen nearly indefinitely. They're kept in liquid nitrogen containers and shipped out when requested. The cost for a vial of donor sperm runs about $150 to $300, or more if you have specific requests, such as a Nobel Peace Prize winner. Most clinics suggest that you order at least three vials at a time.

Testing donors and taking precautions

Here are some common precautions taken to ensure you receive good sperm:

- **Infectious disease testing:** The donor is tested for all infectious diseases as well as certain genetic diseases, depending on his genetic background. He's also required to fill out a very detailed questionnaire about his background, his family background, his interests, and his likes and dislikes. He may be asked to submit a baby picture.

  One center, concerned about donors bringing in a "ringer" to produce a specimen for them, has the donor's hands recorded on a three-dimensional biometric device. The donor then has to "sign in" and match the hand key before he's allowed to produce. Of course, this assures the bank that all of the specimens for a given donor match up with his blood tests, and so on.

- **Use of frozen sperm:** Because the risk of disease transmission is too high, sperm banks no longer use fresh sperm. Instead, sperm are now frozen and the donor retested for infectious disease before the sperm are released for use — usually a waiting period of six months.

> ✔ **Number of children a donor can father:** The American Society for Reproductive Medicine (ASRM) guidelines suggest that a donor be allowed to father no more than ten children, to avoid, it is hoped, unknowing incest between half-siblings 20 years down the road. Sperm banks routinely follow up with questionnaires to centers using donor sperm to ask whether the donation resulted in a live birth.

Ordering sperm

You can choose between sperm that has not been washed, and is therefore only ready for intracervical insemination (ICI ready) or sperm that's already been washed and is therefore ready for intrauterine insemination (IUI ready). The technique for IUI, which injects the sperm directly into the uterus, is more complicated, but most centers report a higher pregnancy rate with IUI than ICI. Pregnancy rates for women under 35 are about 10 to 20 percent per insemination; rates decrease for women over 40 to 5 to 10 percent per insemination. Some fertility centers prefer that the patients bring in ICI sperm, and then do the sperm washing themselves, because they feel that it gives them a better specimen; check with your center before ordering one or the other type.

Remaining anonymous

Estimates show that only one child in ten is ever informed that he or she is the result of donor insemination, but times may be changing. Some donor clinics now advertise that they have donors open to having some contact with any children born — some say after the child reaches age 18, and others are open to an ongoing relationship. Several recent court cases have questioned the sperm donor's right to remain anonymous, and at least one country, Sweden, has made it illegal to keep the donor anonymous.

Asking someone you know to donate

Some parents-to-be choose a donor they know, perhaps a brother or close friend of the intended dad. In these cases, fresh sperm can be used. However, if the insemination is done by a doctor's office, the doctor should insist on having all infectious disease testing up to date.

Fresh sperm have a higher pregnancy rate than frozen, and this fact may be a consideration if you have a relative or friend who's willing to donate. Keep in mind that the donor will need to be tested for infectious diseases. Most clinics will still prefer that the sperm be frozen and quarantined, and in this case there will be a waiting period of six months before the sperm can be used. This gives the clinic time to retest for infectious diseases — many infectious diseases (like HIV) take up to six months to show up in the blood. Many centers won't use fresh sperm at all, but its use is within the new FDA guidelines.

With known-donor insemination, of course, the chance that the child will find out the truth about his conception is much higher, because more people are involved in the process. For some couples, the psychological issues may be too complicated for them to handle. However, couples who want a genetic match that's as close as possible, and who can handle the psychological problems, may find this method to be a good solution.

Although such a topic may be difficult to discuss, some type of legal document should be drawn up. This document should address such issues as how much say the donor will have in the child's upbringing, how much contact he'll have with the child, and whether he'll have legal rights to the child if anything happens to you.

Of course, you may never experience any emotional or legal problems as a result of this donation. The donor may see your child as just another niece or nephew and never give it a second thought. You know your own family best, but covering the possibility of interference down the road is always a good idea.

What if your partner's *father* is interested in being your donor? This happens more often than you might think. He *is* a genetic link, but remember that grandparents in general can be too outspoken about your child's upbringing. (Why do you let that kid have so many cookies? Why do you let him scream like that?) Ask yourself whether his being the silent "parent" as well as the grandparent may cause problems in your relationship.

Using Donor Eggs

Unlike sperm donation, which has been around for decades, the use of donor eggs is a relatively newer phenomenon (the first baby after donor egg was born in 1984). It required the invention and perfection of in vitro fertilization (IVF) in order to become practical. (See Part IV for complete information about IVF.) Egg donation is a growing national trend, with approximately 30,000 babies born in the United States as a result.

The reasons for using donor eggs are similar to those for using donor sperm. The recipient either doesn't make eggs or doesn't make good eggs. This lack of good eggs may be due to premature ovarian failure or age, or the woman may carry a lethal gene or chromosome disorder that she doesn't want to risk passing on. Because female age is so important in fertility, and because egg donation obviates the role of the age of the mother (recipient), egg donation has dramatically altered the fertility potential of women over 40.

Getting donor eggs

Perhaps you're wondering how you can obtain donor eggs. You have several options:

- ✔ **You can be matched with a paid IVF donor at your clinic.** These women donate all their eggs to one or possibly two recipients for a fee.

- ✔ **Use a broker.** Brokers can also be found on the Internet by using a search engine, under "donor eggs." One large site is www.eggdonor.com. Sharon personally likes www.awomans gift.com. This is currently the most common form of egg donation because most clinics have given up recruiting their own donors. The advantage of brokers is that they provide more choice of donors; the disadvantage is that they add considerable cost.

- ✔ **You can be matched with a fellow infertility patient at your clinic.** This woman will agree to share half her eggs with you in exchange for your paying her IVF costs. Few women under 35 are infertile because they have "bad eggs." More often, there are sperm problems or blocked tubes, fibroids, or other uterine abnormalities. The availability of this type of donation varies widely from center to center, with some centers favoring this type of arrangements, while others may not offer it at all.

- ✔ **Find a willing friend or relative.** If you're fortunate enough to have a friend or relative who agrees to donate eggs to you, you'll both be screened through your clinic for infectious diseases, and then your cycles will be coordinated so that you can have a fresh embryo transfer. This is the second most common form of egg donation. The obvious advantage of using a relative is that she shares some fraction of your DNA. In the case of a sister donor, you share 50 percent of your DNA – and the child will have the same grandparents as if you were the genetic parent. Furthermore, because your husband contributes 50 percent of the genes, and your sister the other 50 percent, you can think of the baby as 75 percent genetically "yours" as a couple.

Keeping the facts in mind

Although your reason for using egg donors is similar to that of using sperm donors, differences do exist. Keep the following in mind when thinking about using an egg donor:

- ✔ Using donor eggs is more complicated than using donor sperm; IVF centers usually try to coordinate the menstrual cycles of the egg donor and recipient so that the recipient can transfer into her uterus fresh embryos that were created a few days before in the IVF lab. This transfer requires monitoring at an IVF center to make sure that the uterus is ready to receive the embryos.

✔ Asking someone to be an egg donor is much more complicated than asking someone to be a sperm donor. Egg donation involves several weeks of injections, blood draws, ultrasounds, and, at some clinics, psychological testing. Plus, you'll need to explore the emotional and legal consequences, just as you would if you were using donor sperm. You'll also need a lawyer to draw up a detailed legal contract; you should do this even if you're using someone you know.

✔ One disadvantage of donor eggs is that, unlike donor sperm, you don't know what you're getting in advance. Because the egg donor is doing a stimulated IVF cycle while you're taking medication to be ready for embryo transfer, you won't know how many eggs you'll get or their quality until a few days before your transfer.

✔ Although you may assume that a 22-year-old donor will make a good number of eggs in an IVF cycle, that doesn't always happen. Clinics usually have rules about what happens if your donor doesn't stimulate well, but chances are that you'll still have to pay for the blood tests, medications, and ultrasound examinations that she had before the bad cycle was diagnosed.

Finding donor eggs

Most clinics are still doing traditional donor egg programs; seniority on the recipient list gets you first pick at the donor of your choice, all donors being paid the same. However, a search of the Internet reveals a plethora of near genius beauty queens ready to barter their eggs to the highest bidder.

If you really are looking for something very specific — say, a redhead because everyone in your family has red hair or a biracial donor if you're both biracial — the classifieds may be the way to go. Some centers have very few black donors; others have very few Asian donors. A good place to advertise is the campus newspaper or bulletin board in the student union at a large, diverse college campus.

If you're not looking for an exact match, get on the nearest clinic's waiting list. Eventually, you'll have seniority on the list and will be able to find what you're looking for.

Try some of the broker agencies, and do not assume that you have to restrict yourself to local ones. Many out-of-state agencies are happy to have the donor travel to your fertility center. When you consider the cost of donor eggs (several thousand dollars), the additional cost of a flight and a couple of nights in a hotel is not that much of a premium.

Funding donor eggs

The cost of using donor eggs can vary tremendously, depending on what you're looking for. Are you looking for a Harvard grad with blonde hair and blue eyes who stands 5 feet 7 inches tall and weighs 125 pounds and volunteers at the nursing home once a week and bakes cookies for shut-ins in addition to running her law practice and taking care of her adorable twins, picture available upon request? You may be able to find her, but it will cost you. Some Grade-A egg donors are offering to donate eggs for a mere $5,000 *per egg*.

If you're looking for a normal person, like yourself, you'll probably pay between $5,000 and $10,000 to your donor to do an IVF cycle — with 10 to 15 eggs retrieved, one hopes.

The cost of the IVF cycle itself is between $5,000 and $10,000 in most clinics, and the medications are an additional $3,000 to $4,000.

A donor egg cycle at your average IVF clinic costs from $13,000 to $18,000, including medications, if you don't have insurance. If you're going the designer route, the cost may be much more.

Checking out your donor

Most centers send out donor lists every month or every six weeks. The donor's physical characteristics and family history are listed, as well as education level and current job. Also listed is her childbearing history. Most centers accept anonymous donors only if they're under 35 years old and have no major health issues or inherited family disease. Most centers also have the donor and her partner checked for all infectious diseases, such as HIV, hepatitis B and C, syphilis, and gonorrhea. Some also do psychological screenings to make sure that the donor fully understands the implications of egg donation and is mentally stable enough to handle donating.

If you're bringing a donor that you've found yourself to the clinic, she'll most likely be required to do all the same testing. If your donor is a relative, however, your clinic may allow you to waive some of the testing.

Signing the documents

You and your donor must sign legal consents. The donor signs that she's voluntarily donating her eggs and won't try to claim any parenting rights in the future. This consent is required even if the donor is someone you know.

You sign that you're voluntarily using donor eggs to create a child. You also sign that you and your partner (if you aren't a single parent) agree to be the sole legal parents of the child and assume all costs for bearing and raising the child.

At present, a child born from donor sperm, eggs, or embryos is automatically the child of the recipients and doesn't need to be legally adopted by either parent at birth.

Getting support

You can find numerous support groups on the Internet, not only for egg recipients but also for donors. Go to your favorite search engine, type in "donor eggs," and see what you get! If you have any questions or doubts about donating eggs or receiving donor eggs, you should be able to find plenty of people on the bulletin boards who can help you with your decision. One bulletin board with an active following is found at www.network54.com/Hide/Forum/57451.

If you want a more one-on-one approach, a family counselor who specializes in adoptions or other family situations may be very helpful; the phone book is a good place to look for family counselors, under "Counselors, Human Relations." You can also ask your fertility clinic for recommendations or contact Resolve for suggestions. (We discuss Resolve in more detail in Chapter 8.)

Borrowing a Uterus for the Next Nine Months

Asking someone for the use of her eggs is one thing; she only has to commit to a few weeks of time and discomfort. Asking someone to commit to your cause for nine whole months by being a *gestational carrier* is quite another.

The use of gestational carriers has exploded with the advent of in vitro fertilization. Women with health issues, women who lack a uterus, and women with a history of recurrent miscarriage are among those who are using friends, family, or total strangers to carry and deliver their biological children.

Finding a willing woman

Some people love to be pregnant, and other people love to be pregnant as long as they're getting paid for it. Either type may be suitable as a gestational carrier. Many women ask immediate family members first, but remember that a "no" doesn't mean that person doesn't love you or want to help. Some women see pregnancy as a nine-month misery and wouldn't go through it if you begged them; others truly enjoy being pregnant and welcome the chance to help you out as well.

If your sister and best friend turn you down, you need to look a little further. What if your mom wants to do this for you? Would you feel funny about her giving birth to her grandchildren? How would you handle the local press? (You can assume that there might be some, because this type of human interest story is very popular with the press.)

If all possible friends or relatives are out, you may want to look on the Internet, where gestational carriers place ads and, of course, all sound like the salt of the earth. Again, some women love being pregnant and also don't mind the extra money. Others are just looking for the extra money.

Don't sign up with the first wonderful sounding candidate without doing *a lot* of research. Many women have even hired a private agent to check into the carrier's background. That's not a bad idea; it's easy on paper to say that you're something you're really not!

If you want to go with a woman you don't know, visit her home if possible. And make sure that it *is* her home, not some place that she's borrowed for a few hours to make a good impression. If all this checking sounds sneaky and untrusting, you're right; it is. But the world is full of unscrupulous people who have no problem taking advantage of a desperate couple wanting to have a child. By far, the safest approach is to go with a surrogacy agency, who first makes sure that the surrogate is psychologically screened, and then provides ongoing psychological care. Such agencies also have attorneys who draw up the paperwork and really can provide much-needed peace of mind.

Before a pregnancy occurs, you and your carrier should discuss genetic testing during the pregnancy and pregnancy termination. Even though the baby is genetically yours, the decision to undergo testing and/or end a pregnancy is that of the carrier, *regardless of legal contract*. Make sure that you and your carrier are on the same page on this difficult and touchy issue. If you're not, consider it a deal breaker. Make sure that the contract covers the issue of selective termination as well; many people have very strong feelings, pro and con, and you want to make sure you and your donor feel the same way.

Going through the process

You'll have to do in vitro fertilization to use a gestational carrier because you'll be transferring embryos to her uterus. The carrier will usually take Estrace, an estrogen pill, to thicken her uterine lining, for several weeks. The embryos are then transferred to her uterus. You and your carrier can do synchronized cycles so that the embryos can be transferred to her a few days after your egg retrieval without first being frozen. Or you can do an egg retrieval first, and freeze the embryos to transfer to the carrier a month or even a year down the road. If you need an egg donor as well, the cycle will be coordinated by the clinic using the donor's eggs, your husband's sperm, and the surrogate's uterus. This is more complex than traditional surrogacy (see below) but is easier from a legal point of view because the surrogate is not genetically related to the offspring.

Once the carrier gets pregnant, her pregnancy and delivery will proceed just like any other. Most couples are in fairly close contact with the carrier during the pregnancy, so that any problems that arise can be dealt with jointly. If you've hired a carrier rather than using a friend or relative, you should have a payment plan agreed on before doing the embryo transfer.

In most cases, the carrier agrees to let you be present for the delivery, so you can see the baby right away. You need to know your state's rules for petitioning to have your names on the birth certificate as the biological parents of the baby. Your lawyer will be instrumental in getting the affidavits you'll need from the IVF center, verifying that the baby is your biological child.

After a short hospital stay, you take the baby home with you.

Traditional Surrogacy — the Road Less Traveled

Unlike gestational carriers, surrogates are both the egg donors and the pregnancy carriers. The good thing about traditional surrogacy is that it often doesn't require doing in vitro fertilization. The bad news is that you're asking for more than nine months out of a woman's life — you're also asking for her biological child. Because the child born is the natural child of the surrogate, you could find yourself without a leg to stand on legally if the surrogate decides to keep the baby. Legal agreements, no matter how complete, may not hold up in court if this happens.

If the surrogate is a relative, you may have a greater trust in her to keep her promise to give the baby to you after she delivers. But keep in mind that if she does change her mind, you're looking at a family nightmare from which you may never recover.

States have different laws about the legality of surrogacy, and some states specify that no money may change hands except to cover reasonable expenses. You'll most likely need to go through an adoption process after delivery, which may involve a home study by an adoption agency.

Because of the risks of surrogacy, many couples use donor eggs from one person and hire another to be the gestational carrier, in order to avoid the risks of using a traditional surrogate. This route is more expensive, but it may buy you some peace of mind about the likelihood of your carrier changing her mind and keeping the baby.

Adopting at the Cellular Level — Embryo Donation

Some clinics maintain lists of couples who want to donate their embryos to another couple, usually because the donating couple has one or more children through IVF and doesn't want any more. Brokers also match unwanted embryos with prospective parents via the Internet or through organizations dedicated to egg and embryo donation. Screening ranges from no more than infectious blood testing to a full-blown home study done by an adoption agency; you also receive information about the donating parents and usually some type of family genetic history.

When you use donor embryos, you're essentially adopting a child; the difference between this and traditional adoption is that you get to experience the pregnancy and delivery just as if this were your genetic child. Your name is on the birth certificate, and unless you give out the information, no one will know that you used donor embryos. Some couples find it easier emotionally to have a child who's not related to either one of them, rather than using donor eggs or sperm.

Of course, this method again brings up the possibility of legal questions, moral issues, and possible complications a few years down the road. At the time of this writing, no cases have been filed of biological parents going to court to get their children back after their birth. But that doesn't mean that it couldn't happen in the future, despite the paperwork that parents sign when they donate their embryos.

Using donor embryos is fairly simple from a medical point of view. The procedure requires doing a frozen embryo transfer at an IVF clinic. This cycle requires minimal medication, usually just estrogen pills before the transfer and progesterone after the transfer to maintain the pregnancy. However, the legal issues associated with donor embryos can be quite complex; for example, if the child should be born with an abnormality, the potential for a lawsuit is considerable. For this reason, many fertility clinics have shied away from embryo donation.

Telling the Family or Keeping It to Yourself

Will you tell your family? That depends on you, your family, and a host of other factors that only you know. Some people don't even tell their families that they're doing IVF, much less tell them that they're using donor eggs.

Donor sperm have been utilized for more than 30 years, and evidence shows that most parents *do not* tell the child that his father isn't his biological parent. It seems likely that some families won't talk about using donor eggs, either, although in a recent study, just over half the parents surveyed indicated that they planned to tell the child eventually.

It's possible that somewhere down the line, your child will find out that he's the product of donor eggs or sperm, even if you don't want him to. It may happen in high school biology, where students often test their blood types. Or it may happen when your child develops a rare inherited disease, and you need to go back to his biological family for information.

Keeping a secret like this is difficult, but dealing with negative family reactions, if there are any, is difficult too. If you tell your child, you'll cry inside every time he says, "You're not my *real* mother!" and if you don't tell, you'll cringe every times he says, "I wish I had a different mother!" All children say things like this, whether they're adopted, biological, or whatever; take it with a grain of salt!

Utilizing a Registry

You've seen the show one hundred times. Mothers, fathers, brothers, sisters meeting in a tearful on-air display of how technology can help locate and reunite long-lost relatives. Will this become commonplace in the case of donor eggs, sperm, and embryos in the future? Most gamete donors in the past had no intention of maintaining any contact with their future offspring, and most parents of children conceived through donor gametes weren't interested in future contact, either. Is this changing? Will everyone be able to maintain anonymity in the future, when information once secreted away in confidential files is available to anyone who can hack into a computer?

Today, you can find thousands of internet sites under sibling registry, parent registry, donor registry, and so on. Donors, parents, siblings, and children can be registered with agencies that will put interested parties together in the future. While these sites have traditionally been utilized mostly for adopted children and the biological parents, the future may find gamete donors and their offspring being reunited as well.

The downside to all of this? Plenty! Many parents who choose donor options desire to remain in the "No Tell" camp. This could be challenging if/when a half sibling or a biological relative comes to call. At the moment, both parties, for example, parent/relative and child must be searching to find one another. But with the improvement of tracking tools on the internet, this caveat might cease to exist. Some men who assumed that the details of their donation to a sperm bank a few decades ago were permanently locked away have been surprised to find that the women to whom they donated to feel that they, and their children, have a right to know who they are.

For this reason, donor and adoption agencies are being forced to be crystal clear regarding the issue of disclosure. The exception to the "closed at all costs" status has sometimes been used when the issue of medical necessity arises. Should a donor be found to have a hereditary or genetic condition, requiring notification or treatment for his/her offspring, some agencies will contact the recipients and inform them without putting the two parties in contact with one another directly.

Getting Pregnant When You're Single or Gay

It's never been easier to have a child if you're a single parent or in a same sex relationship, with sperm banks available to single or gay women and the use of gestational carriers and egg donors available to single or gay men. (See the section "Borrowing From the Bank — The Sperm Bank, That Is" for info on finding donor sperm.)

Finding sperm

If you're a single or gay woman, you're going to find it easier to have a baby than a single man — you've got the right equipment! All you need is the sperm, and sperm is something that's readily available, whether you want to use an anonymous donor or a close friend.

If you're considering using a friend as your donor, here are some of the benefits:

- ✔ You're most likely aware of the person's personality traits.
- ✔ You know what he looks like.
- ✔ You probably like the person, or you wouldn't be asking him to do this for you.

Alas, where you find pros, you also find cons. Here are some of the potential complications that come from using a donor you know over one who remains anonymous:

- ✔ How involved will he be in your child's life? No involvement, holiday visits, or heavy involvement?
- ✔ If your parenting techniques differ, how much input will he have on how you raise your child?
- ✔ If something happens to you, will he be the legal guardian?

If you're thinking of using an anonymous donor, consider the following pros:

- ✔ You won't have to worry about the father wanting to be involved with the child.
- ✔ You can be very picky about physical characteristics and other attributes.

On the con side, consider these issues:

- ✔ You'll have to rely on what the catalog says about the donor, with no way of knowing how accurate the information really is.
- ✔ You won't be able to tell your child much about his paternal heritage.
- ✔ It may be difficult for your child to be able to contact his birth father, if he wants to.

Even if you don't foresee any complications down the road, writing up a legal document to cover your bases is always a wise idea.

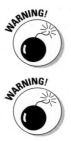

If you're using fresh sperm from a known donor, you need to be aware of the risk of contracting an infectious disease such as HIV or hepatitis. It's much wiser to use a frozen specimen after having your donor tested at the time the specimen is frozen, and then tested again six months later. If he's still negative, you can use the frozen specimen.

Never try to do an intracervical or intrauterine insemination at home! You can place the sperm near the cervix but not inside it!

Finding eggs and a uterus

Things are certainly more complicated if you're a guy or gay couple trying to have a baby without a female partner. You just can't do it alone! If you want to be a dad, the first thing you need to find is a mother. You may want to ask a friend, or you may want to hire a surrogate who'll carry the baby for you and then relinquish all parental rights to you. A *traditional surrogate* is both the biological mother of the baby and the person who carries the baby throughout the pregnancy; a *gestational carrier* is not the biological mother. (See "Borrowing a Uterus for the Next Nine Months" for more on surrogates.)

If your surrogate is married, the child, when born, may be presumed to be legally her husband's in some states. You may have to adopt your own child.

Legal issues should be written up by a lawyer who's well versed in surrogacy in the state where the baby will be born, because that state's laws will govern your experience. Many of the laws that govern gay parent surrogacy also cover a single male's use of a surrogate or carrier, with California being the most liberal state.

Your lawyer will need to submit affidavits to the court from your clinic, your carrier or surrogate, and you to help establish paternity for the birth certificate. Some states require DNA testing to establish paternity; others don't.

If you want to use a gestational carrier, you'll have to utilize IVF; the eggs of one woman can be fertilized (see the "Using Donor Eggs" section for all the details on donor eggs), and the resulting embryo can be transferred to the gestational carrier. This method, of course, is much more expensive than traditional surrogacy, because you have to pay both the gestational carrier and the egg donor, not to mention the IVF center. You're looking at spending $40,000 or more.

Finding the right clinic

Not all fertility clinics will work with singles or gays. One place to look for information is the National Center for Chronic Disease and Health Promotion's "Reproductive Health Information Source" (www.cdc.gov/nccdphp/drh/ART99/index99.htm). Under the section "Clinic Services and Profiles," you find basic information as to whether the clinics work with donor egg patients, gestational carriers, or singles. If you live in a rural or particularly conservative area, you may have to travel to get the job done. The American Fertility Association (www.theafa.org) now has a gay/lesbian resource section on their website (under "LGBT family building").

After you have your list of possibilities, mention your specific circumstances during your first phone call. You want to make sure that your doctor is supportive of your situation before you make an appointment.

Chapter 19

Moving On

For some people, the road to biological childbearing closes early. A severe male factor (such as a total absence of sperm), lack of a uterus or ovaries, or other structural problems may make biological parenthood impossible. Other couples invest months or years, along with huge sums of money, seeking biological parenthood, only to end up at the same roadblock.

How you get to this point isn't important. What matters is making decisions about what road to take next. You may choose to adopt, and after you make that decision, you need to make many more. Do you want to adopt internationally, interracially, through a public agency, or from a private source? Do you want a newborn or an older child?

You may choose instead to work with children as a teacher or social worker, or as a foster parent. Or you may decide that you can live a fulfilling life without children. In this chapter, we show you how to evaluate your choices and find the path that's right for you — when you're ready.

Deciding to Let Go of the Dream

Jackie was sure that she had finally had enough. This realization came about three weeks prior to the start of the successful cycle that brought Jackie her beautiful daughter Ava. Less than halfway through that cycle, which she referred to as a "goat rodeo" for all that went wrong, Jackie had decided that she *could not take another step*. She fought with her doctor, nurse (also known as coauthor Sharon Perkins), husband, and anyone else who would listen to her complain. She knew that she had reached her endpoint. Luckily, the light at the end of the tunnel wasn't a train. But then again, it generally never is.

Everyone reaches points in their lives when they instinctively know that they can't take another step. The process of infertility is no exception. The trick is knowing when you have reached the end of the line, or when a well deserved break may be in order (we discuss ways to take a respite in Chapter 9).

But if you have truly gotten to that point of no return where you can't fathom another test, another shot, another phone call — regardless of the outcome, it's time to do something different.

Letting go is never easy, and the higher the stakes, the more difficult the process.

Going through the grief process

Grief is one of life's most difficult emotions. Despite the fact that you may have many people around who are willing and able to help, grief can cause you to feel isolated, desperate, and hopeless. Either extreme of avoiding grief or immersing yourself in it can lead to depression, which actually stops you from moving through, and beyond, the grief process. As clichéd as it may sound, you can get through it, and time will help.

Perhaps the best way to deal with the morass of emotions brought on by the loss of the dream of a biological child is by looking at the grief process. Elisabeth Kubler-Ross, the author of *On Death and Dying,* identified the five stages of grief following the death of a loved one: denial, anger, bargaining, depression, and acceptance. The death of a dream is much the same.

You may go through these stages of grief more than once. You may skip a stage or repeat it twice before you come to accept what has happened. Working through the grief process of not having a biological child takes time. And unfortunately, it's hard to hurry up the process no matter how much you want it to be over. The only way past grief is through it. But you don't have to do it alone.

Knowing when to get help

While grief is a process to move through, many people can get stuck in it as well. Figuring out whether you are stuck or not can be tricky and often requires the input of your friends, family, and even colleagues who might be more objective in offering you a reality check. Asking your partner or a trusted friend to help you figure out if you're dealing with your grief or dwelling on it too much can help give you clarity on what to do next. Friends, family, support groups, and books can help to buoy you through the process.

It's easy to isolate yourself when you're feeling the kind of pain brought on by grief. If you find that you can't even bring yourself to check in with those around you, you could probably use some guidance. If you are beset with the 'Why Me's?' that have you questioning yourself, your faith, and life as you know it, you would likely benefit from the wisdom that a pastor, priest, rabbi, or cleric may be able to provide. If your feelings of grief have become feeling of despair and hopelessness, particularly of the type that have you contemplating doing harm to yourself or someone else, you need help, and fast.

Professional help is a wonderful option for those whose hope switch is temporarily stuck in the off position. You might ask your family physician, fertility specialist, or nurse to recommend a therapist to help you work through your emotions. It's not about finding someone to tell you that your dreams can come true; it's working to re-tool those dreams to better fit your circumstances. You can be happy again and you will, provided you deal with that which ails you. Don't be alarmed if a professional suggests antidepressants. This treatment, like your depression, may be a temporary situation. Whether medication or talk therapy, you *can* find relief during this difficult time.

Opting to Adopt

A life without biological children doesn't mean a life without any children. Many children, both in the United States and abroad, need parents to love and care for them. Adoption is a tree with many branches, and you need to first decide for what kind of child you're looking. Are you open to adopting an older child or one with physical handicaps? Are you interested in a child of another race? Or are you willing to keep all your options open and try several different routes at one time?

More than 120,000 children are adopted each year in the United States. Nearly half, about 40 percent, are adopted by step-parents or other relatives. Ninety percent of adoptions are domestic, and the other 10 percent come from foreign adoptions. Some adoptions are *open* adoptions, meaning that the adoptive and birth parents meet and continue to have some involvement in one another's lives. Other adoptions are arranged through established public agencies and usually don't include any contact between birth and adoptive families. Adoption can cost anywhere from a few dollars to thousands of dollars. We look briefly at different types of adoption.

Web sites such as `www.adoption.com` also contain adoption forums, waiting children information, and ads for prospective adoptive parents. The National Adoption Information Clearinghouse (NAIC) can be found at `www.calib.com/naic` and also contains information on every aspect of adoption.

Traditional domestic adoption

When most people think about adoption, they think about traditional domestic adoption. An old movie, *Penny Serenade,* details the typical scenario: A couple is unable to have children, so they go through the process of adopting a Caucasian infant. The film contains the traditional themes — parents-to-be are evaluated by a strict social worker, and the baby is almost taken away because the hopeful father lost his job and income before the adoption was finalized. This type of adoption is becoming rarer today because more birth mothers are choosing to place their children through private adoption, which gives them more control over who will adopt their child (see the next section, "Private domestic adoption" for more information on private adoptions). Some agencies still doing traditional adoptions are Catholic charities and county and state adoption agencies. Two well-known established private adoption agencies, Gladney (`www.adoptionsbygladney.com`) and Spence-Chapin (`www.spence-chapin.org`), have large Internet Web sites.

In a traditional adoption, the adoptive parents usually have no contact with the birth parents. A social worker conducts a home study to make sure that you're financially and emotionally able to support a child. The children adopted are usually infants, although more older and special-needs children are starting to be adopted, especially through state and public agencies.

If you're older, have any type of criminal record, or aren't reasonably financially secure, the agency may turn you down. The number of people looking to adopt an infant far outweighs the number of infants available, so agencies can afford to be picky.

Private domestic adoption

You've probably seen the ads, and maybe you've even written one: "Loving, financially secure couple wants to give your child a home." Newspapers and many Internet Web sites contain these ads, written to appeal to young women looking to give their children up for adoption. If you really want a newborn, this method is probably your best route to adoption.

These adoptions are handled by a lawyer who may be your source for a baby in addition to being your legal advisor. You may also find an infant through an organization specializing in finding newborns. Your source for a baby may also be your pastor or your doctor.

Private adoption is expensive — you can pay between $8,000 and $30,000 to adopt privately. Legitimate payable expenses in private adoption include lawyers' fees, birth mom's living costs, pregnancy, delivery, and newborn care costs.

To be successful at a private adoption, tell everyone you know that you're looking. Write the most emotionally appealing ad you can, and send it to as many newspapers as you can afford. (Make sure the state in which you're advertising allows this type of ad — not all do.) Many prospective adoptive parents spend up to $5,000 in advertising costs alone. Also, post a Web site on the Internet and make sure that you, your house, and your lifestyle are pictured in as appealing a manner as possible.

Get a good lawyer, even before you start looking. If you find a baby, you want to have all the legal issues taken care of as soon as possible.

After you find a possible candidate, keep your guard up all the time. Go slow, and don't commit to anything right away. And, most importantly, don't give anyone money without having a lawyer review everything.

A private adoption can be as open as you want it to be. Some couples have the birth mother live with them before she delivers; others just have a few meetings at a neutral location. Some never meet the birth parents at all. You may be able to be at the delivery and take the baby home from the hospital, if the birth mother agrees. Many experts today argue that open adoption is better for the adopted child and his family because his origins are never hidden and are often well known. However, you must do what you feel is best for all involved.

If you're normally a trusting person, you'd better learn to be wary and cautious during this process. We've heard of many cases of women pretending to be pregnant, taking money from more than one couple, or just reneging on the deal after the baby is born. You can't be too careful.

For information about the legalities of adoption, check the Web site www.adoption.about.com.

Private international adoption

Harry Holt became an adoption pioneer when he and his wife headed off for Korea to help find families for the mixed-race children of the Korean War. (The sidebar "Molly's adoption," later in this chapter, tells you one of his success stories.) Now, Holt is one of many agencies placing children from Korea, China, Russia, South America, and India, among others. (His Web site can be found at www.holtintl.org.)

Ten percent of adoptions (or more than 10,000) each year are international adoptions. Not all are done through agencies; some are private. The cost of adopting internationally is seldom less than a domestic adoption and, sometimes, is much more. Besides the costs for a home study, lawyers' fees, and agency services, there's the cost of travel and doing business in a foreign country.

Some parents feel more secure with a foreign adoption, because the chances of the birth parents showing up and asking to take their child back are perceived as lower than with a stateside adoption.

Some of the children up for adoption are younger than 6 months, but the red tape of international adoptions means that your baby may be closer to a year by the time you get him or her home. Some countries want you to stay in the country for several weeks; others let you pick your child up at the airport.

Children adopted from foreign countries may arrive sicker than those adopted from the United States. Medical care ranges from excellent to nearly nonexistent, depending on from where your child came. More countries are trying to place children in foster care rather than keep them in orphanages, to help their social and emotional development. Some children come with serious attachment disorders, and others may have undiagnosed medical conditions.

Adopting a special-needs child

Plenty of children up for adoption, in this country and abroad, are classified as *special-needs children*. Usually, they have a physical handicap, but they may also have a mental or emotional handicap. Some children are classified as special-needs kids because they're not infants or toddlers, or because they're members of a racial minority.

Back in the heyday of adoption, before abortion was legal and having a child out of wedlock was a social stigma, children were plentiful, and older children (older being anyone over 1 year old back then), racially mixed children, and handicapped children were rarely adopted. Now, prospective parents are applying to adopt Down syndrome babies, children with serious emotional and physical disabilities, and children of a different race.

Sometimes, people are tempted to adopt special-needs children because they're more easily available. Other couples are drawn by a picture of a child on a TV program or in a magazine. Sharon remembers thinking seriously about adopting a child with handicaps while her family was waiting for their referral; *OURS Magazine* had pictures every month of hard-to-place children who were waiting for homes, and every one of the pictures appealed to her. However, she realized that her family wasn't really emotionally prepared to handle a child with serious problems.

Although it's easy to be caught up emotionally in the idea of raising a special-needs child, look realistically at your lifestyle and personalities before making a decision.

Social workers in the United States are still somewhat hesitant to place an African-American or Native American child in a family of a different race. Many Native American groups are vehemently opposed to their children being placed in white families, and many African-Americans feel the same way, saying the children won't develop a proper racial identity if they aren't raised by parents of the same race.

Foster parenting first?

Some couples look at foster parenting as a way to get a foot in the door, so to speak. Although you may possibly be allowed to adopt a foster child, the majority of children in foster care aren't available for adoption.

However, some foster children are released for adoption. If they do become available for adoption, 64 percent will be adopted by their former foster family, so in some cases you may be able to adopt your foster child.

Foster parents usually need to take classes to qualify. They're also subject to home inspections and supervision from social workers. Foster parents receive a monthly stipend of anywhere from $300 to $700 a month, depending on where they live.

Foster parenting can be very rewarding, but it can also be heartbreaking to see children you've come to care about go back to environments that were harmful to them in the first place. However, there's a real need for good foster parents, and if you want to be truly instrumental in the life of a child — or more than one — foster parenting can be a good place to start.

Deciding to Live Child Free

So here you are. You've tried and tried to conceive your child, and you've run out of money, time, hope, or all the above. Third-party reproduction (donor eggs or sperm) isn't an option for you. Adoption is neither financially nor emotionally feasible at this time. What do you do?

Take stock in your life as a child-free individual or couple. Think that living a life without children sounds depressing? Well, consider a few benefits of being child free:

- ✔ **Extra money.** Can you figure out a fun way to spend $250,000? We thought so! We discuss the costs of child rearing at the beginning of this book, but, in short, child-free couples have a "spare" quarter million to play with. Maybe you've always wanted a second home, for winter or summer, or maybe you'll decide to take a trip around the world. And maybe you just like the idea of being able to go out to dinner whenever you want and not worry about whether you can afford the extra appetizer or bottle of wine.

- ✔ **Extra time.** Most parents today find themselves in a time crunch that forces them to skip many former activities, such as hobbies and working out.

  Former pleasures, such as putting your feet up after a long day at work or enjoying a relaxing dinner with your partner, quickly become a thing of the past for most parents, new and old. And sleeping in on Saturdays? Forget about it!

Even after considering the extra money and time, along with the ability to be spontaneous, your mind may still be filled with 101 romantic notions of life with baby. Do you dream of watching your young charge score the winning touchdown for your collegiate alma mater? Consider that the chances of your child becoming a star athlete are probably about equal to him or her spending time in prison. Do you dream about you and your partner sharing blissful moments with your baby? Keep in mind that many couples spend far more time fighting over child rearing than they do reveling in it.

And also keep in mind that not having children of your own doesn't mean that you have no children in your life whatsoever. You probably have nieces or nephews or friends' children to spoil and care for. And the best part is, at the end of the day when they get tired and grouchy, you can give them back!

Chapter 20

Hello, Dolly! New Advances, New Concerns in Fertility

*Y*ou probably remember hearing about Dolly, the famous cloned sheep who had to be put to death in 2003 at the age of 6 as the result of a progressive lung disease. (For more on Dolly, see the sidebar "The creation of Dolly," later in this chapter.) Now, if you believe the tabloids, cloned human babies are already a reality. Every week you see a story about one wealthy person or another harboring a little "Mini Me" created by scientists working secretly in some exotic place.

Whether or not you believe the tabloids and all the hype, one thing is certain: technology is a double-edged sword. Every scientific advance brings questions about what technology *can* do versus what it *should* do. Some of the newest advances — sex selection, preimplantation genetic diagnosis, and stem cell research — have come under heavy fire by ethicists and others concerned about the consequences of tinkering with potential human beings.

In this chapter, we look at some of the hottest fertility debates and how they may affect you.

Looking Down the Road: Long-Term Health Effects of Fertility Medication

Fertility medications, or *gonadotropins,* are natural hormones, normally produced by the body. And when you go through menopause, the blood levels of all of these hormones are going to be far higher than anything that can be attained by injecting fertility medication. However, when given to women of reproductive age, whose ovaries can and do respond, they are powerful stuff. Anyone who takes them through even one cycle can attest to the physical and emotional effects of having one's hormones surging at a much higher level than nature ever intended. Do people suffer long-term effects 2 or 20 years down the road? No one knows for sure, but here are the most recent conclusions on the safety of taking gonadotropins.

Effects on the mother

At this time, experts have no solid proof that taking gonadotropins has any long-term effect on women. Some studies have shown a possible link to fertility medications and ovarian cancer, but other studies have not supported these findings.

One thing most studies have agreed upon is that the risk of ovarian cancer is higher in all women who've never become pregnant, regardless of whether or not they've taken fertility medications. So if you've taken fertility drugs for any amount of time and never had a child, make sure to do your yearly gynecological checkup — no skipping a year or being a few months late. This is especially important if other women in your family have had ovarian cancer because doctors have established a genetic link for this type of cancer, among others. (Of course this recommendation applies to all women, regardless of whether or not they have had fertility treatment, but if this warning gets you to take the doctor visits seriously, it will all be for the best.)

Effects on the baby

No one is sure whether fertility medications will have a long-term effect on the children conceived through their use — the children born through high-tech methods such as in vitro fertilization (IVF) aren't old enough yet. The oldest IVF baby, Louise Brown, is only in her twenties. Techniques such as ICSI (intracytoplasmic sperm injection) and assisted hatching are even newer; they've only been used extensively since the 1990s.

Because research is ongoing even as children are being born, high-tech treatment has an element of risk simply because the jury's still out on long-term effects. Some studies have suggested that high-tech babies have lower birth weight and developmental delays. What is not known at this point is whether it is the treatment or the condition of infertility that puts the patients at high risk.

However, more twins and triplets are born to moms using fertility meds, and multiples more commonly have low birth weight and developmental delays. Also, more babies are born to older mothers through high-tech treatment, and older women tend to have more complicated pregnancies than women under age 35.

It's important to note that up to this point, no effect of fertility medications on the babies has been shown. Furthermore, fertility medications are natural hormones, normally present in the body. And even though they may be present at higher than normal values during the stimulation phase, they're all well out of your system by the time the embryo implants. So whatever effect these medications might have would have to be on the egg and these effects are purely hypothetical. Still, only time will tell for sure.

Because some men who need ICSI to conceive have part of a chromosome missing, which results in their infertility, some of their sons may have the same chromosomal abnormality and may also need to do ICSI (or whatever high-tech methods are available in 30 years) to have children.

Sex Selection: When You Absolutely, Positively, Want a Boy (Or a Girl)

There are lots of old wives' tales about having a boy versus a girl — where to sleep, what to eat, what to wear, and so on. But if you already have five boys and would dearly love a girl, or if you carry a genetic link to a sex-determined disease, such as hemophilia, you're probably looking for something a little more scientific. Until recently, 50-50 odds were the best you could do, but newer advances have made it possible to increase the odds of taking home the boy or girl for which you're hoping.

Many years ago, a doctor named Shettles wrote an entire book on how to select the gender of your child based on early observations of sperm, which indicated that male sperm were smaller, faster, more sensitive to an acidic environment, and more prone to early death. In contrast, female sperm were thought to be larger, slower, more hardy, and lived longer. Many different methods were based on these assumptions, including advice that women douche with vinegar (acid) if they wanted a girl, timing intercourse for close to ovulation if they wanted a boy (since male sperm were "faster"), and so on. Unfortunately, these early observations of sperm behavior have not been borne out and there is not a shred of evidence that any of these methods are any more successful than thinking masculine thoughts or wearing cowboy boots to bed!

About 40 years ago, a small scientific study purported to show that a method based on density and speed of swimming could separate sperm into males and females. This method, called the Erickson method, was actually patented, and was successfully marketed for many years. Unfortunately, there has never been a large study substantiating the claims of successful gender selection, and this method, too, has fallen by the wayside. Remember that "successfully marketed" doesn't necessarily mean "successful"!

The trouble with statistics like these is that they can be quite misleading. First, you have to remember that nature gives you odds of about 53 percent to 47 percent in favor of males, so a 65 percent chance of a boy is only 12 percent more than nature gives you already. Furthermore, small studies that show, say 7 out of 10 boys versus 3 out of 10 girls to technically demonstrate a 70% boy rate, but it is easy to see how this could have happened by chance alone. That is why studies need to be scrutinized by professional editors, and undergo peer review, before they are published. Until a study is published in a reputable journal, you should take any reported results as hearsay and take with a large grain of salt!

The one method of sperm selection for gender determination that appears to have promise is *MicroSort,* first done at Genetics and IVF in Fairfax, Virginia. One vial of MicroSorted sperm costs about $3,400 (and you have to bring your own sperm!), and one vial is enough for only one IVF cycle; you can buy a second vial from the same sample for $700, which sounds like a bargain! And don't forget to add travel costs to the deal. This is one package the post office can't deliver. The sperm sample must be produced on site, although after it's washed and processed, you can take it back to your local clinic for insemination purposes. One disadvantage of MicroSort is that some doctors feel that it lowers the number of sperm available, so you may need to do IVF, although IUI can also be used.

MicroSort uses the fact that female sperm contain slightly more DNA (3% more to be exact, too little to allow for separation by standard means, such as density gradients or swimming contests. In the MicroSort technique, individual sperm are stained with a fluorescent dye that binds to the DNA. The males show up green, and the females show up red/pink. The sample is sorted using an instrument called a flow cytometer.

Female MicroSorted sperm will result in a girl 91 percent of the time, and male MicroSorted sperm will give you a boy about 76 percent of the time.

Of course, the merchandise is nonrefundable. You should note that these numbers refer to the percentage of sperm separated, not necessarily to live births. There has as yet not been any large series proving that these ratios will actually be reflected in the percentage of boys versus girls (although logically, this would make sense; remember that a lot of "logical" things in medicine don't turn out that way!)

At the moment, the most secure way to determine a baby's sex is to do *preimplantation genetic diagnosis* (PGD), in which a cell taken from an already created embryo can be analyzed to see if the baby will be a boy or a girl (see Chapter 16 for more on PGD). This method is more than 95percent accurate, and its accuracy is only limited by the technical limits of the PGD methodology itself. Of course, this procedure requires doing IVF, which is a little inefficient, because an IVF cycle is expensive (about $10,000) and may give you only a few embryos to test.

The Promises — and Pitfalls — of Preimplantation Genetic Diagnosis (PGD)

Right now, PGD is mainly used to screen for genetic diseases or to check for sex if the parents are carriers of a disease that affects only a child of one sex; however, geneticists and other specialists in genetic-borne illnesses hope that the coming years bring an ever improved rate of success for distinguishing healthy embryos to implant. Most agree that this is the best use of PGD, a process that is expensive, technologically challenging and labor intensive for all those involved (including the patient!). (See Chapter 16 for more information about PGD and its uses.)

Currently, PGD can test for a wide variety of genetic diseases, including hemophilia, Huntington's, muscular dystrophy, sickle cell disease, and Tay-Sachs, as well as chromosomal defects, such as Down syndrome and Turner syndrome.

However, the technology is there to determine the sex of the potential infant, although it's still very expensive. One can imagine PGD being used routinely in a few years for couples who want only a boy or a girl. In fact, it's already available in many clinics in the United States. A quick search of the Internet will reveal many clinics offering these services.

As genetic mapping advances, it's not hard to imagine parents screening embryos not only for sex or genetic diseases but also for hair and eye color, intelligence, and personality traits. Although it's possible that none of these traits will ever be able to be accurately determined by PGD, they may be. This possibility has ethicists concerned about where PGD is headed.

Ten years from today, will parents be routinely selecting the child of their choice, picking height, IQ, hair and eye color, and left- or right-handedness? Or will they even go one step further and have the potential to insert genes that they themselves don't possess into their children, with short parents having tall children, or brunettes having blondes?

The potential for gene tinkering is limitless, after certain traits have been mapped out and identified. The positive aspect of such manipulation could be the elimination of certain diseases or handicaps.

The negative side is that we could end up with populations skewed in one direction only, such as a nation full of tall, blonde, genius baseball players. Or we could find the male-to-female ratio off balance, as is happening in China with its one-child-only rule.

Although the potential for using gene selection for good purposes is high, the potential for abuse is just as high. However, many experts feel that such fears are overstated. They point out that if people really wanted a tall blonde baby, they could already go to a sperm bank and get the sperm from a tall blonde sperm donor, and then match it with the egg of a tall blonde egg donor. The reality is that individuals are shaped by many factors, both genetic and environmental. Even identical twins, who have identical genes, and were carried in their mother's womb at the same time, are not identical individuals.

Freezing Eggs: The Next Big Technology?

Sperm has been frozen for decades. Embryos have been frozen for 20 years. Eggs haven't caught up yet, although a lot of clinics are working on it. Egg freezing would be a boon for women, whose eggs are all present at the time of birth and age along with their carrier, as well as those with illnesses that require them to undergo chemotherapy before their childbearing years are over. Many women are marrying later and/or deciding to have children later — in their 30s and beyond — only to find that their eggs have used up their expiration limit.

The trouble is, eggs don't freeze well. They contain a lot of water, which crystallizes when it freezes. Ice crystals can damage the chromosomes or ruin the inner workings of the cell. Antifreeze solutions could be used to prevent the water inside from freezing, but antifreeze agents tend to be *cytotoxic*, which means damaging to cells, and will damage the egg. Also, frozen eggs can only be fertilized by using ICSI, which adds to the cost of doing an embryo transfer.

However, several clinics devoted to egg freezing claim that their survival rate of frozen eggs has reached 80 percent, and that nearly 60 percent of those eggs fertilize normally — almost as high as the percentage of fresh eggs that fertilize.

Undoubtedly, the next few years will bring improvements to egg freezing. One day freezing your own eggs for later or using frozen donor eggs will eliminate the need to synchronize donor and recipient cycles, as well as bring a wider choice of donors because eggs can be shipped around the world.

Caution: Beware of "Freeze Eggs Quick" promises by organizations, particularly those that are not medical in nature. As with all new opportunities, there are those who may look to take advantage of them . . . and you in the process. There's nothing guaranteed about egg freezing at this time, but the process is getting better all the time. Just remember that "successfully marketed" is not the same as "successful"!

The American Society for Reproductive Medicine maintains that egg freezing is considered experimental and should only be performed under approval and oversight by a research committee. If you are considering freezing eggs, make sure that the institution with which you decide to work has such oversight in place before you start.

Transplanting ovaries

Other experimental techniques that may hold promise for freezing eggs for future use involve freezing a portion of the ovary and transplanting it back to the original owner or to another woman. This has been done for women undergoing chemotherapy; once the treatment is finished and the risk of recurrence is low, the tissue is transplanted either back to the pelvis or to the forearm. Follicles have developed in the ovary after it was transplanted.

The first baby was born after ovary transplantation from one identical twin to another in 2004; when this technique is refined, it could bring hope of delivering a genetic child to women who undergo chemotherapy.

Posthumous Conception: Legal and Ethical Issues

It's not difficult or expensive to do. It creates a child. It usually helps heal wounds that come from the death of a loved one. So why is there so much controversy over posthumous conception?

Posthumous collection of sperm — removing sperm from the testes after a man has died — has been done on just about every continent. The legal issues have been discussed almost as much as the ethical issues. And there's still little legal or moral consensus about using a deceased man's sperm to create a child.

The person using the sperm is usually the spouse or partner of the dead man. Sometimes, but not always, she has advance written permission to collect and use the sperm at the time of his death. Legal issues have revolved around inheritance of the dead man's property and the payment of Social Security to the children who are born after a man's death — more than 300 days after his death.

The waters become murkier when the man has given no written permission for the sperm extraction. Can a spouse or partner legally request this be done? How does she know that it's what the man would want done? Does it matter?

One widow used a videotape in which her husband, who had been killed in a car accident, expressed a desire to have children someday as support for her request to have sperm removed at the time of his death.

Most recently, a case in which a man left frozen sperm to his fiancée came under scrutiny because she didn't want to use the sperm, but the man's parents did. They wanted to use donor eggs and a gestational carrier to create a child of their child, which they presumably would then raise.

In England, a widower is trying to find a surrogate to carry embryos created right before his wife's death; she had an egg retrieval done while she was waiting for a heart-lung transplant.

In another case of motherhood after death, the parents of a dead woman were searching for a gestational carrier to give birth to their dead daughter's children, created from their daughter's eggs and donor sperm.

Cases like these and even more complex ones will be popping up in courts all over the world in the next few years.

Dividing Up the Leftover Embryos

A few years ago, England found itself with more than 3,000 embryos in storage tanks that weren't being used or paid for by the people who created them. Because English law stipulated that frozen embryos must be used within five years, unless the parents were granted an extension, the embryos were destroyed.

In the United States, an estimated 100,000 embryos are frozen in storage tanks. Some will be used for another pregnancy attempt by their parents, but others will be left frozen, unpaid for and unused. In the United States, clinics who have documented proof that they tried to contact parents can destroy embryos after five years, according to guidelines from the American Society for Reproductive Medicine (ASRM).

The United States still has no hard and fast rules for frozen embryos. Each state rules differently when the cases go to court.

Infertility centers try to prevent these types of lawsuits by having couples sign a form at the time of egg retrieval stating what they want done with their embryos if they die or are divorced. Recently, though, a judge ruled that the decisions made at the time of retrieval were meaningless under changed circumstances.

Frozen embryos have been at the center of other types of lawsuits. Even in 1983, when IVF was a brand-new technology, frozen embryos made the news when their wealthy parents were killed in a plane crash, leaving no heirs. Technically, their only offspring were two frozen embryos. Of course, many women offered to carry the embryos and raise them — as long as their inherited fortune came with them! In the end, the embryos were treated as property and were destroyed.

Even if parents don't divorce or die, the decision of what to do with frozen embryos is a tough one because the choices are limited. Parents can donate the embryos to research, donate them to another couple, or have them destroyed. Not liking any of the choices, many parents just keep the embryos in storage, postponing any decision on what to do with them.

Frozen embryos have survived and created healthy children after a ten-year freezing period, so most centers aren't anxious to destroy embryos after five years.

In an ideal world, couples would use up all their embryos, having one baby initially and then one or more a few years later. However, for various reasons, that often doesn't happen. Leftover embryos then become a huge emotional and legal headache for most IVF centers. It takes space to store them and costs money to maintain the storage tanks. Few centers want to make decisions about potential human beings without some input from their parents, even if the parents haven't been seen or heard from in years.

When parents separate or divorce with embryos still in storage, frozen embryos can become a bitter battleground. In more than one case, divorcing couples have fought publicly over what should be done with their unused embryos. One ex-husband wanted to implant the embryos in his new wife!

The recent debates about using "leftover embryos" for stem cell research has created heated debates among ethicists. Is it ethically justifiable to destroy embryos — that many argue will be destroyed anyway — to potentially save other people? Or is the destruction of human embryos — potential people in their own right — wrong even if it's done for a good cause? Whose life takes precedence? These are hard questions with hard answers that many ethicists are still debating, and that many IVF patients agonize over on a personal level.

Saving Stem Cells for Research: Raising Ethical Concerns

Stem cells are cells that can be grown into any type of tissue or organ. In other words, they're not specific.

Human embryos are a good source of stem cells, and it could be possible to substitute DNA from a living person into a human egg after the egg's DNA was removed. The egg could then be "shocked" to get it to grow, and after two weeks or so, the stem cells would be removed. Of course, in the process, the embryo would cease to exist.

The stem cells would then be grown into whatever the adult needed — organs, skin, or other tissue. Because the genetic match would be exact, the person's body wouldn't reject the new organ or tissue. People needing organ transplants or new skin after a burn may find this type of science valuable.

Some doctors feel that the surplus of embryos destroyed every year should be used for stem cell development. Others feel that the potential life of the embryo shouldn't be sacrificed to save an already living person. Many people with frozen embryos would like to see something positive done with embryos that they donate for research, and would rather have them used for stem cell development than just be destroyed.

Parents with sick children have already been in the news for trying to create embryos for the specific purpose of donating stem cells to their living child. Others have had a baby specifically for the purpose of donating blood or tissue to a sick child. Whether it's morally and ethically acceptable to give birth to a child so that that child can save another's life is a question that's still under debate.

Animal cloning from an adult hasn't been very successful, but separating cells at an early embryonic stage has worked fairly well. The trouble with this technique is that it doesn't have much practicality in humans. Although identical twins, triplets, or more could be created, few families are looking to have an army of identical children.

Cutting the cord — but saving it

Stem cells can be obtained from other places besides human embryos. Many parents are now banking blood from their child's umbilical cord in case the child needs stem cells at a later date. Unfortunately, the utility and/or cost-effectiveness of such an approach has not yet been evaluated. One possible strategy would collect all of the umbilical blood in a given community, with the idea of setting up a stem cell bank. It has been estimated that 10,000 specimens would be required to have a sample of every possible combination of HLA genes. When someone needed stem cells, say for a bone marrow transplant, such stem cells would then be available. As with so many aspects of this new science, only time will tell.

Cloning and Human Concerns

People talk about cloning as if all cloning is the same thing. In reality, there are three different types of cloning; some have been successful, some have been partially successful, and some haven't been done at all yet as far as we know. We discuss all three in this section.

The cloning causing the most controversy is the type that produced Dolly the sheep. It involves taking a healthy embryo, removing its DNA, and putting the DNA from another person into the embryo. Any cell contains DNA, so obtaining DNA isn't difficult. If the embryo continues growing normally, it can be placed into a host uterus to grow for nine months.

There are numerous concerns about cloning. Many of the offspring cloned so far have had serious abnormalities. There is also concern that cloned individuals might age much faster than normal because their DNA was obtained from a mature adult.

People wanting an exact copy of themselves may be disappointed because cloned animals aren't totally identical. Environmental influences can change certain characteristics and alter appearance.

Another type of cloning that could be used to create human beings has been done pretty successfully in animals. It involves taking a cell from an embryo and allowing it to grow into a second, identical embryo. This is how identical twins occur in nature.

It would be possible to give birth to identical twins several years apart by using this technique, which is done frequently in farming. It would also be possible to do genetic testing on the "cloned" embryo while freezing the original. If the clone passed the genetic tests, the "original" could then be thawed and implanted.

The creation of Dolly

The cloning technique that created Dolly, the well-known cloned sheep, involved taking a cell from another sheep and putting it into a sheep embryo. The genetic material was removed from the embryo, so that the only DNA was from the donor sheep, which was about 6 years old at the time. Dolly was the only successful clone born out of about 300 original attempts. Dolly started to develop arthritis when she was almost 6 years old, causing concern that she was aging faster than normal. In early 2003, Dolly had to be euthanized at the age of 6 after being diagnosed with a progressive lung disease. Sheep usually live to be 12 to 14 years old. Calf cloning has been mildly successful; 73 percent of pregnancies end in miscarriage, and 20 percent die soon after birth. Some are born oversized, with enlarged tongues, with immune deficiencies, or with diseases such as diabetes.

Forcing Clinics to Decide Who's Fit to Parent

If you're fertile, you can become a parent anytime you want. No one is in your bedroom rating your ability to raise children. And after children are born, they're taken only from parents who've crossed far over the line of normal parenting behavior.

People who do IVF are no better or worse as parents than anyone else; the potential for child abuse or neglect exists just as it does in any other population. Some clinics require psychological screening for their patients, trying to weed out those who are psychologically unprepared to raise children; others do not.

Not long ago, a father was arrested for beating his infant son to death. The father had used IVF with donor eggs and a gestational carrier to create his son. This case raised questions about how aggressive clinics should be in evaluating patients for parenthood. Should potential parents be turned away because they don't fit a typical social mold? In Australia, for example, gay women aren't allowed to do IVF. Should IVF parents be required to have a certain income level or be of a certain intelligence level?

At this time, most clinics set their own rules for evaluating patients. One prime example is the use of donor eggs or embryos for older women — older as in over 55. Many centers use 55 as an arbitrary cutoff age. Why 55 and not 65? Some centers do strict testing on patients over 40 to make sure that they're healthy enough to carry a pregnancy. Yet some 45-year-olds are much healthier than some 25-year-olds.

IVF isn't well regulated in the United States. Although most centers follow guidelines set by ASRM and the Society of Assisted Reproductive Technology (SART), guidelines are only that. A patient denied treatment at one center may be accepted at another. Should IVF centers be in the business of choosing who will be good parents? Are they guilty if an IVF parent harms his child?

Making Mistakes in the Lab: When Saying You're Sorry Isn't Enough

Black children born to white couples. Embryos misplaced while in storage. A clinic in California charged with more than 100 cases of taking one woman's eggs and giving them to another and of selling embryos left in storage. These are just a few of the mistakes (whether accidental or intentional) that fertility clinics have made.

Most clinics are careful not to work on eggs or embryos belonging to two different people at the same time. They label everything that they're working on to prevent mix-ups, yet mix-ups do sometimes occur.

When a clinic makes these kinds of mistakes, saying sorry isn't nearly good enough. Most of the highly publicized cases of parents ending up with the wrong children have come to light only because the parents and children were of different races. It's hard to say whether similar errors have been made and not discovered because parents and children were all of the same race.

In one instance involving black children and white parents, the error was made in the andrology lab; sperm from a black man was used instead of the sperm from the Caucasian spouse. In this case, the birth mother was also the biological mother, making the children genetically hers.

In another case, embryos from a black couple were implanted along with a white couple's own embryos. The woman gave birth to one biological child and one unrelated child, who was then returned to his biological parents by the courts.

It's hard to safeguard yourself against errors like these. The errors aren't made purposely; they're the result of fallible human beings making mistakes. You can help keep mistakes to a minimum by reading everything you're given to sign, and making sure that your name is properly spelled on everything. When you leave a semen specimen, make sure that it's labeled properly. When the embryologist hands your embryos over for transfer, make sure that she says your proper name.

If you have questions at any point about your eggs or embryos, ask them at that time. If there's any question of error, getting to the bottom of it right then is much easier than getting to the bottom of it nine months later. Monetary compensation is never going to be adequate enough to fix the heartbreak caused by an error in an embryology lab.

Injecting Immune Therapy

If standard fertility methods have failed you, you may be interested in moving on to some of the more controversial methods:

- Leukocyte immune therapy (LIT)
- Intravenous immunoglobulin (IVIG)
- Enbrel or Remicade

These methods are considered controversial because only a few doctors support them or because they're considered to be risky in some way. Immune issues are generally believed to be responsible for less than 5 percent of infertility, but some doctors feel that this condition is under-diagnosed because the testing for immune factors is expensive and done only in a few labs.

However, mainstream organizations have been quite uniform in rejecting these therapies. Very few university centers offer them, and if a doctor goes out of his or her way to recommend them, you should become suspicious and seek a second opinion. As with other unproven therapies, there are several dangers:

- You waste time with unproven therapy instead of using something that can actually work.
- There may be quite serious side effects from the therapy. The potential dangers of many of these immunotherapies far exceed the potential dangers of fertility medications.
- They are expensive.

Leukocyte immune therapy

The idea that some women's bodies reject an embryo isn't a new one, but the methods for overcoming rejection are fairly new. One method, leukocyte immune therapy (LIT), was halted by the U.S. Food and Drug Administration and shows no signs of being reapproved at this writing. LIT was fairly simple: White blood cells from the woman's partner or a donor were washed and injected under the woman's skin. The theory behind LIT is that some women don't have the right amount of blocking antibodies, which keep them from rejecting a growing fetus as a foreign piece of tissue. By giving proteins from your partner or another person, some of the proper blocking antibodies are introduced into your body, and the embryo will, one hopes, not be rejected.

The FDA currently bans the use of LIT in the United States, but some women have gone abroad to have LIT done. If you choose this option, you and your partner need up-to-date infectious blood testing.

There are no studies showing that this therapy is safe. Since it is banned by the FDA, there is no other requirement for studies showing safety.

Investing in IVIG

Because LIT has been banned, some doctors recommend intravenous immunoglobulin (IVIG) therapy as a substitute. Unfortunately, IVIG must be administered as an intravenous infusion, which takes two to four hours, and must be done by a doctor or nurse. By way of comparison, LIT is a subcutaneous (under the skin) injection that takes just a few minutes to give.

IVIG has two major drawbacks:

- ✔ A single infusion may run between $3,000 and $4,000, and if you get pregnant, your doctor will most likely recommend at least two or three infusions.

- ✔ Unlike the proteins injected from your partner in LIT, IVIG is a commercially produced blood product from strangers, so there is a small chance of transmission of HIV or hepatitis through the infusion.

Use of IVIG therapy in infertility is extremely controversial. Many doctors don't see any benefit at all to IVIG; other doctors believe that good prospective (set up in advance) studies on IVIG treatment in infertility are few and inconclusive.

Side effects of IVIG can be severe; anaphylactic shock is a small risk. Rash, fever, headache, dizziness, and nausea are fairly common side effects. A publication by the practice committee of SART has specifically denounced the use of IVIG.

Enbrel and Remicade

The newest drugs proclaimed by some doctors to help pregnancies implant are Enbrel and Remicade, drugs that decrease levels of TNF, or tumor necrosis factor.

In larger than normal amounts, TNF can cause pain and inflammation seen in autoimmune diseases such as Crohn's disease and rheumatoid arthritis; Enbrel and Remicade help relieve the inflammation and pain by decreasing concentrations of TNF.

Some doctors use TNF fighters to decrease immune responses that may keep pregnancies from implanting and growing. A number of deaths and lawsuits have resulted from patients taking Enbrel and Remicade. To date, Enbrel and Remicade have been implicated in the following:

- ✔ Development of lymphoma, a type of cancer
- ✔ Neurological damage
- ✔ An increase in the development of systemic lupus erythematosus, an autoimmune disease
- ✔ Serious infections
- ✔ Blood disorders, including severe anemia

Part VI
The Part of Tens

The 5th Wave   By Rich Tennant

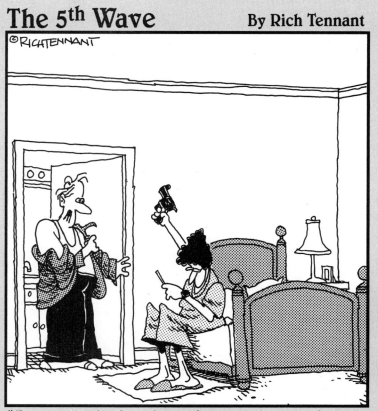

"I never realized trying to have a baby would mean replacing the soft music and candle light with an ovulation strip, a thermometer, and a starter pistol."

In this part . . .

Want to know the ten most annoying things people say when you're trying to get pregnant? Want to know where to find fertility medications for reasonable prices and find out exactly what a gonadotropin is? Need to navigate your way through an infertility chat board? Then this is the part for you.

Chapter 21

The Ten-Plus Most Annoying Things to Hear When You're Trying to Get Pregnant

- -

In This Chapter
- ▶ "Supportive" statements
- ▶ Unbelievable utterances
- ▶ Direct from the doctor

- -

As if trying to get pregnant wasn't stressful enough, anything to do with reproduction seems to be fair game for comment by friends, relatives, and complete strangers. In this chapter, we list some of the most common and most annoying things you'll hear on the road to pregnancy. Feel free to tear this chapter out and throw darts at it!

Helpful Hints

"Just *relax,* and you'll get pregnant." (Who hasn't said this to you by now?)

"My friend Bootsy adopted a child and got pregnant the next day. Have you considered this?"

"Have you tried . . . ?" "Have you read . . . ?" "Have you heard . . . ?" (These questions all usually refer to harebrained schemes for getting pregnant.)

"Dr. Perfect has the best stats around. He can get anyone pregnant, well almost anyone." (Of course, you usually hear this after your first, second, third, or later unsuccessful attempt.)

"I Know How You Feel"

"I know how you feel. It took us *four* months to conceive our third child."
(There should be a law against comments like this.)

"I can't believe you're having such a tough time! I get pregnant every time my partner walks in the door!" (See response to preceding comment.)

"Things could be worse." (No, really?)

"I bet this experience has brought you and your partner a lot closer."
(Of course, brain surgery would, too, but I'm sure there's an easier way.)

Comments You Can't Believe You Heard

"Are you pregnant yet?"

"You're *still* not pregnant?" (Yes folks, people really *do* say the dumbest things!)

"Do you have a good doctor?" (Actually, I'm using a vet, but thanks for asking.)

"Trying to conceive is *really* hard work." (You may hear this from your spouse, whose contribution involves monthly ejaculations while watching and/or reading pornography in your doctor's office.)

"Plenty of people live happy lives without children." (Thanks for sharing!)

Straight from Your Doctor's Mouth

"Your chances of conceiving are 2.6786 percent, about the same as getting hit by lightning." (This statement is obviously taken from the table of famous statistics that doctors pull out of thin air.)

"You're not having much of a response, are you?" (Doctors generally say this when you're lying in a prone position with an ultrasound wand in position.)

"You need to be very aggressive, considering your age."

"Maybe you shouldn't have waited so long to start trying." (Hmmm, let's spend some time flogging ourselves over that!)

"Guess you and your partner will just have to keep 'practicing'." (With a wink, wink, nudge, nudge from the doctor who continues to "practice" his skills, or lack thereof, on you!)

Leaving You Speechless

"Why do you think God is doing this to you?" (I dunno, maybe you could ask for me.)

Chapter 22

Ten (Okay, Seven) Groups of Fertility Medications and Where to Find Them

In This Chapter

▶ Categorizing fertility medications

▶ Locating fertility medications

Although fertility medications come with a bewildering array of names, these medications fit into only a few categories. The different names are brand name-only differences, in most cases. In this chapter, we describe the different categories and list the most common brand names of each.

Sorting the Medications

Fertility medications are often sold in boxes of five or ten vials or in multidose bottles or syringes. There's no logical reason for fertility medications to be sold in multiple units; the main reason, of course, is profit. Pharmacies that specialize in fertility medications will break up a box and sell you one or two, but usually your local Cost-Cut Pharmacy won't.

Gonadotropins

These drugs are the mainstay of fertility treatment. Gonadotropins (*gonad* meaning reproductive organ; *tropin* being Greek for "turning towards," in this case, a hormone which has an affinity for the gonad) stimulate follicle growth. All gonadotropins are manufactured in the lab, and are generally divided into two broad categories according to the raw material from which they are extracted. *Recombinant* gonadotropins are extracted from a protein product that is generated by cells in culture. The cells are Chinese hamster ovary cells that have been injected ("transfected") with the DNA for the gonadotropins, and therefore produce the hormones (which are proteins) from the DNA blueprint.

Urinary gonadotropins are extracted from protein extracted from the urine of postmenopausal women. Postmenopausal women have very high FSH levels, and their bodies excrete all of this FSH in the urine. Urinary products generally contain both FSH and LH (although the LH can be removed), and recombinant products generally contain only FSH (although recombinant LH has also recently been brought to the market).

Side effects of gonadotropins are generally caused by the hormones that are produced by the ovary in response to the gonadotropins, (rather than due to direct effects of the gonadotropins themselves) and include bloating, headache, and mood swings.

Recombinant gonadotropins

Recombinant drugs contain relatively few other human proteins and are considered to be nearly free from impurities. These drugs are follicle-stimulating drugs; they contain nearly pure FSH, so they encourage the growth of many follicles rather than just one in an in vitro fertilization (IVF) or stimulated cycle. Because they're purified and unlikely to cause a skin reaction, they can be given subcutaneously with a very small needle; women with a body mass index over 30 should receive the drug intramuscularly for best absorption. Two brands are currently available: Follistim and Gonal-F.

Follistim

Follistim is made by Organon, a large manufacturer of several fertility medications. It comes in a prefilled, premixed multidose syringe containing 300IU, 600IU, or 900 IU of medication. You turn a dial to choose the amount of medication you want to inject, and then change the needle for your next dose.

Gonal-F

Gonal-F is produced by Serono Labs, another large manufacturer of fertility medications. Gonal-F is sold in three types of packaging:

✔ **In a multidose vial containing 450 IU of medication.** The advantage is that you mix it with a small amount of water and have only a tiny amount to inject at a time; plus you have to mix a new batch only every couple of days. The disadvantage is that you can't save the unused portion for another cycle. As a result, you may waste a lot of medication or have to buy a combination of multidose and single-dose vials.

> ✔ **In single vials of 75IU**, which must be mixed with sterile water before being injected subcutaneously. If you only need a dose or two of medication, this method may be cheaper to purchase.
>
> ✔ **In a prefilled, premixed pen** containing 300IU, 450IU, or 900IU of medication.

Urinary FSH

One purified FSH alone product made from urine is available. The advantage to a product made from human products rather than lab-manufactured ones is that the cost is less.

Bravelle

Bravelle is made by Ferring, another large manufacturer of fertility medications. Although Bravelle is made from purified urine, it's nearly as pure as recombinant FSH and tends to be somewhat cheaper. It comes in 75 IU vials and is given subcutaneously with a small needle after being mixed with sterile water.

Recombinant LH

There's only one recombinant LH product on the market at the moment. Luveris, manufactured by Serono, is a recombinant LH preparation that administers 75IU of LH after being mixed with 1 cc of sterile water. The drug is given subcutaneously.

Urinary LH/FSH

These were the earliest gonadotropins on the market. They're made from purified urine from menopausal women and contain nearly equal amounts of LH and FSH. Some doctors now believe that some LH is helpful in a stimulated cycle and may prescribe these along with a pure FSH product.

Menopur

Menopur is manufactured by Ferring, and contains equal amounts of LH and FSH. It comes in 75 IU vials. Because it is highly purified, it is given subcutaneously after being mixed with 1 cc of water. More than one vial can be mixed with the 1 cc of sterile water. Menopur should be given within 15 minutes after mixing.

Repronex

Repronex is also manufactured by Ferring. It is the last of the "traditional" gonadotropin preparations. These preparations undergo considerably less purification, and therefore contain much more in the way of foreign proteins. This is not dangerous, and in fact, some doctors feel that some patients respond better to this less purified version of the natural FSH and LH hormones. Some centers give Repronex subcutaneously, but others have found skin rashes to be fairly common (10 to 20%) unless given intramuscularly. It comes in 75 IU vials and is mixed with 1 cc diluent if given subcutaneously, 2 cc if given intramuscularly. Repronex tends to be cheaper than the other medications. If it is prescribed for you, consider trying to inject it subcutaneously (which is easier and less painful), and if you get a rash, change to intramuscular.

GnRH agonists

Leuprolide acetate, more commonly known as Lupron, is a gonadotropin-releasing hormone agonist, meaning that it suppresses hormones such as LH and FSH. It's manufactured by TAP Pharmaceutical Products and sold in a 14-day kit, which contains a 2.8 ml multidose vial of premixed Lupron and 14 syringes. Lupron first causes a stimulation of the pituitary, which makes extra FSH and LH, which can then stimulate your ovaries, but then after a few days starts to suppress the pituitary and causes what you will hear the nurses and doctors call "down-regulation." This means that your normal menstrual cycle, which matures only one egg at a time, will be shut off. More importantly, this allows many follicles to be stimulated with gonadotropins. If taken for more than a few weeks without any other medications, Lupron causes low estrogen levels, which can result in hot flashes, headaches, and bone pain.

Some centers use a smaller dose of Lupron, called a microdose Lupron, which can be purchased premixed from pharmacies that specialize in fertility medications. Microdose Lupron is used exclusively for stimulation as part of a protocol called a "microdose flare." This means that the Lupron is used for its stimulatory properties, and the gonadotropins are started either at the same time, or two days later. The lower dose of Lupron means that the down-regulation takes longer to achieve and thus the stimulatory properties of the Lupron are maximized. The microdose flare is an example of a "poor responder" protocol, which means that it's used for women who either have a history of, or are anticipated to have a poor response to stimulation.

GnRH antagonists

A newer category of medication called GnRH antagonists was designed to keep women from releasing eggs early during an IVF cycle without the initial stimulatory effects of Lupron. (For this reason, the antagonists do not have to be administered ahead of time, and can simply be given near the end of the stimulation to prevent the body from releasing the eggs before the doctors can get to them during an egg retrieval procedure). It's manufactured by Organon as Antagon and by Serono as Cetrotide. Cetrotide is manufactured as a 3 mg one-time injection and also as a 250 mcg (which is the same as 0.25 mg) daily injection; Antagon is only sold as a daily 250 mcg injection. The daily injection usually starts around day six of an IVF cycle (when the lead follicle is around 14 mm in diameter). Antagon is sold in a prefilled syringe that requires no mixing. Cetrotide comes with a syringe prefilled with diluent, which needs to be injected into a powder; the mixture is then drawn back into the syringe and injected.

hCG (human chorionic gonadotropin) intramuscular

Several different brands of hCG are sold; all contain 10,000 IU of hCG. They're packaged with more water than is needed for a single injection, usually 10 cc; the hCG is generally mixed with 2 cc of water and then injected intramuscularly. (Several recent studies have confirmed that these medications are absorbed equally well when injected subcutaneously. Therefore, some clinics are using them with the small sub-cu injection. Ask your doctor what his recommendation is. Common brand names are:

- ✔ Novarel (Ferring)
- ✔ Pregnyl (Organon)
- ✔ Profasi (Serono)

hCG subcutaneous recombinant

Ovidrel is a lab-manufactured subcutaneous dose of hCG packaged as 250 mcg equivalent to 5,000 to 10,000 IU; it comes with a 1 cc vial of water for mixing. Serono makes Ovidrel.

Progesterone

Progesterone can be given in intramuscular injections (the highest blood levels), vaginal suppositories, vaginal gel, vaginal pills, or oral pills (the lowest blood levels).

- ✔ **Injections:** The intramuscular injection form of progesterone comes in multidose vials of 50 mg/ml. Progesterone in oil needs to be mixed under a special hood, so it's made only by pharmacies that compound medications; these are usually pharmacies that specialize in fertility medications, such as those found at the end of this chapter.

- ✔ **Vaginal suppositories:** These suppositories are made in several strengths and must be made by the pharmacy, so they can be hard to find; they're not commercially manufactured. They're little bullets that must be inserted manually and come in 100 mgm, 200 mgm, and 400 mgm strength. Vaginally administered progesterone produces blood levels that are lower than those achieved with the injections, but much higher tissue levels of progesterone in the uterine lining. This is because there appears to be a special uptake mechanism for medications from the vagina into the uterus.

- ✔ **Gel:** Crinone is a gel manufactured by Serono; it comes in prefilled applicators of 90 mg. Some patients have fewer problems with yeast infections and irritation with Crinone than with vaginal suppositories.

- ✔ **Capsules:** These are manufactured as Prometrium by Solvay and are available in 100 mg and 200 mg. Compounding pharmacies also make their own micronized progesterone capsules.

- ✔ **Micronized tablets:** These are also compounded by pharmacies. If they are taken orally, they absorb well but are then rapidly metabolized in the liver, leading to low serum levels of progesterone and low effectiveness. Oral progesterone is not generally recommended during fertility procedures, (but may be adequate for menopausal replacement therapy). Oral progesterone also causes considerable sleepiness, as some of its metabolites act as sedatives.

- ✔ **Micronized tablets taken vaginally:** The same tablets can be taken vaginally. The progesterone absorbs much better this way and produces excellent tissue levels in the uterus. Some centers prefer the vaginal tablets to suppositories because they're less messy and the powder inside the capsules stays in the vagina for 24 hours or more, thus producing a steady supply of progesterone during the day, as opposed to suppositories which melt quickly and are quickly gone.

Ovulation induction medications

Clomiphene citrate is more commonly called Clomid even though it's sold as Clomid by several manufacturers and Serophene by Serono Labs. Clomid is a 50 mg pill that stimulates the ovaries and increases the release of follicle-stimulating hormones. Side effects include hot flashes, bloating, headache, and blurred vision.

Femara (Leterozole) was originally used in the treatment of breast cancer. Some clinics are also using it for ovulation induction, although its use as an ovulation induction drug is considered "off label" by the FDA, meaning it's not approved for this use. Be sure to discuss all the possible pros and cons with your doctor before taking this drug.

Mail-Order Pharmacies

Although medications such as Clomid and hCG are fairly easy to find at your local pharmacy, gonadotropins and progesterone can be harder to find. A whole industry of mail-order pharmacies that specialize in fertility drugs has evolved, and there are some advantages to using them over your local pharmacy:

✔ They charge less for fertility medications than most pharmacies

✔ They mail the medications directly to your home

✔ They offer overnight delivery

✔ They take a wide variety of insurances

✔ They may have special programs to help low income women afford medications

✔ Many produce injection instruction tapes and have hotlines you can call with medication questions 24 hours a day

This list of mail-order pharmacies is by no means complete; the area in which you live may have similar pharmacies with which your clinic deals on a regular basis.

✔ **Alexander's Twin Pharmacy:** Trenton, New Jersey; 1-877-750-7222

✔ **Apothecary Pharmacy:** Scottsdale, AZ; 1-877-792-7684; www.theapothecaryshop.com

✔ **Apthorp Pharmacy:** New York, New York; 1-800-775-3582

✔ **FertilityMeds:** Alpine, California; 1-800-346-9660

✔ **Franklin Drug:** Philadelphia, Pennsylvania; 1-800-537-3788

✔ **Freedom Drug:** Lynnfield, Massachusetts; 1-800-660-4283

✔ **IVPcare:** Carrollton, Texas; 1-800-483-8001

✔ **King's Pharmacy:** New York, New York; several locations in the city; 1-800-RXKINGS

✔ **MDR Pharmacy:** Encino, Los Angeles, CA; 1-800-515-DRUG; www.mdrusa.com

✔ **Metro Drug:** New York, New York; several locations in the city; 1-212-627-2300

✔ **Poet's Pharmacy:** Freehold, New Jersey; 1-800-427-POET

✔ **Reses Pharmacy:** Pomona, New Jersey; 1-609-646-3600

✔ **Schraft's:** Livingston, New Jersey; 1-800-876-4545

✔ **Stadtlander's:** Pittsburgh, Pennsylvania; 1-800-218-6315

Index

• J •

• K •

• L •

• *P* •

BUSINESS, CAREERS & PERSONAL FINANCE

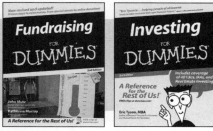

0-7645-9847-3   0-7645-2431-3

Also available:
- Business Plans Kit For Dummies
  0-7645-9794-9
- Economics For Dummies
  0-7645-5726-2
- Grant Writing For Dummies
  0-7645-8416-2
- Home Buying For Dummies
  0-7645-5331-3
- Managing For Dummies
  0-7645-1771-6
- Marketing For Dummies
  0-7645-5600-2

- Personal Finance For Dummies
  0-7645-2590-5*
- Resumes For Dummies
  0-7645-5471-9
- Selling For Dummies
  0-7645-5363-1
- Six Sigma For Dummies
  0-7645-6798-5
- Small Business Kit For Dummies
  0-7645-5984-2
- Starting an eBay Business For Dummies
  0-7645-6924-4
- Your Dream Career For Dummies
  0-7645-9795-7

HOME & BUSINESS COMPUTER BASICS

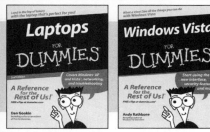

0-470-05432-8   0-471-75421-8

Also available:
- Cleaning Windows Vista For Dummies
  0-471-78293-9
- Excel 2007 For Dummies
  0-470-03737-7
- Mac OS X Tiger For Dummies
  0-7645-7675-5
- MacBook For Dummies
  0-470-04859-X
- Macs For Dummies
  0-470-04849-2
- Office 2007 For Dummies
  0-470-00923-3

- Outlook 2007 For Dummies
  0-470-03830-6
- PCs For Dummies
  0-7645-8958-X
- Salesforce.com For Dummies
  0-470-04893-X
- Upgrading & Fixing Laptops For Dummies
  0-7645-8959-8
- Word 2007 For Dummies
  0-470-03658-3
- Quicken 2007 For Dummies
  0-470-04600-7

FOOD, HOME, GARDEN, HOBBIES, MUSIC & PETS

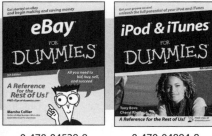

0-7645-8404-9   0-7645-9904-6

Also available:
- Candy Making For Dummies
  0-7645-9734-5
- Card Games For Dummies
  0-7645-9910-0
- Crocheting For Dummies
  0-7645-4151-X
- Dog Training For Dummies
  0-7645-8418-9
- Healthy Carb Cookbook For Dummies
  0-7645-8476-6
- Home Maintenance For Dummies
  0-7645-5215-5

- Horses For Dummies
  0-7645-9797-3
- Jewelry Making & Beading For Dummies
  0-7645-2571-9
- Orchids For Dummies
  0-7645-6759-4
- Puppies For Dummies
  0-7645-5255-4
- Rock Guitar For Dummies
  0-7645-5356-9
- Sewing For Dummies
  0-7645-6847-7
- Singing For Dummies
  0-7645-2475-5

INTERNET & DIGITAL MEDIA

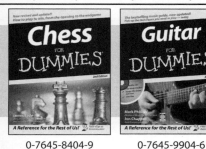

0-470-04529-9   0-470-04894-8

Also available:
- Blogging For Dummies
  0-471-77084-1
- Digital Photography For Dummies
  0-7645-9802-3
- Digital Photography All-in-One Desk Reference For Dummies
  0-470-03743-1
- Digital SLR Cameras and Photography For Dummies
  0-7645-9803-1
- eBay Business All-in-One Desk Reference For Dummies
  0-7645-8438-3
- HDTV For Dummies
  0-470-09673-X

- Home Entertainment PCs For Dummies
  0-470-05523-5
- MySpace For Dummies
  0-470-09529-6
- Search Engine Optimization For Dummies
  0-471-97998-8
- Skype For Dummies
  0-470-04891-3
- The Internet For Dummies
  0-7645-8996-2
- Wiring Your Digital Home For Dummies
  0-471-91830-X

* Separate Canadian edition also available
† Separate U.K. edition also available

Available wherever books are sold. For more information or to order direct: U.S. customers visit www.dummies.com or call 1-877-762-2974.
U.K. customers visit www.wileyeurope.com or call 0800 243407. Canadian customers visit www.wiley.ca or call 1-800-567-4797.

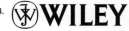 **WILEY**

SPORTS, FITNESS, PARENTING, RELIGION & SPIRITUALITY

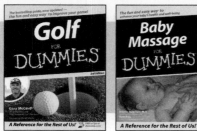

0-471-76871-5

0-7645-7841-3

Also available:
- Catholicism For Dummies
  0-7645-5391-7
- Exercise Balls For Dummies
  0-7645-5623-1
- Fitness For Dummies
  0-7645-7851-0
- Football For Dummies
  0-7645-3936-1
- Judaism For Dummies
  0-7645-5299-6
- Potty Training For Dummies
  0-7645-5417-4
- Buddhism For Dummies
  0-7645-5359-3

- Pregnancy For Dummies
  0-7645-4483-7 †
- Ten Minute Tone-Ups For Dummies
  0-7645-7207-5
- NASCAR For Dummies
  0-7645-7681-X
- Religion For Dummies
  0-7645-5264-3
- Soccer For Dummies
  0-7645-5229-5
- Women in the Bible For Dummies
  0-7645-8475-8

TRAVEL

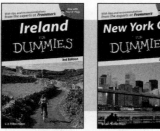

0-7645-7749-2

0-7645-6945-7

Also available:
- Alaska For Dummies
  0-7645-7746-8
- Cruise Vacations For Dummies
  0-7645-6941-4
- England For Dummies
  0-7645-4276-1
- Europe For Dummies
  0-7645-7529-5
- Germany For Dummies
  0-7645-7823-5
- Hawaii For Dummies
  0-7645-7402-7

- Italy For Dummies
  0-7645-7386-1
- Las Vegas For Dummies
  0-7645-7382-9
- London For Dummies
  0-7645-4277-X
- Paris For Dummies
  0-7645-7630-5
- RV Vacations For Dummies
  0-7645-4442-X
- Walt Disney World & Orlando
  For Dummies
  0-7645-9660-8

GRAPHICS, DESIGN & WEB DEVELOPMENT

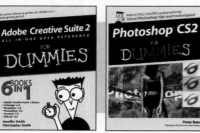

0-7645-8815-X

0-7645-9571-7

Also available:
- 3D Game Animation For Dummies
  0-7645-8789-7
- AutoCAD 2006 For Dummies
  0-7645-8925-3
- Building a Web Site For Dummies
  0-7645-7144-3
- Creating Web Pages For Dummies
  0-470-08030-2
- Creating Web Pages All-in-One Desk
  Reference For Dummies
  0-7645-4345-8
- Dreamweaver 8 For Dummies
  0-7645-9649-7

- InDesign CS2 For Dummies
  0-7645-9572-5
- Macromedia Flash 8 For Dummies
  0-7645-9691-8
- Photoshop CS2 and Digital
  Photography For Dummies
  0-7645-9580-6
- Photoshop Elements 4 For Dummies
  0-471-77483-9
- Syndicating Web Sites with RSS Feeds
  For Dummies
  0-7645-8848-6
- Yahoo! SiteBuilder For Dummies
  0-7645-9800-7

NETWORKING, SECURITY, PROGRAMMING & DATABASES

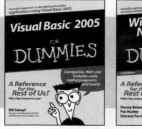

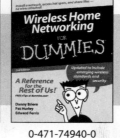

0-7645-7728-X

0-471-74940-0

Also available:
- Access 2007 For Dummies
  0-470-04612-0
- ASP.NET 2 For Dummies
  0-7645-7907-X
- C# 2005 For Dummies
  0-7645-9704-3
- Hacking For Dummies
  0-470-05235-X
- Hacking Wireless Networks
  For Dummies
  0-7645-9730-2
- Java For Dummies
  0-470-08716-1

- Microsoft SQL Server 2005 For Dummies
  0-7645-7755-7
- Networking All-in-One Desk Reference
  For Dummies
  0-7645-9939-9
- Preventing Identity Theft For Dummies
  0-7645-7336-5
- Telecom For Dummies
  0-471-77085-X
- Visual Studio 2005 All-in-One Desk
  Reference For Dummies
  0-7645-9775-2
- XML For Dummies
  0-7645-8845-1

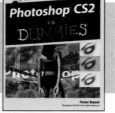